Caring for Children
with Cerebral Palsy

This book is printed on recycled paper. ♻ Recycled Paper

Caring for Children with Cerebral Palsy

A Team Approach

edited by

John P. Dormans, M.D.

The Children's Hospital of Philadelphia
University of Pennsylvania School of Medicine
Children's Seashore House
Philadelphia, Pennsylvania

and

Louis Pellegrino, M.D.

University of Medicine and
Dentistry of New Jersey
Robert Wood Johnson Medical School
New Brunswick, New Jersey

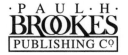

·P A U L·H·
BROOKES
PUBLISHING C^O

Baltimore • London • Toronto • Sydney

Paul H. Brookes Publishing Co.
Post Office Box 10624
Baltimore, Maryland 21285-0624

www.brookespublishing.com

Typeset by Edington-Rand, Cheverly, Maryland.
Manufactured in the United States of America by
The Maple Press Co., York, Pennsylvania

Illustrations by Lynn Reynolds, Ars Medica.

The suggestions in this book are not intended as a substitute for professional medical consultation. The volume editors and publisher disclaim any liability arising directly or indirectly from the use of this book.

The individuals and situations described in this book are completely fictional or are based on composites of various people and circumstances, in which cases pseudonyms have been used. Any similarity to actual individuals or circumstances is coincidental, and no implications should be inferred.

Second printing, March 2000.

Library of Congress Cataloging-in-Publication Data

Caring for children with cerebral palsy : a team approach / [edited]
   by John P. Dormans and Louis Pellegrino.
      p.   cm.
   Includes bibliographical references and index.
   ISBN 1-55766-322-X
   1. Cerebral palsied children—Rehabilitation.   2. Cerebral palsied children—
Life skills guides.   I. Dormans, John P.   II. Pellegrino, Louis.
   [DNLM: 1. Cerebral palsy—infancy & childhood.   2. Cerebral Palsy—
rehabilitation.   3. Activities of Daily Living.   4. Patient Care Team.
WS 342 C277 1998]
RJ496.C4C34   1998
618.92'836—dc21
DNLM/DLC
for Library of Congress   97-23367
                                                                                 CIP

British Library Cataloguing in Publication data are available from the British Library.

Contents

About the Editors

John P. Dormans, M.D., is Chief of Orthopaedic Surgery at The Children's Hospital of Philadelphia and Associate Professor of Orthopaedic Surgery at the University of Pennsylvania School of Medicine. He holds The Children's Hospital of Philadelphia Endowed Chair in Pediatric Orthopaedic Surgery and is Research Associate of the Stokes Research Institute at The Children's Hospital of Philadelphia. Dr. Dormans is Co-director of the Cerebral Palsy Program at The Children's Hospital of Philadelphia and Children's Seashore House, a regional children's hospital for specialized care and rehabilitation of children.

Dr. Dormans did a pediatric orthopedic fellowship at the Hospital for Sick Children in Toronto, Ontario, Canada, and during that time spent time at the Hugh MacMillan Rehabilitation Center in Toronto. Dr. Dormans has been at The Children's Hospital of Philadelphia and the University of Pennsylvania School of Medicine since 1990 and has been the recipient of both the Jesse T. Nicholson Award for Excellence in Clinical Teaching (awarded by the senior Orthopaedic Residency Class of 1993) and also the Dean's Award for Excellence in Clinical Teaching from the University of Pennsylvania School of Medicine in 1995. He is also the Co-director of the Pediatric Orthopaedic Fellowship at The Children's Hospital of Philadelphia. He was a Kashawegi Suzuki traveling fellow to Japan in 1996.

Dr. Dormans has published more than 70 articles and has authored more than 25 chapters in various contributed books. Dr. Dormans is a Fellow of the American Academy of Orthopaedic Surgeons, the American Board of Orthopaedic Surgeons, the American College of Surgeons, the Pediatric Orthopaedic Society of North America, the Scoliosis Research Society, and the American Academy of Cerebral Palsy and Developmental Medicine.

Dr. Dormans has a strong interest in orthopedic care of children in developing countries. He is Chairman of the International Affairs Committee for the American Academy of Cerebral Palsy and Developmental Medicine and also serves on the International Affairs Committee of the American Academy of Orthopaedic Surgeons. He has worked in various countries, including Ethiopia, Bulgaria, and Indonesia and currently serves on the Board of Directors for Orthopaedics Overseas and as Program Director for the Indonesian Program through

Orthopaedic Overseas. He serves as an advisory editor to *Clinical Orthopaedics and Related Research*. Dr. Dormans lives in Gladwyn, Pennsylvania, with his wife and four children.

Louis Pellegrino, M.D., is a pediatrician who completed subspecialty training in Neurodevelopmental Pediatrics at the University of Rochester, New York. Following his fellowship training, he joined the faculty at the University of Pennsylvania School of Medicine as an assistant professor and was Medical Director of the Cerebral Palsy Program at The Children's Hospital of Philadelphia and Children's Seashore House. He is now Assistant Professor of Clinical Pediatrics at the University of Medicine and Dentistry of New Jersey, Robert Wood Johnson Medical School. He has written extensively on the subject of cerebral palsy and maintains cerebral palsy as a primary focus in his clinical, teaching, and academic pursuits, working in a variety of medical and educational settings in collaboration with many different professionals who devote themselves to the care of children with developmental disabilities.

Dr. Pellegrino is board-certified in pediatrics and is a fellow of the American Academy of Pediatrics. He is a member of the American Academy of Pediatrics, the American Academy of Cerebral Palsy and Developmental Medicine, and the Society for Developmental Pediatrics. He lives in Hillsborough, New Jersey, with his wife, Joan, and daughter, Elizabeth.

Contributors

Jennifer Rauck Burstein, M.A., CC/SLP
Senior Speech Pathologist
The Children's Hospital of
   Philadelphia
Children's Seashore House
3405 Civic Center Boulevard
Philadelphia, PA 19104

Lynette E. Byarm, M.S., OTR/L, BCP
Clinical Specialist
Occupational Therapy
Voorhees Pediatric Facility
1304 Laurel Oak Road
Voorhees, NJ 08043

Lawson A. Copley, M.D.
Major
Unites States Air Force
96 Medical Operation Squadron
Eglin Air Force Base, FL 32542

Johanna E. Deitz Curry, M.S., PT
Physical Therapist
The Children's Hospital of
   Philadelphia
Children's Seashore House
3405 Civic Center Boulevard
Philadelphia, PA 19104

Ann-Christine Duhaime, M.D.
Associate Neurosurgeon
The Children's Hospital of
   Philadelphia
Children's Seashore House
3405 Civic Center Boulevard
Philadelphia, PA 19104

Susan K. Effgen, Ph.D., PT
Director
Pediatric Physical Therapy
Allegheny University of the Health
   Sciences
MS 502, Department of Physical
   Therapy
Philadelphia, PA 19102

Peggy S. Eicher, M.D.
Professor of Pediatrics
The Children's Hospital of
   Philadelphia
Children's Seashore House
3405 Civic Center Boulevard
Philadelphia, PA 19104

Lesley A. Geyer, M.A., OTR/L, BCP
Pediatric Coordinator
Austill's Rehabilitation Services
105 Coeway Lane
Exton, PA 19341

Adadot Hayes, M.D.
Developmental Physician Consultant
State of Tennessee
266 Lake Terrace Drive
Hendersonville, TN 37075

Linda Hock-Long, Ph.D.
Manager
Ambulatory Care and Day Hospital
The Children's Hospital of
　Philadelphia
Children's Seashore House
3405 Civic Center Boulevard
Philadelphia, PA 19104

Lisa A. Kurtz, M.Ed., OTR/L, BCP
Director of Occupational Therapy
The Children's Hospital of
　Philadelphia
Children's Seashore House
3405 Civic Center Boulevard
Philadelphia, PA 19104
Assistant Clinical Professor
Thomas Jefferson University

Sandy McGee, PT
Assistant Director of Physical Therapy
The Children's Hospital of
　Philadelphia
Children's Seashore House
3405 Civic Center Boulevard
Philadelphia, PA 19104

Gretchen Meyer, M.D.
Neurodevelopmental Surgeon
United States Navy
Naval Medical Center Portsmouth
1108 Brandonet
Chesapeake, VA 23320

Freeman Miller, M.D.
Pediatric Orthopaedic Surgeon
Alfred I. DuPont Institute of the
　Nemours Foundation
1600 Rockland Road
Post Office Box 269
Wilmington, DE 19899

Stephanie Ried, M.D.
Medical Director for Rehabilitation
Driscall Children's Hospital
3511 S. Almeda
Corpus Christi, TX 78411

Christine F. Rouse
Executive Director
Kids are Kids
71 Tunbridge Road
Haverford, PA 19041

Shirley Albinson-Scull, M.S., PT
Service Line Director
Pediatric Rehabilitation
The Children's Hospital of Philadelphia
Children's Seashore House
3405 Civic Center Boulevard
Philadelphia, PA 19104

Cynthia B. Solot, M.A., CCC
Senior Speech-Language Pathologist
The Children's Hospital of
　Philadelphia
Children's Seashore House
3405 Civic Center Boulevard
Philadelphia, PA 19104

Meg Stanger, M.B., PT
Director of Pediatric Occupational
　Therapy/Physical Therapy
The Children's Institute
6301 Northumberland Street
Pittsburgh, PA 15217

**Symme W. Trachtenberg, M.S.W.,
　LSW**
Director Social Work/Community
　and Government Liaison
The Children's Hospital of
　Philadelphia
Children's Seashore House
3405 Civic Center Boulevard
Philadelphia, PA 19104
Clinical Associate of Pediatrics
University of Pennsylvania Medical
　School

James S. Walker, B.S.
Orthotist
National Orthotic and Prosthetic
    Corporation
The Children's Hospital of
    Philadelphia
Children's Seashore House
Clinical Consultant to Children's
    Seashore House
3405 Civic Center Boulevard
Philadelphia, PA 19104

Audrey Wood, M.S., PT
Physical Therapy Supervisor
The Children's Hospital of
    Philadelphia
Children's Seashore House
3405 Civic Center Boulevard
Philadelphia, PA 19104

Mary Lisa Wright-Drechsel, OTR/L
OT Education Coordinator
The Children's Hospital of
    Philadelphia
Children's Seashore House
3405 Civic Center Boulevard
Philadelphia, PA 19104

Foreword

Cerebral palsy is defined as a disorder of movement and posture that is a result of a nonprogressive abnormality of the immature brain. However, this definition hides the complexity of the disorder and its tendency to change over time. Furthermore, despite advances in modern medicine, there is little evidence that the prevalence of this disorder is decreasing. Thus, the needs for care of children with cerebral palsy are likely to remain unchanged for the foreseeable future.

It was recognized many years ago that the complexity of cerebral palsy warranted a team approach to care. The Maternal and Child Health Bureau provided financial resources to support "Crippled Children's Services" that included multidisciplinary clinics for children with cerebral palsy. One such clinic was set up at The Children's Hospital of Philadelphia and Children's Seashore House. Since its inception, this idea of a team approach has evolved into the program that forms the basis for this book. A mission of The Children's Hospital of Philadelphia and Children's Seashore House has been to identify children with cerebral palsy early, provide comprehensive evaluations, promote community interventions, and provide long-term follow-up services.

In *Caring for Children with Cerebral Palsy: A Team Approach,* the team members of the cerebral palsy program—pediatricians, orthopedic surgeons, physical and occupational therapists, speech-language pathologists, social workers, educators, and administrators—have combined forces to become a team of authors. In this new resource, they describe the collaborative approach they use to provide care for children with cerebral palsy. In reading this book, you gain detailed information on the diagnosis, treatment, and support of children with cerebral palsy, within the context of team-based caregiving. This book is useful for physicians, occupational therapists, physical therapists, nurses, speech-language pathologists, and educators, as well as for social workers, home visitors, and family members.

Caring for Children with Cerebral Palsy: A Team Approach is divided into four sections. The first provides an introduction to cerebral palsy and emphasizes the importance of an interdisciplinary team approach. Definitions, etiology, epidemiology, and diagnostic criteria are discussed. The basics of interdisciplinary and well-child care are also covered. In the second section, the management of associated deficits, including spasticity, other musculoskeletal impairments, and feeding disorders, is explained. Within this section, orthopedic and neurosurgical interventions are emphasized. The third section discusses optimizing function and preventing disability. Mobility, daily living skills, communication, and orthotics are described in detail. The final section of the book addresses opportunities for children with cerebral palsy. The importance of family, school, advocacy, and transitions to adulthood is discussed. Together, these chapters provide guideposts of care from diagnosis in infancy to entry into adulthood.

In these days of change in health care delivery, it is the children who are most likely to be at a disadvantage. Individuals with cerebral palsy fall into this group. It must be our role as health care professionals, teachers, and family members to advocate for the needs of the children we care for and love. This can most effectively be accomplished by providing a care management plan that is clear and effective. *Caring for Children with Cerebral Palsy: A Team Approach* provides the background you need to develop such an individual care plan. It helps you advocate for a level of services appropriate for your child or patient's need.

You might well ask, "What is the use of a book on a team approach to caring for children with cerebral palsy in the new managed care environment?" If one takes the optimistic view, managed care, with an emphasis on prophylaxis and care management, should be supportive of a team approach. The early identification of complications of cerebral palsy, such as contractures, may lead to interventions that delay or prevent surgery or hospitalizations. Improved nutrition is likely to lead to fewer significant illnesses, and support of the family is likely to help maintain an intact family with all of the related financial and emotional benefits. In addition, managed care will demand that we show benefit from our interventions; interdisciplinary teams should be most able to develop outcomes research that will help guide cost-effective care in the future.

Thus, I am hopeful that many of you will continue to be part of team structures in caring for children with cerebral palsy. However, this book is also meant for those of you who will have to be an interdisciplinary team by yourself and for others of you who will need to decide whether referral to a cerebral palsy clinic is warranted. It is hoped that this volume provides each of you with the information you need to deliver optimum and efficient care to these wonderful children. I wish you well and thank you for toiling in these fields; by working together, we will continue to provide effective care for our children with cerebral palsy.

Mark L. Batshaw
Physician-in-Chief
The Children's Hospital of Philadelphia
Children's Seashore House
Philadelphia, Pennsylvania

Caring for Children
with Cerebral Palsy

Introduction to Cerebral Palsy and the Interdisciplinary Team Approach

CHAPTER 1

Definitions, Etiology, and Epidemiology of Cerebral Palsy

Louis Pellegrino and John P. Dormans

"The act of birth does occasionally imprint upon the nervous and muscular systems of the nascent infantile organism very serious and peculiar evils . . . . premature birth, difficult labours, mechanical injuries during parturition to the head and neck, which were apt to be succeeded by a determinate affection of the limbs of the child that I designated . . . spastic rigidity from asphyxia neonatorum."

William John Little (1862/1966)

"One has to consider that the anomaly of the birth process, rather than being the causal etiologic factor, may itself be the consequence of the real prenatal etiology [of infantile cerebral paralysis]."

Sigmund Freud (1897/1968)

"Our present ability to recognize the important antecedents of cerebral palsy and to predict the occurrence of the disorder failed to account for a majority of cases . . . [we] probably do not know what causes most cases of cerebral palsy."

Nelson and Ellenberg (1986)

THE EMERGENCE OF CEREBRAL
PALSY AS A CONCEPT: HISTORICAL NOTES

William John Little presented a paper in 1862 entitled "The Influence of Abnormal Parturition, Difficult Labours, Premature Birth, and Asphyxia Neonatorum on the Mental and Physical Condition of the Child, Especially in Relation to Deformities" to the Obstetrical Society of London. Little described 47 children with, what he termed, *spastic rigidity* (now called spastic diplegia) and proposed that this motor impairment syndrome was a consequence of adverse events at the time of birth. Little linked the term *asphyxia neonatorum* (which literally means "oxygen deprivation caused by respiratory failure in newborns") with the later appearance of spastic rigidity, thus memorializing the idea that birth-related brain injury and what later became known as cerebral palsy were two sides of the same coin—one being the cause, the other the effect. The identification of birth-related brain injury with cerebral palsy has been remarkably resilient; it is only since the early 1980s, more than a century after Little's original proposal, that the concept has been seriously and successfully challenged.

One of the earliest and most celebrated challenges to Little's theory came from Sigmund Freud. Freud, whose training and early work was in the field of neurology, published a series of monographs, culminating in a work entitled "Infantile Cerebral Paralysis." Freud described several types of "paralysis in childhood due to cerebral causes" (1897/1968, p. 17). He specifically challenged Little's theory, proposing that antecedent prenatal abnormalities (i.e., abnormalities of the fetus or the placenta) result in difficulties both at the time of birth and with subsequent neuromotor dysfunction. In other words, problems at the time of birth were a marker, rather than the cause, of cerebral palsy.

The term *cerebral palsy* was originally introduced and popularized in the writings of Sir William Osler (1889/1987), one of the founding fathers of modern medicine. Osler's strong interest in pathology and the pathophysiology of disease is evident in his treatment of cerebral palsy. The decades that followed Osler's seminal contributions on cerebral palsy were marked by a strong emphasis on the neurological abnormalities and pathological features of cerebral palsy. Individuals with cerebral palsy and other chronic neurological conditions were placed in hospitals and other institutional settings (e.g., the Infirmary for Nervous Diseases in Philadelphia, where Osler gathered the material for his case studies) for clinical scrutiny and ongoing provision of care. Cerebral palsy came to be conceptualized as a "static encephalopathy," a nonprogressive, incurable medical condition caused by a brain-damaging event. Whether Osler intended it, his emphasis on the pathological features of cerebral palsy lent implicit support to Little's original identification of cerebral palsy with birth-related brain injury.

The second half of the 20th century has witnessed three developments that have significantly affected thinking about cerebral palsy. The first development relates to the advent of modern epidemiological science, which is concerned with the prevalence of disease in populations and uses statistical techniques to uncover clues to the causes of disease. Several epidemiological studies, which culminated in a landmark paper by Nelson and Ellenberg in 1986 (see section on "The Prenatal Period" in this chapter), have cast serious doubt on the overly simplistic link between birth asphyxia and cerebral palsy and tend to support the notion that prenatal factors (which often cannot be specified) predominate in the pathogenesis of cerebral palsy.

The second development is the emergence of the neurosciences and medical genetics, which have given scientists and doctors a greater appreciation of the complexity and diversity of circumstances that may lead to cerebral palsy. The advent of neuroimaging techniques such as *computed tomography (CT)* and *magnetic resonance imaging (MRI)* has, in particular, provided an unprecedented "window" on brain structure and development.

The third development is the emergence of *developmental disability* as a concept, which is a result of societal and intellectual currents that have also supported the rise of interdisciplinary care (see Chapter 3). Developmental disabilities—as the term itself suggests—are defined in terms of developmental and functional considerations and include conditions such as mental retardation, autism, and learning disabilities. Within this new framework, cerebral palsy has been reconceptualized as a developmental disability. This has several important implications. The one-dimensional understanding of cerebral palsy as a "static encephalopathy" has been replaced with a dynamic diagnostic entity that more accurately reflects the real experiences of individuals with this motor impairment syndrome. In other words, cerebral palsy is a developmental disability that is defined in terms of its functional consequences, rather than in terms of its neurological causes. The definition of cerebral palsy provided in this chapter (see section on "Cerebral Palsy: A Definition" in this chapter) is sufficiently flexible to accommodate both aspects of the cerebral palsy diagnosis. Current understanding of the definitions, subtypes, and causes of cerebral palsy is summarized in this chapter; the diagnosis of cerebral palsy as a developmental disability is considered in Chapter 2.

CEREBRAL PALSY: A DEFINITION

The definition and classification of cerebral palsy have been a source of great confusion and controversy ever since the concept was introduced. The term itself is somewhat misleading: Whereas *"cerebral"* appropriately emphasizes the importance of the brain in the genesis of the condition, *"palsy"* is an anachronism that in modern parlance is usually associated with *paralysis,* which suggests a complete loss of movement (not typical of cerebral palsy). Many professionals and individuals outside of the discipline have advocated that the term *cerebral palsy* should be abolished and replaced with a term (or terms) that is either scientifically more satisfying or at least less jarring to contemporary sensibilities.

In their seminal work *The Natural History of Cerebral Palsy* originally published in 1954, Crothers and Paine (1959) suggested that the remarkable resilience of the term cerebral palsy relates to its administrative and pragmatic utility. Despite the many pejorative connotations that have come to be associated with the term cerebral palsy over the years, the term has persisted primarily because it is useful. It is useful in the design of medical and therapeutic programs targeting a group of individuals with similar functional and medical issues, in the design of scientific studies, as a means of gaining access to special education services, and in creating priorities for legislation and for other forms of advocacy at the societal level. Despite its drawbacks, the term cerebral palsy has come to have a life of its own and will most likely be with us for years to come.

In the many definitions of cerebral palsy that have been put forward since the mid-1980s, there are three recurrent elements that provide the basis for a concise definition. The first element is that there is a significant problem with motor function. The second element is that this motor impairment results from something that "went wrong" with the brain during its early development. The third element is that the disturbance of typical brain development occurred over a discrete period of time and does not represent a continuing, recurrent, or progressive process.

Cerebral Palsy Is a Motor Impairment Syndrome

Regardless of the specific cause, or *etiology,* all people with cerebral palsy have a significant problem with controlling *movement* and *posture.* Although abnormalities of *muscle tone* (defined as the resistance of a muscle to passive stretch) are important in classifying specific subtypes of cerebral palsy, they are not part of the actual definition. The emphasis on cerebral palsy as a motor impairment syndrome also differentiates it from other conditions that result from anomalies of brain development and function, such as mental retardation and autism (although problems such as mental retardation are often associated with cerebral palsy; see section on "Cognitive Impairments, Mental Retardation, and Learning Disabilities" in this chapter).

Cerebral Palsy Is a Result of a
Disturbance or Anomaly in Early Brain Development

The major events in the development of the brain and their timing are outlined in Table 1.1. The brain grows most rapidly and develops most profoundly during the prenatal period and continues to grow rapidly during the early postnatal years. Insults to the brain that occur after 8 years of age result in neurological impairments reminiscent of those observed in adults; similar insults prior to 3 years of age (including during the prenatal period) result in neurological impairments and motor outcomes—such as cerebral palsy—that are characteristic of injury to the immature brain (Chugani, 1993). From 3 to 8 years, mixed

Table 1.1.   Major events in the development of the central nervous system

Event	Description	Timing
Dorsal induction	Formation of the neural tube (primordium of the central nervous system)	1/2–1 month postconception
Ventral induction	Elaboration of the primary subdivisions of the central nervous system	1–2 months postconception
Neuronal proliferation	Multiplication of neurons	2–4 months postconception
Neuronal migration	Movement of neurons to their final locations in the central nervous system	3–5 months postconception
Organization/ synaptogenesis	Elaboration and organization of connections among neurons	6 months postconception to 8 years postnatal
Myelination	Elaboration of nonneuronal brain and nerve elements	Birth to early adulthood

Adapted from Volpe (1995).

patterns of neurological impairment are observed. An arbitrary upper age limit of 5 or 6 years has been suggested for assigning the diagnosis of cerebral palsy; however, in practice, the determination is typically made on a case-by-case basis.

The emphasis on the complicity of the brain in the genesis of cerebral palsy helps to differentiate this motor impairment syndrome from others that result from disturbances in other domains of the neuromotor apparatus (see Chapter 2).

Cerebral Palsy Is a Result of Nonprogressive Insults or Anomalies

A number of *progressive* or *degenerative* (i.e., worsening) disorders of the nervous or muscular systems can result in motor impairment syndromes that share some of the features of cerebral palsy. The critical distinction is that although the motor impairment and functional consequences of cerebral palsy may change and even worsen with time, the underlying brain anomaly that initially caused the motor impairment does not. This distinction is especially important because the *prognoses* (i.e., expectations for outcome) of progressive conditions are often very different from those of *static* conditions such as cerebral palsy. Progressive conditions may have specific implications for genetic counseling (e.g., a family may be at high risk for recurrence of the condition in future offspring) and may be amenable to specific drug and dietary interventions that could slow or reverse the degenerative process. The definition of cerebral palsy may therefore be summarized as follows:

> Cerebral palsy is an umbrella term covering a group of nonprogressive, but often changing, motor impairment syndromes secondary to lesions or anomalies of the brain arising in the early stages of its development. (Mutch, Alberman, Hagberg, Kodama, & Perat, 1992)

TYPES OF CEREBRAL PALSY

Many attempts have been made to derive a consistent classification scheme for cerebral palsy based on motor impairment subtypes (Stanley & Alberman, 1984). As described previously, the types of motor impairment associated with cerebral palsy are defined in terms of abnormalities of movement, muscle tone, and posture.

- *Abnormalities of movement* may be manifested as disturbances of voluntary movements or the presence of involuntary movements.
- *Muscle tone* may be increased (i.e., *hypertonia)* or decreased (i.e., *hypotonia).*
- *Posture* refers to the motion and the positioning of one body part or body segment relative to another. Posture represents the integration of movement patterns as these occur within the context of altered muscle tone.

By invoking these qualitative aspects of motor function, professionals are, in effect, classifying cerebral palsy by *physiological type* (see Table 1.2).

The motor impairments associated with cerebral palsy may also be classified according to their *geographic distribution* or the extent of the body's musculoskeletal system that is involved. Most schemes use limb involvement as an index for the geographic extent of the motor impairment (see Table 1.3). *Total body cerebral palsy* and *quadramembral cerebral palsy* are terms occasionally used to emphasize global involvement of the musculoskeletal system in abnormalities of muscle tone and movement.

Some classification schemes also attempt to incorporate statements about the severity of the motor impairment into descriptions of subtypes, but these schemes run the risk of confounding aspects of musculoskeletal impairment with functional disability (Blair & Stanley, 1985; see Chapter 3). Finally, cerebral palsy may be classified according to the presumed neuroanatomical substrate of the observed motor impairment. The term *pyramidal* refers to a well-defined system of neuronal pathways that originates in the cerebral gray matter and terminates at various levels of the brain stem and spinal cord (see Figure 1.1). The spastic forms of cerebral palsy are often associated with abnor-

Table 1.2. Cerebral palsy by physiological type

Physiological type	Description
Spasticity	Velocity-dependent resistance to stretch, clasp-knife response, increased deep tendon reflexes, clonus
Athetosis	Involuntary writhing movements, often with chorea (i.e., involuntary jerky movements)
Rigidity	"Lead-pipe" hypertonia, fluctuating tone, prominent primitive reflexes
Ataxia	Problems with balance and controlling position of body in space
Hypotonia	Low muscle tone, normal or increased deep tendon reflexes
Mixed	Evidence of two or more physiological types

Note: See Chapters 2 and 5 for detailed descriptions of physical findings.

malities or disruptions of these pathways; hence, *spastic cerebral palsy* and *pyramidal cerebral palsy* are often used synonymously. In contrast, types of cerebral palsy in which rigidity or hypotonia predominate or in which involuntary movements or ataxia are prominent are associated with abnormalities of the brain's motor control system (especially the *basal ganglia* and the *cerebellum*) that lie outside of the pyramidal tracts and are therefore referred to as *extrapyramidal*. In practice, *extrapyramidal cerebral palsy* refers to all cases of cerebral palsy that do not meet the criteria for pyramidal or spastic cerebral

Table 1.3. Cerebral palsy by distribution

Distribution	Description
Hemiplegia	Arm and leg on same side involved, arm usually more than leg
Monoplegia	One limb, usually arm, affected (a variant of hemiplegia)
Diplegia	Both sides of body involved, legs more than arms
Quadriplegia	Both sides of body involved, both legs and arms significantly affected
Triplegia	Both sides of body involved, but one limb (usually arm) relatively spared
Double hemiplegia	Both sides of body involved, but one side more than other; arms usually more affected

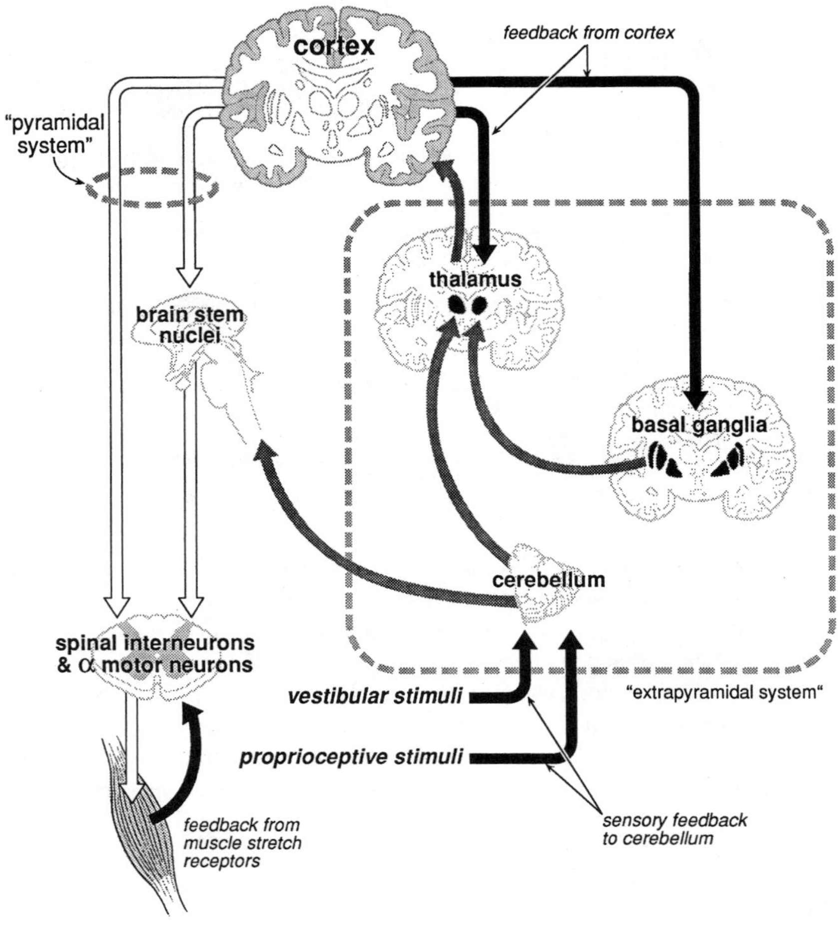

Figure 1.1. Schematic representation of the components of the motor control system. The "pyramidal system" refers to descending pathways originating in the cerebral cortex and terminating in the brain stem and spinal cord. These pathways ultimately determine the timing and degree of muscle contraction and regulate muscle tone. The "extrapyramidal system" consists of deep-brain structures that influence motor activity by modulating neuronal activity in the cortex and brain stem, hence, indirectly affecting the output of descending motor pathways.

palsy. The advantages of the pyramidal/extrapyramidal classification scheme are its simplicity and its reference to the neurological basis of motor impairments. However, these classifications also are the scheme's disadvantages. This system tends to oversimplify to the point of obscuring the subtle and important variations in motor functions seen in cerebral palsy. In fact, the physiological mechanisms suggested by these terms, although suggesting a firm scientific basis for their use, are presumptive and, in some cases, controversial (Young, 1994). For the purposes of this book, a classification scheme that combines physiological and geographical descriptions is used (Hagberg, Sanner, & Steen, 1972). The relationships among various aspects of different classification schemes are summarized in Figure 1.2.

Spastic cerebral palsy is the most common motor impairment type, accounting for approximately 70%–80% of all cases of cerebral palsy, and is categorized according to the distribution of limbs involved. Approximately 25%–35% of children with spastic cerebral palsy have *spastic diplegia,* with their legs clearly more affected than their arms. Approximately 35%–40% of children with spastic cerebral palsy have *spastic hemiplegia,* with one side of their body more affected than the other side (the arm is usually more affected than the leg). Because the motor neurons that control one side of the body are located in the opposite cerebral cortex, a right-side hemiplegia implies damage to, or dysfunction of, the left side of the brain and vice versa. In *spastic quadriplegia* (40%–45% of those with spastic cerebral palsy), all four limbs and usually the trunk and muscles that control the mouth, tongue, and pharynx are affected. The severity of the motor impairment in spastic quadriplegia implies wider cerebral dysfunction and worse prognosis than the other forms of spastic cerebral palsy. Mental retardation, seizures, sensory impairments, and medical complications are commonly observed in spastic quadriplegia.

Dyskinetic cerebral palsy (accounting for approximately 10%–15% of all cases of cerebral palsy) is characterized by tonal abnormalities that involve the whole body. Patterns of muscle typically change from hour to hour and day to day. Children with dyskinetic cerebral palsy often exhibit rigid muscle tone while awake and typical or decreased muscle tone while asleep. Involuntary movements are often present—although sometimes difficult to detect—and are the hallmark of this type of cerebral palsy. Rapid, random, jerky movements (i.e., chorea) and slow, writhing movements (i.e., athetosis) are seen in *athetoid cerebral palsy,* a subtype of dyskinetic cerebral palsy. Rigid posturing centered in the trunk and neck is also characteristic of dystonic cerebral palsy.

Ataxic cerebral palsy (accounting for less than 5% of all cases of cerebral palsy) is characterized by abnormalities of voluntary movement involving balance and position of the trunk and limbs. For children who can walk, this abnormality is most often noted as a wide-based, unsteady gait. Difficulties with controlling the hand and arm during reaching (e.g., overshooting or past-pointing) and problems with the timing of motor movements are also seen in children with ataxic cerebral palsy. In addition, ataxic cerebral palsy may be associated with increased or decreased muscle tone in particular children. The term *mixed cerebral palsy* is used when more than one type of motor pattern is present; however, this term should be used only when one pattern does not clearly dominate another.

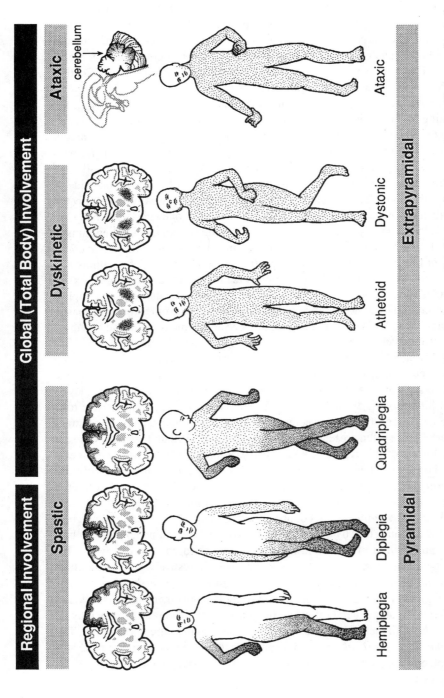

Figure 1.2. The classification of cerebral palsy. Although overlaps in terminology are shown, cerebral palsy may be classified according to the distribution (i.e., regional versus global involvement; hemiplegic, diplegic, or quadriplegic), physiological type (i.e., spastic, dyskinetic/dystonic, dyskinetic/athetoid, or ataxic), or by presumed neurological substrate (i.e., pyramidal versus extrapyramidal). (From Pellegrino, L. [1997]. Cerebral palsy. In M.L. Batshaw [Ed.], *Children with disabilities* [4th ed., p. 502]. Baltimore: Paul H. Brookes Publishing Co.; reprinted by permission.)

THE EPIDEMIOLOGY AND ETIOLOGY OF CEREBRAL PALSY

Epidemiology—literally, "the study of epidemics"—is the branch of medicine concerned with describing and tracking diseases and disorders as they occur in populations. *Etiology* refers to the cause (or causes) of a particular disorder. In the case of cerebral palsy, advances in epidemiology have led to a fundamental shift in understanding the probable causes of the disorder; it is these insights that provide the foundation for further advances. These advances are fueled by improvements in brain imaging technology and by advances in our understanding of brain development and the genetics of the nervous system. A better understanding of the causes of cerebral palsy will, we hope, create new opportunities to prevent or ameliorate the condition in its early stages of formation.

Trends in the Epidemiology of Cerebral Palsy

A basic requirement in establishing the causes of a disability such as cerebral palsy is to determine how common it is in the general population and to establish a clear sense of the conditions in which it arises. These are difficult tasks that require both a centralized system of health care delivery and a long-term commitment to data collection supported by public policy. These conditions exist primarily in countries with systems of socialized medicine or in large but relatively isolated populations served by a single health care delivery system. General understanding of trends in the prevalence of cerebral palsy mostly comes from studies in Scandinavia, the United Kingdom, Western Australia, and Japan. In the United States, epidemiological trends have been more difficult to track, but work using special statistical techniques (Bhushan, Paneth, & Kiely, 1993) has provided a glimpse into trends in the United States, which in general mirror those in evidence in other developed countries.

The *prevalence* of a disorder refers to its frequency in a population. The *incidence* of a disorder refers to its rate of appearance in a given period of time (e.g., new cases per year). Because the signs and symptoms of cerebral palsy are not fully manifest until 2–3 years of age, it is usually not possible to assign an accurate estimate of incidence; therefore, prevalence figures are generally used. Since the late 1950s, estimates of the prevalence of all forms of cerebral palsy in the general world population have varied from 0.6 to 2.4 per 1,000, with 2 per 1,000 being the frequently quoted approximation. Figures from Sweden provide an illustration of the trends in the prevalence of cerebral palsy since 1980 (Hagberg, Hagberg, & Olow, 1984, 1993; Hagberg, Hagberg, Olow, & Von Wendt, 1989; Hagberg, Hagberg, & Zetterstrom, 1989; see Figure 1.3). Following a small decline in the rates of cerebral palsy in the late 1960s and early 1970s, the childhood prevalence of cerebral palsy has increased steadily. A consensus exists that this increase is a result of improved survival of very low birth weight (VLBW) infants (those born weighing less than 1,500 grams, which

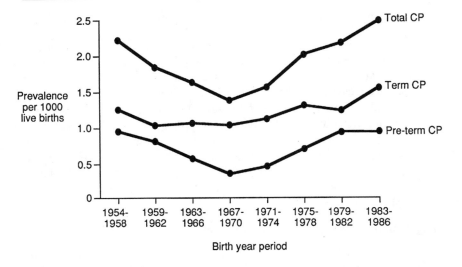

Figure 1.3. The prevalence of cerebral palsy. Although the prevalence of cerebral palsy for infants born at term has remained fairly constant since the 1970s, the proportion of children with cerebral palsy represented by prematurely born infants has increased. This increase is probably a result of the increased survival rate of infants with very low birth weight (less than 1,500 grams). As a result, there has been an overall increase in the prevalence of cerebral palsy. (From Hagberg, B., Hagberg, G., & Olow, I. [1993]. The changing panorama of cerebral palsy in Sweden: VI. Prevalence and origin during the birth year period 1983–1986. *Acta Paediatrica, 82,* 388; reprinted by permission.)

is approximately 3 pounds, 5 ounces). Prematurely born children with VLBW now represent nearly half of the childhood cases of cerebral palsy (Cummins, Nelson, Grether, & Velie, 1993). The decline in the cerebral palsy rate in the 1960s and 1970s probably represents a hiatus when improvements in obstetrical care resulted in fewer intrapartum complications but advances in neonatal care had not yet resulted in increases in the survival figures for VLBW infants. Another factor in the early decline of rates of cerebral palsy may have been improvements in the diagnosis and treatment of maternal–fetal Rh factor incompatibility, which in years past resulted in severe newborn jaundice caused by high blood bilirubin levels and a neurological condition called *kernicterus,* which was an important cause of dyskinetic cerebral palsy.

The Prenatal Period

The fact that improvements in obstetrical care have not resulted in steady declines in the rate of cerebral palsy has surprised many people; this probably represents a failed expectation based on a false assumption. It is still widely believed that adverse conditions at the time of birth, resulting in oxygen deprivation and birth asphyxia, are the primary causes of cerebral palsy. However, landmark epidemiological studies from the 1970s and 1980s (Nelson &

Ellenberg, 1985, 1986) strongly challenge this assumption, suggesting that prenatal factors predominate in the genesis of cerebral palsy (see Table 1.4).

The prenatal period is defined as spanning from conception to the onset of labor. Prenatal factors include maternal factors, constitutional (i.e., genetic) or familial factors, and pregnancy-specific or gestational factors. It is important to recognize that although the risk factors listed in Table 1.4 are statistically significant antecedents of cerebral palsy for a group of individuals, none of the factors robustly predicts cerebral palsy in an individual child. For example, although twins and triplets are overrepresented among children with cerebral palsy, the large majority of children produced from multiple-gestation pregnancies do not develop cerebral palsy.

It is sometimes possible to identify a specific prenatal cause of cerebral palsy for a specific child. A careful medical history and a physical examination are the cornerstones of establishing such a diagnosis, and these practices have been greatly enhanced by advances in brain-imaging technology and by improvements in our understanding of the genetic basis of nervous system

Table 1.4. Risk factors for cerebral palsy in populations

Maternal and familial factors
Mother
 Thyroid disorder
 Menstrual cycle more than 36 days
 Previous pregnancy loss
 Previous loss of newborn
 Mental retardation
 Seizure disorder

Prior-born child
 Less than 2,000 grams
 Motor deficit
 Mental retardation
 Sensory deficit

Factors related to current pregnancy
 Polyhydramnios (i.e., increased amniotic fluid)
 Treatment of mother with thyroid hormone
 Treatment of mother with estrogen or progesterone
 Fetus with congenital malformations
 Maternal seizure disorder
 Severe proteinuria (i.e., protein in urine), high blood pressure
 Bleeding in third trimester

Adapted from Nelson (1996).
Note: Risk factors apply to groups with cerebral palsy, not to individuals.

development. The specific causes of cerebral palsy include developmental brain abnormalities, genetic or chromosome abnormalities, radiation exposure, prenatal infections, erythroblastosis fetalis, congenital malformations, illicit drug use, and fetal alcohol syndrome. For example, genetic abnormalities may lead to brain malformations or abnormalities in the early stages of embryonic development. Erythroblastosis fetalis is caused by Rh incompatibility between the mother and the fetus and results in damage to the developing midbrain, particularly the basal ganglion, which results in a functional impairment called *athetosis*. Intrauterine infection may damage the developing central nervous system (CNS) of the fetus. TORCHES (an acronym for toxoplasmosis, rubella, cytomegalovirus infection, herpes, and syphilis) is a useful way of remembering types of infections that can occur in the intrauterine environment.

The Perinatal Period and Birth Asphyxia

The *perinatal period* begins with the onset of labor and extends into the early days of postnatal life. The *intrapartum period* begins with the onset of labor and ends at birth. The birthing process represents a dramatic series of events during which the child must make a rapid transition from an intrauterine to an extrauterine environment. However, this transition is not always accomplished successfully. Problems associated with birth or around the time of birth may result in oxygen deprivation (i.e., hypoxia) or insufficient blood flow to the brain (i.e., cerebral ischemia). *Birth asphyxia* is a term used more loosely to describe the circumstances that lead to and the consequences that derive from hypoxic-ischemic insults. The apparent precision of the terms used to describe these events belies the fact that true hypoxia-ischemia as a cause of subsequent cerebral palsy is notoriously difficult to document. Birth asphyxia can be documented as the definitive cause of cerebral palsy in no more than 10% or fewer cases of cerebral palsy (Nelson & Ellenberg, 1986). Even when birth asphyxia seems a likely antecedent to cerebral palsy, a significant percentage of children show evidence of preexisting abnormalities, such as congenital malformations or *intrauterine growth retardation*. In general, birth asphyxia should not be considered the cause of cerebral palsy unless there is clear evidence of oxygen deprivation (e.g., severely decreased blood pH, which indicates an accumulation of lactic acid as an end product of anaerobic metabolism) and subsequent evidence of organ system damage related to tissue hypoxia (e.g., damage to the kidneys resulting in renal dysfunction). Hypoxic-ischemic encephalopathy (HIE) as manifested by hypotonia, paucity of spontaneous movement, and seizures in the neonatal period is especially important to document (Nelson & Emery, 1993). Apgar scores (see Table 1.5) provide a method for documenting the newborn's cardiopulmonary and neuromotor status in the first minutes following birth (Apgar, 1953). Low Apgar scores may reflect adverse circumstances unrelated to birth asphyxia, including infections and other preexisting prenatal conditions, and cannot be used as an independent indicator of birth asphyxia.

Table 1.5. Apgar scores for newborns

Sign	Score		
	0	1	2
Heart rate	Absent	Less than 100 per minute	Greater than 100 per minute
Respiratory effort	Absent	Weak cry	Strong cry
Muscle tone	Limp	Some flexion	Good flexion
Reflex irritability	No response	Some motion	Cry
Color	Blue/pale	Body pink, extremities blue	Body and extremities pink

Note: Total minimum score = 0; total maximum score = 10.

Birth trauma resulting in direct injury to the brain is not a common cause of cerebral palsy in developed countries, which is a direct result of improvements in obstetrical care in the past several decades. This observation is supported by the fact that, although the overall prevalence of cerebral palsy has increased, there is a low rate of cerebral palsy among infants who weigh more than 4 kilograms and who are considered at the greatest risk for birth-related brain trauma (Cummins et al., 1993). The complex relationship that exists between perinatal events and the issue of prematurity is discussed in the section on "Prematurity, Low Birth Weight, and Cerebral Palsy" in this chapter.

The Postnatal Period

The *immediate postnatal period* refers to the first few hours or days following birth; the *neonatal period* refers to the first few weeks following birth (definitions for these periods vary from author to author). The postnatal period includes both the immediate postnatal period and the neonatal period and, strictly speaking, defines all years subsequent to birth (although "*postnatal*" usually refers only to the first few years after birth). In the early postnatal epochs, neonatal illness, especially if complicated by infections with such agents as *Group B Streptococcus* or other bacteria (e.g., herpes simplex virus), may be a factor or primary cause in the development of cerebral palsy. Beyond the newborn period, the most frequent causes of cerebral palsy are *traumatic brain injury (TBI)* and infections resulting in *meningitis* (i.e., infection of the membranes covering the brain) or *encephalitis* (i.e., infection of the brain itself) (Molnar, 1992). TBI may be the result of an accidental injury (e.g., a consequence of a motor vehicle accident), or it may be the result of abuse (e.g., shaken impact syndrome). A decline in meningitis, which is a result of the introduction of immunization against *Hemophilus influenza Type B,* should result in a decline in cases of cerebral palsy resulting from postnatal infection. Hypoxic-ischemic injury caused by near-drowning episodes is a problem (similar to TBI) that has a seasonal variation of occurrence, being more common in the summer. Brain tumors are a relatively rare cause of cerebral palsy and may occur as a result of direct disruption of motor pathways by the tumor or as a consequence of surgical intervention, chemotherapy, or radiation therapy. Strictly speaking, when a tumor is in its progressive stage, the resulting motor impairment should not be called cerebral palsy; however, it would be correct to refer to residual motor impairment following successful treatment as cerebral palsy.

Prematurity, Low Birth Weight, and Cerebral Palsy

As mentioned previously, the most dramatic epidemiological trend since the mid-1980s has been the rapid increase in the proportion of prematurely born infants who subsequently develop cerebral palsy. Infants with birth weights less than 1,500 grams are especially vulnerable to cerebral palsy, with a childhood prevalence of 60 per 1,000 as compared with an overall prevalence of 2 per 1,000 (Stanley, 1992). However, it should be remembered that although the incidence of other developmental problems in prematurely born infants is still very high, the vast majority of VLBW infants do not develop cerebral palsy. The relationship of premature birth to cerebral palsy is only beginning to be understood.

First, the premature infant has fragile blood vessels deep within the brain (in an area called the *germinal matrix*) that may bleed into the brain's internal fluid spaces (known as *ventricles*), and this may result in a condition known as *intraventricular hemorrhage (IVH),* also referred to as *periventricular hemorrhage.* Refer to Table 1.6 for the grading system for IVH. Grades III and IV are associated with an increased risk for neurological sequelae, including hydrocephalus (caused by the blockage of flow of cerebrospinal fluid), mental retardation, and cerebral palsy.

Second, the area of the brain near the lateral ventricles is especially vulnerable to injury between 26 and 32 weeks' gestation (Volpe, 1995). Disturbances in regional blood flow and oxygen supply may result in damage to the adjacent white matter, an area that is composed of neuronal connections that are important in many aspects of motor control. Damage to these areas results most

Table 1.6.   Grading system for intraventricular hemorrhage

Grade	Pathology
I	Bleeding confined to germinal matrix
II	Bleeding extends into ventricles
III	Bleeding is complicated by dilatation of ventricles
IV	Bleeding extends into substance of the brain

commonly in problems of motor control and muscle tone in the legs. These problems are called *spastic diplegia*. Therefore, abnormalities that disrupt the typical regulation and the maintenance of the latter stages of pregnancy may set in motion a series of pathological events, which results in preterm birth, IVH, periventricular white matter injury (i.e., periventricular leukomalacia [PVL]), and subsequent cerebral palsy (Adinolfi, 1993; Leviton, 1993; see Figure 1.4).

Because the perinatal period is characterized by rapid fluctuations of physiology and environment, it is often assumed that perinatal events are the primary cause of cerebral palsy in premature, VLBW infants. However, it must be recognized that the immature condition of the preterm infant's brain also makes it vulnerable to disturbances in late gestation that may predate the onset of labor

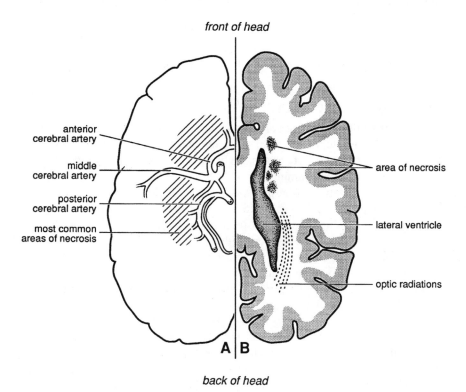

Figure 1.4. Periventricular leukomalacia. In this schematic, cross-sectional view, the blood vessels that supply the brain with blood are shown in section "A," and brain structures are shown in section "B." The area surrounding the ventricles contains "white matter," which includes the descending neuronal pathways of the motor control system (see Figure 1.1). This area—especially farther forward in the brain—is susceptible to damage in premature infants because of a relative paucity of blood vessels. Fluctuations in blood flow, blood oxygen, or blood glucose levels can cause damage (i.e., necrosis) in this area, resulting in a disturbance of the motor control system and subsequent (usually spastic) cerebral palsy.

(e.g., placental insufficiency, which is an infection of the membranes surrounding the fetus [chorionitis]). Inflammation of the placenta has been reported in 50%–80% of extremely premature births (Steer, 1991). It has been suggested that such conditions may lead to premature labor and brain injury via independent mechanisms, which is reminiscent of Freud's (1897/1968) suggestion that prenatal conditions may independently result in cerebral palsy and in problems at the time of birth. The premature infant also is vulnerable to insults to the periventricular region as a result of neonatal illness, which may be complicated by hypoxic episodes, infections, alterations in blood pressure (and consequently cerebral blood flow), low blood sugar (i.e., hypoglycemia), and infection. For the prematurely born infant, it may be impossible to specify the time or origin of his or her cerebral palsy. Likewise, a specific inciting agent (e.g., infection, hypoxia) may not be identifiable. It may be that cumulative or synergistic effects are required to exceed some threshold of vulnerability that results in subsequent cerebral palsy, with the specific sequence of events or combination of inciting agents varying from child to child (Petterson, Stanley, & Garner, 1993).

The Full-Term Infant and Cerebral Palsy

Although the full-term infant is at considerably less risk than the prematurely born infant for developing cerebral palsy, the much larger number of full-term infants accounts for the fact that a slight majority of children with cerebral palsy are born at term (Cummins et al., 1993). Among full-term infants who subsequently develop cerebral palsy, there is an increased incidence of non–CNS malformations (Kuban & Leviton, 1994); there is also an increased incidence of stunted intrauterine growth, termed *intrauterine growth retardation,* in these children (Uvebrant & Hagberg, 1992) that suggests a greater importance of prenatal, and possibly genetic, factors in the etiology of their cerebral palsy. Full-term infants also predominate among those children who develop cerebral palsy as a consequence of true HIE. *Meconium aspiration syndrome* (i.e., aspiration of the first bowel movement during labor and delivery, with subsequent respiratory compromise) and *persistent pulmonary hypertension of the newborn* (also known as *persistent fetal circulation,* which results in severe hypoxia) are among the causes of HIE in the full-term infant. Developmental differences between the premature and the full-term brain make the latter more vulnerable to injury of the basal ganglia, and this results in an increased rate of dyskinetic cerebral palsy in full-term children who experience HIE (Krageloh-Mann, Hagberg, et al., 1995).

As mentioned previously, direct brain injury caused by trauma during birth is not a common cause of cerebral palsy in developed countries as a result of improvements in obstetrical practice since the 1970s.

Multiple Gestations and Cerebral Palsy

Twins and triplets are significantly overrepresented among children with cerebral palsy (Petterson, Nelson, Watson, & Stanley, 1993; Petterson, Stanley, & Henderson, 1990). This overrepresentation is probably a result of the fact that children who are the product of a multiple gestation are born prematurely more often than singleton children; in other words, multiple gestations do not, by themselves, create an added risk for cerebral palsy (Grether, Nelson, & Cummins, 1993). An exception to this rule occurs when one twin dies: The surviving twin has a 100 times greater chance than a singleton of developing cerebral palsy (Grether et al., 1993). This may relate to problems that develop as a result of shared placental circulation between some twin pairs (Nelson, 1996).

Cerebral Palsy Subtypes and Etiology

Spastic cerebral palsy, especially spastic diplegia, has long been associated with prematurity (Kuban & Leviton, 1994), regardless of the fact that spastic cerebral palsy is the most prevalent subtype across all gestational groups and conditions. Among children with spastic cerebral palsy, the most common finding on brain imaging is PVL (Krageloh-Mann, Petersen, et al., 1995). Hemiplegic cerebral palsy is more often associated with asymmetric congenital vascular or developmental anomalies of the brain; but even in this group, PVL is still the most common finding on brain imaging (Nieman, Wakat, Krageloh-Mann, Grodd, & Michaelis, 1994). Spastic quadriplegia is often seen in the context of prematurity, and it is also one of the main sequelae of HIE (Krageloh-Mann, Hagberg, et al., 1995).

The incidence of dyskinetic cerebral palsy is also increased among children who have experienced true HIE. Slowly progressive metabolic and neurodegenerative diseases that mimic cerebral palsy may also present *dyskinetic* or extrapyramidal cerebral palsy. Care must be taken in these cases to rule out this possibility (see Table 1.7).

Ataxic cerebral palsy is uncommon; is difficult to diagnose; and, in many ways, may seem clinically "out of place" with respect to the other forms of cerebral palsy. This is in part true because of the strong association between several genetic and metabolic conditions and *congenital ataxia* (Hughes & Newton, 1992; see Table 1.8).

Diagnosing the Etiology of Cerebral Palsy in the Individual Child

Epidemiological studies are useful in helping to understand the predominant factors in the etiology of cerebral palsy for whole groups; however, this does not easily translate into well-defined rules or guidelines for establishing the diagnosis of etiology for the individual child. It is also important to distinguish between diagnosing cerebral palsy as a developmental disability, which relies

Table 1.7. Selected progressive/metabolic conditions mistaken for cerebral palsy

Syndrome/condition	Description and implications
Glutaric aciduria Type 1	Dystonia or ataxia; episodic deterioration; *preventive therapy may prevent disability if child can reach adolescence without major deterioration*
Arginase deficiency	Slowly progressive ataxia or spasticity; *rate of progression can be slowed with a low-protein diet and sodium benzoate therapy*
Sjögren-Larsson syndrome	Scaly skin, mental retardation, spastic diplegia, or quadriplegia
Ceretendinous xanthomatosis	Yellow lesions on tendons, cataracts, mental retardation; *therapy with oral chenodeoxycholic acid is effective in arresting and possibly reversing progression*
Metachromatic leukodystrophy	Progressive ataxia or spasticity; *bone marrow transplantation may help*
Pelizaeus Merzbacher disease	Sex-linked (males affected); slowly progressive spasticity, nystagmus (i.e., involuntary eye movements)
Lesch-Nyhan syndrome	Uric acid in urine; self-mutilation
Peroxisomal disorders	Mild forms associated with slowly progressive spasticity, deafness, retinal abnormalities, and enlarged liver

Adapted from Moser (1994).

primarily on an analysis of developmental, functional, and physical data, and diagnosing the cause of cerebral palsy, which relies primarily on historical medical data (see Chapter 2). Epidemiological studies do provide some clues that may guide medical history; however, cerebral palsy, by definition, originates in the early epochs of the brain's development. Thus, careful attention must be paid to establishing a clear understanding of the sequence of events characterizing the pregnancy, the birth, and the newborn period. It is particularly important to remember the differences that arise in the context of premature births and those that arise in children born at term. Cerebral palsy that results from discrete postnatal events is usually identified relatively easily. Knowing the particular motor impairment subtype (i.e., spastic, dyskinetic, or ataxic) may also help in directing diagnostic efforts.

Table 1.8.   Selected examples of congenital ataxia

Syndrome/condition	Description
Joubert syndrome	Hypotonia, mental retardation, breathing abnormalities, extra digits, abnormal eye movements, retinal findings, small cerebellum
Chiari malformation Type 1	Small cerebellum, hydrocephalus
Dandy-Walker syndrome	Small cerebellum, cyst of fourth ventricle of brain
Angelman syndrome	Mental retardation, small mid-face, inappropriate laughing, chromosome 15 deletion
Gillespie syndrome	Small or absent iris, mental retardation
Marinesco-Sjögren syndrome	Mental retardation, cataracts, skeletal abnormalities, progressive[a]
Ataxia telangiectasia	Small cerebellum, telangiectasias (i.e., birth marks composed of small blood vessels), progressive[a] ataxia, immune deficiency
Hexosaminidase A and B deficiency	Progressive[a], metabolic
Behr syndrome	Optic atrophy, loss of proprioception, peripheral neuropathy, possibly progressive[a]
Ataxia with hearing loss, mental retardation, and hypogonadism	Genital anomalies, possibly progressive[a]
Ataxia with hearing loss, amyotrophy, and intellectual deterioration	Progressive[a], muscle atrophy

[a]Progressive conditions with ataxia that are mistaken for ataxic cerebral palsy.

Brain-imaging techniques are available to help define the anatomical differences of the CNS seen in infants and children with cerebral palsy, and these are especially helpful adjuncts in the diagnosis of etiology (Barnes, 1992). Ultrasonography is used for fetal and neonatal screening and can distinguish gross malformations of the brain and abnormalities related to brain hemorrhage (e.g., IVH, PVL, hydrocephalus). CT and MRI in particular provide more detailed resolution of anatomical structures and can help to define the cause of cerebral palsy in individual cases. New techniques, such as positron emission tomography scanning and single photon emission computed tomography, complement CT and MRI by providing information about brain function, which in some cases is abnormal even when the brain structure appears to be normal (Chugani, 1993).

Perhaps the most important and most daunting issue in the diagnosis of the etiology of cerebral palsy is ascertaining with certainty that the motor impairment that is manifested is not a result of a slowly progressive neurological condition that mimics cerebral palsy. Although most serious metabolic conditions are fairly dramatic in their presentation and would not be mistaken for a nonprogressive condition, a growing list of slowly progressive disorders is being recognized and require special vigilance to identify (see Tables 1.7 and 1.8). A special urgency is connected with this effort because some of these conditions are potentially treatable, and subsequent impairments and disabilities may be prevented as a result of the treatment (Batshaw, 1997).

ASSOCIATED IMPAIRMENTS AND DISABILITIES

Although cerebral palsy is defined according to impairments of motor control, it is widely recognized that a number of impairments and disabilities that affect other aspects of the nervous system also are frequently associated with cerebral palsy. *Impairments* refer to fundamental anatomical, physiological, or psychological deficits. *Disabilities* refer to compromises in functioning that a person experiences as a consequence of an impairment (World Health Organization, 1980; see Chapter 3). In some children, impairments are limited to the motor system and the functional disability relates to deficits only in mobility. However, in many children with cerebral palsy, other types of associated impairments and disabilities are present and may have a significant or even decisive impact on their ultimate prognosis.

Vision

Approximately 40% of all children with cerebral palsy have some abnormality of vision or oculomotor control, and at least 7% have a severe visual deficit (Evans, Elliot, Alberman, & Evans, 1985). Commonly encountered visual impairments include *myopia* (i.e., nearsightedness), *amblyopia* (i.e., loss of vision related to disuse, sometimes referred to as *lazy eye*), loss of vision in segments of the visual field (called *visual field defects,* which are especially seen in children with hemiplegia), and *cortical blindness* (i.e., loss of vision caused by abnormalities of the brain rather than abnormalities of the eye or the optic nerve). Children born prematurely may sustain visual loss, including blindness, as a consequence of *retinopathy of prematurity,* which is caused by oxygen-related damage to vulnerable blood vessels in the immature retina (Avery, 1991). Oculomotor disturbances (e.g., strabismus) are also common and may lead to the development of amblyopia (Menacker, 1993). Many of the visual and oculomotor problems in children with cerebral palsy can be remediated with corrective lenses, eye patching, or surgery. Given the high incidence of visual problems in children with cerebral palsy, it is particularly urgent to ensure that these children undergo a complete ophthalmological examination as soon as neurodevelopmental problems are identified, preferably during infancy. In addition, regular reevaluations should be scheduled every year thereafter.

Hearing

Estimates of hearing loss in children with cerebral palsy range from 3% to 10% (Evans et al., 1985); however, as a result of the difficulty in identifying hearing problems, particularly with unilateral or high-frequency hearing loss, the true incidence is probably 20%–25% (Mowat, 1961). Children born prematurely are at a higher risk for hearing loss than children born at term (Thiringer, Kankkuren, Liden, & Niklasson, 1984). There are special techniques available that allow for the evaluation of hearing loss in early infancy (see Chapter 4), and these should be considered in all children with a suspected or established diagnosis of cerebral palsy.

Other Sensory Impairments

In addition to impairments of hearing and vision, many children with cerebral palsy have somatosensory deficits (e.g., abnormalities of proprioception, awareness of position of limbs in space) (Molnar, 1992); however, these are difficult to test and quantify, and the benefits of intervention strategies for these deficits are still unclear. *Somatosensory-evoked potentials* involve assessment of the response of sensory nerves to an electrical stimulus via neurophysiological techniques. Although such measures may yield some prognostic information (e.g., the likelihood that a child with hemiplegic cerebral palsy will make good use of the affected side of the body), the clinical utility of this procedure is generally uncertain (Scher, 1994). Aspects of somatosensory function are assessed through standardized measures of fine and gross motor function performed commonly by physical and occupational therapists (see Chapters 12 and 13).

Cognitive Impairments, Mental Retardation, and Learning Disabilities

Cognitive impairments refer to specific aspects of higher cortical function, such as memory, language processing, problem solving, and attention. These impairments are often evaluated by standardized tests such as the intelligence quotient (IQ) test or the Wechsler Intelligence Scale for Children–Revised (Wechsler, 1974). Significant cognitive impairments are more frequent in children with cerebral palsy than they are in the general population, and they result in a diagnosis of mental retardation or learning disability in approximately 75% of these children (Evans et al., 1985). The prevalence of mental retardation is approximately 50%, with 25%–30% of children with cerebral palsy having lower IQ scores than typically developing children or having discrete learning disabilities, such as abnormalities of visual perception or problem solving (Evans et al., 1985; Murphy, Yeargin-Allsopp, Decoufle, & Drews, 1993). The frequency of more severe cognitive disabilities (e.g., severe mental retardation) is directly related to the severity of the motor impairment—children with spastic quadriplegia or with *mixed* cerebral palsy (i.e., dyskinetic and spastic features) are at an especially high risk for severe cognitive disabilities (Lipkin, 1996).

Neurological, Orthopedic, and Other Physiological Impairments

Children with cerebral palsy have an increased incidence of medical and surgical problems that may be thought of as either *associated impairments* or *secondary impairments.* Seizure disorders may occur in as many as 46% of children with cerebral palsy (Murphy et al., 1993) and are usually the result of the same brain anomalies that caused the cerebral palsy. Thus, seizure disorders are an example of an associated impairment. Muscular contractures, hip dislocation, and scoliosis are examples of secondary impairments; they are a consequence of underlying abnormalities in muscle tone that result in chronic shortening of muscle-tendon units and deformities caused by persistent abnormal and unbalanced forces across joints (see Chapters 6 and 7). Children with cerebral palsy are also subject to a number of other significant medical problems related to respiratory, gastrointestinal, and urinary tract dysfunction (see Chapter 4).

LIFE EXPECTANCY

Although most children with cerebral palsy will live to adulthood, their projected life expectancy is somewhat less than that of the typical population (Crichton, Mackinnon, & White, 1995; O'Grady, Nishimura, Kohn, & Bruvold, 1985). Life expectancy varies with the type of cerebral palsy. For example, although a child with severe spastic quadriplegia may not live beyond age 40, a child with a mild right hemiplegia will likely live a typical life span (i.e., 70–90 years of age) (O'Grady et al., 1985). Life expectancy is also strongly related to the presence of specific medical and surgical conditions (see Chapter 4). Respiratory, gastrointestinal, and nutritional issues are of particular concern as these account for a large amount of the morbidity and the mortality experienced by individuals with cerebral palsy.

SUMMARY

Cerebral palsy is defined as a nonprogressive motor impairment syndrome that results from lesions or anomalies affecting the immature brain. Cerebral palsy subtypes are classified according to the types of motor impairments observed and by the geographical distribution (i.e., total body versus regional) of these impairments. Historically, cerebral palsy has been attributed to anomalies of the birth process, especially birth asphyxia. However, epidemiological evidence since the mid-1980s suggests that, in most cases, prenatal factors predominate in the pathogenesis of cerebral palsy. Children born prematurely are at an especially high risk for developing cerebral palsy as a consequence of a special vulnerability of the periventricular region of the immature brain in the early part of the third trimester of pregnancy. Full-term infants who subsequently develop cerebral palsy are slightly more likely to have experienced significant birth asphyxia, but an increased incidence of non–CNS anomalies and intrauterine growth retardation in this group suggests predisposing factors of prenatal origin.

Although cerebral palsy is defined strictly in terms of motor impairments and deficits in functional mobility, it is associated with a number of other impairments and disabilities, including sensory abnormalities, cognitive disabilities, and medical and surgical problems that may have a significant impact on health, well-being, and functional independence. Prognosis is affected by the severity of the motor impairment, by the presence of associated impairments and disabilities, and by societal conditions that may either provide opportunities or present barriers to fuller independence and greater participation. Although some individuals with more severe forms of cerebral palsy may have a reduced life span, the majority of individuals experience typical life expectancy. The goal of this book is to describe the dimensions of this complex disability and to invoke an interdisciplinary process, or team approach, as a means of enhancing the lives and, we hope, improving the prognosis of children with cerebral palsy.

REFERENCES

Adinolfi, M. (1993). Infectious diseases in pregnancy, cytokines and neurological impairment: An hypothesis. *Developmental Medicine and Child Neurology, 35,* 549–558.

Apgar, V. (1953). A proposal for new method of evaluation of the newborn infant. *Anesthesia Analog, 32,* 260–267.

Avery, G.B. (Ed.). (1991). *Neonatology: Pathophysiology and management of the newborn* (4th ed.). Philadelphia: J.B. Lippincott.

Barnes, P.D. (1992). Imaging of the central nervous system in pediatrics and adolescence. *Pediatric Clinics of North America, 39*(4), 743–776.

Batshaw, M.L. (1997). PKU and other inborn errors of metabolism. In M.L. Batshaw (Ed.), *Children with disabilities* (4th ed., pp. 389–404). Baltimore: Paul H. Brookes Publishing Co.

Bhushan, V., Paneth, N., & Kiely, J.L. (1993). Impact of improved survival of very low birth weight infants on recent secular trends in the prevalence of cerebral palsy. *Pediatrics, 91*(6), 1094–1100.

Blair, E., & Stanley, F. (1985). Interobserver agreement in the classification of cerebral palsy. *Developmental Medicine and Child Neurology, 27,* 615–622.

Chugani, H.T. (1993). Positron emission tomography scanning applications in newborns. *Clinics in Perinatology, 20*(2), 395–409.

Crichton, J.U., Mackinnon, M., & White, C.P. (1995). The life-expectancy of persons with cerebral palsy. *Developmental Medicine and Child Neurology, 37,* 567–576.

Crothers, B., & Paine, D.S. (1959). *The natural history of cerebral palsy.* Cambridge, MA: Harvard University Press.

Cummins, S.K., Nelson, K.B., Grether, J.K., & Velie, E.M. (1993). Cerebral palsy in four northern California counties, births 1983 through 1985. *Journal of Pediatrics, 123*(2), 230–237.

Evans, P., Elliot, M., Alberman, E., & Evans, S. (1985). Prevalence and disabilities in 4 to 8 year olds with cerebral palsy. *Archives of Disease in Childhood, 60,* 940–945.

Freud, S. (1968). *Infantile cerebral palsy.* Coral Gables, FL: University of Miami Press. (Original work published 1897)

Grether, J.K., Nelson, K.B., & Cummins, S.K. (1993). Twinning and cerebral palsy: Experience in four northern California counties, births 1983 through 1985. *Pediatrics, 92*(6), 854–858.

Hagberg, B., Hagberg, G., & Olow, I. (1984). The changing panorama of cerebral palsy in Sweden: IV. Epidemiological trends 1959–78. *Acta Paediatrica Scandinavia, 73,* 433–440.

Hagberg, B., Hagberg, G., & Olow, I. (1993). The changing panorama of cerebral palsy in Sweden: VI. Prevalence and origin during the birth year period 1983–1986. *Acta Paediatrica, 82,* 387–393.

Hagberg, B., Hagberg, G., Olow, I., & Von Wendt, L. (1989). The changing panorama of cerebral palsy in Sweden: V. The birth period 1979–82. *Acta Paediatrica Scandinavia, 78,* 283–290.

Hagberg, B., Hagberg, G., & Zetterstrom, R. (1989). Decreasing perinatal mortality-increase in cerebral palsy morbidity. *Acta Paediatrica Scandinavia, 78,* 664–670.

Hagberg, B., Sanner, G., & Steen, M. (1972). The disequilibrium syndrome in cerebral palsy. *Acta Paediatrica Scandinavia, 73,* 433–440.

Hughes, I., & Newton, R. (1992). Genetic aspects of cerebral palsy. *Developmental Medicine and Child Neurology, 34,* 80–86.

Krageloh-Mann, I., Hagberg, G., Meisner, C., Haas, G., Eeg-Olofsson, K.E., Selbmann, H.K., Hagberg, B., & Michaelis, R. (1995). Bilateral spastic cerebral palsy: A collaborative study between South-West Germany and Western Sweden: III. Aetiology. *Developmental Medicine and Child Neurology, 37,* 191–203.

Krageloh-Mann, I., Petersen, D., Hagberg, G., Vollmer, B., Hagberg, B., & Michaelis, R. (1995). Bilateral spastic cerebral palsy: MRI pathology and origin: Analysis from a representative series of 56 cases. *Developmental Medicine and Child Neurology, 37,* 379–397.

Kuban, K.C., & Leviton, A. (1994). Cerebral palsy. *New England Journal of Medicine, 330*(3), 188–195.

Leviton, A. (1993). Preterm birth and cerebral palsy: Is tumor necrosis factor the missing link? *Developmental Medicine and Child Neurology 35,* 549–558.

Lipkin, P.H. (1996). Epidemiology of developmental disabilities. In A.J. Capute & P.J. Accardo (Eds.), *Developmental disabilities in infancy and childhood: Neurodevelopmental diagnosis and treatment* (Vol. 1, pp. 137–156). Baltimore: Paul H. Brookes Publishing Co.

Little, W.J. (1966, May–June). The influence of abnormal parturition, difficult labours, premature birth, and asphyxia neonatorum on the mental and physical condition of the child, especially in relation to deformities. *Clinical Orthopaedics and Related Research, 46,* 7–22. (Original work published 1862)

Menacker, S.J. (1993). Visual function in children with developmental disabilities. *Pediatric Clinics of North America, 40*(3), 659–675.

Molnar, G.E. (1992). *Pediatric rehabilitation* (2nd ed.). Baltimore: Williams & Wilkins.

Moser, H.W. (1994, March). *Metabolic masqueraders.* Paper presented at The Spectrum of Developmental Disabilities Conference XVI: Cerebral palsy: Neuroscience into Practice, Baltimore.

Mowat, J. (1961). Ear, nose and throat disorders: Deafness. In J. L. Henderson (Ed.), *Cerebral palsy in childhood and adolescence.* Edinburgh, Scotland: E & S Livingstone Ltd.

Murphy, C.C., Yeargin-Allsopp, M., Decoufle, P., & Drews, D.C. (1993). Prevalence of cerebral palsy among ten-year old children in metropolitan Atlanta, 1985 through 1987. *Journal of Pediatrics, 123*(5), S13–S20.

Mutch, L., Alberman, E., Hagberg, B., Kodama, K., & Perat, M.V. (1992). Cerebral palsy epidemiology: Where are we now and where are we going? *Developmental Medicine and Child Neurology, 34,* 547–555.

Nelson, K.B. (1996). The epidemiology and etiology of cerebral palsy. In A.J. Capute & P. J. Accardo (Eds.), *Developmental disabilities in infancy and childhood: The spectrum of developmental disabilities* (Vol. 2, pp. 73–79). Baltimore: Paul H. Brookes Publishing Co.

Nelson, K.B., & Ellenberg, J.H. (1985). Antecedents of cerebral palsy: I. Univariate analysis of risks. *American Journal of Diseases of Children, 139,* 1031–1038.

Nelson, K.B., & Ellenberg, J.H. (1986). Antecedents of cerebral palsy: Multivariate analysis of risk. *New England Journal of Medicine, 315,* 81–86.

Nelson, K.B., & Emery, E.S. (1993). Birth asphyxia and the neonatal brain: What do we know and when do we know it? *Clinics in Perinatology, 20*(2), 327–344.

Nieman, G., Wakat, J., Krageloh-Mann, I., Grodd, W., & Michaelis, R. (1994). Congenital hemiparesis and periventricular leukamalacia: Pathologic aspects on magnetic resonance imaging. *Developmental Medicine and Child Neurology, 36,* 943–946.

O'Grady, R.S., Nishimura, D.M., Kohn, J.G., & Bruvold, W.H. (1985). Vocational predictions compared with present vocational status in 60 young adults with cerebral palsy. *Developmental Medicine and Child Neurology, 27,* 775–784.

Osler, W. (1987). *The cerebral palsies of children.* Philadelphia: J.B. Lippincott. (Original work published 1889)

Pellegrino, L. (1997). Cerebral palsy. In M.L. Batshaw (Ed.), *Children with disabilities* (4th ed., pp. 499–528). Baltimore: Paul H. Brookes Publishing Co.

Petterson, B., Nelson, K.B., Watson, L., & Stanley, F. (1993). Twins, triplets, and cerebral palsy in births in Western Australia in the 1980's. *British Medical Journal, 307,* 1239–1243.

Petterson, B., Stanley, F.J., & Garner, B.J. (1993). Spastic quadriplegia in Western Australia: II. Pedigrees and family patterns of birthweight and gestational age. *Developmental Medicine and Child Neurology, 35,* 202–215.

Petterson, B., Stanley, F.J., & Henderson, D. (1990). Cerebral palsy in multiple births in Western Australia: Genetic aspects. *American Journal of Medical Genetics, 37,* 346–351.

Scher, M.S. (1994). Pediatric electroencephalography and evoked potentials. In K. Swaiman (Ed.), *Pediatric neurology* (pp. 75–122). St. Louis: C.V. Mosby.

Stanley, F.J. (1992). Survival and cerebral palsy in low birthweight infants: Implications for perinatal care. *Pediatric Perinatal Epidemiology, 6,* 298–310.

Stanley, F.J., & Alberman, E. (1984). *The epidemiology of the cerebral palsies.* Philadelphia: J.B. Lippincott.

Steer, P.J. (1991). Premature labor. *Archive of Disease in Childhood, 66*(10), 1167–1170.

Thiringer, K., Kankkuren, A., Liden, G., & Niklasson, A. (1984). Perinatal risk factor in the aetiology of hearing loss. *Developmental Medicine and Child Neurology, 26,* 799–807.

Uvebrant, P., & Hagberg, G. (1992). Intrauterine growth in children with cerebral palsy. *Acta Paediatrica, 81,* 407–412.

Volpe, J.J. (1995). *Neurology of the newborn.* Philadelphia: W.B. Saunders.
Wechsler, D. (1974). Wechsler Intelligence Scale for Children–Revised. New York: The Psychological Corporation.
World Health Organization. (1980). *International classification of impairments, disabilities and handicap.* Geneva, Switzerland: Author.
Young, R.R. (1994). Spasticity: A review. *Neurology, 44*(Suppl.), S12–S20.

CHAPTER 2

Making the Diagnosis of Cerebral Palsy

Louis Pellegrino and John P. Dormans

The diagnosis of cerebral palsy rests on a clear understanding of the dimensions defined in Chapter 1. There are three components to this definition. First, cerebral palsy is a *disorder of movement and posture.* This component clearly focuses attention on the aspects of central nervous system (CNS) function that are related to the development of motor skills and functional mobility. Second, cerebral palsy is a result of *abnormalities in the early development of the brain.* This component is a reminder that there may be an underlying cause, or etiology, in cases of cerebral palsy that can be identified. It also underscores the need to identify other nonmotor impairments and disabilities related to abnormal brain development. Third, the definition of cerebral palsy stipulates that the disorder must be *nonprogressive.* This component means that the clinician must be able to recognize when functional deterioration is related to ongoing deterioration in the brain (i.e., the brain abnormalities that lead to cerebral palsy occur during early development, often before birth, and occur only once; see Chapter 1). The different aspects of diagnosing cerebral palsy—as they relate to the three components of its definition—are presented in Table 2.1. This chapter primarily focuses on the diagnosis of cerebral palsy as it relates to the delayed development of motor skills and functional mobility. This chapter also intro-

Table 2.1. Relationship between the definition of cerebral palsy and the aspects of diagnosis

Components of definition	Aspects of diagnosis
Cerebral palsy is a disorder of movement and posture.	• Analysis of abnormalities in motor development leads to the diagnosis of cerebral palsy.
Cerebral palsy is a result of abnormalities in the development of the immature brain.	• Medical evaluation and testing lead to a diagnosis of the cause (i.e., etiology) of cerebral palsy. • Medical, cognitive, and sensory evaluations lead to diagnosis of associated impairments and disabilities.
Cerebral palsy is nonprogressive.	• Medical evaluation rules out progressively worsening (i.e., neurodegenerative) conditions.

duces some of the impairments and disabilities associated with cerebral palsy. The diagnosis of the cause of cerebral palsy for a particular child is also discussed briefly; however, a detailed review of the causes, along with a discussion of progressive neurological conditions that mimic cerebral palsy, is discussed in Chapter 1. For more detailed discussions regarding disabilities associated with cerebral palsy, see Chapters 1, 4, and 11.

THE DIAGNOSIS OF CEREBRAL PALSY: A DEVELOPMENTAL DISABILITY

Cerebral palsy is a developmental disability and, as such, falls into a diagnostic category that includes mental retardation, autism, learning and language disorders, and disorders of attention and impulse control. *Development* can be defined operationally as the characteristic ways in which human behavior changes during the life cycle and, particularly, during childhood. *Disability* refers to a decrement in skills or function resulting from a physical or a psychological impairment that disrupts the typical development process. The hybrid term *developmental disability* emphasizes the interdependence of developmental processes and the acquisition of meaningful skills and abilities.

The diagnosis of a developmental disability is based on an analysis of the behavioral and the functional characteristics of a particular child. This is best accomplished by partitioning the developmental process into several functional domains (see Figure 2.1). These functional domains fall into two major groupings: basic physiological and psychological processes and integrated functional processes. The basic physiological and psychological processes include sensory function, cognitive processes, and motor function. Problems with the basic

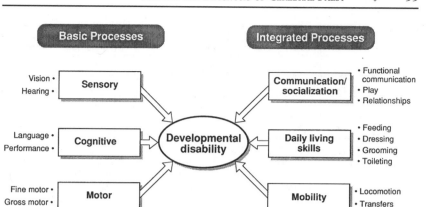

Figure 2.1. Functional domains that characterize a developmental disability. Basic physiological/psychological processes include sensory, cognitive, and motor functions. Integrated functional processes include communication/socialization skills, daily living skills, and mobility skills.

physiological and psychological processes are called *impairments* (see Chapter 3). The integrated functional processes are based on the basic functional domains and include communication/socialization skills, daily living skills, and mobility skills. Problems with the integrated processes are called *functional limitations* and *disabilities* (see Chapter 3). The basic physiological and psychological processes most directly relate to specific aspects of CNS function and are intrinsic to the individual child. These processes can be evaluated in the time frame of a typical professional office visit (e.g., performing a hearing test). The integrated functional processes are the concrete expression of development that is functionally and socially meaningful in real-life settings; for example, being able to play a board game, being able to dress, or being able to walk to school are all meaningful, integrated activities that depend on the adequate development of sensory, cognitive, and motor functions. Integrated functional processes are best observed and best described over an extended period of time and in different settings, and it is most efficient to gather this information through detailed interviews with the child's parents, family members, and teachers.

A detailed analysis of the content of these functional domains can lead to the diagnosis of a developmental disability for a particular child. As a result, this analysis can yield a developmental/functional profile (see Figure 2.2) that is characteristic of each type of developmental disability. In the case of cerebral palsy, the developmental disability is defined in terms of decrements in motor function and functional mobility. It should be emphasized that the developmental/ functional profile of cerebral palsy does not mean that children with the disorder do not have problems with sensory and cognitive function or with daily living skills and communication/socialization skills. Rather,

	Sensory	Cognitive	Motor	Commu-nication	Daily living skills	Mobility
Cerebral Palsy			✓			✓
Mental Retardation		✓			✓	
Autism		✓		✓		
Deafness	✓			✓		

Figure 2.2. Developmental profile across functional domains. A specific pattern of functional deficits characterizes an exact developmental disability. For cerebral palsy, motor processes and mobility functions are impaired.

this profile emphasizes that cerebral palsy is defined simply in terms of motor function and mobility—separate from other deficits, which are defined as associated impairments and disabilities. For example, a child's problems with motor function and mobility may lead to a diagnosis of cerebral palsy; however, the child may also demonstrate deficits in cognition and daily living skills that result in a second, independent diagnosis of mental retardation. Although cerebral palsy is commonly associated with mental retardation, mental retardation is not a part of the diagnosis of cerebral palsy.

The term *dissociation* has been applied to specific children when particular functional domains stand out as problematic (see Figure 2.3). The expectation is that the various "streams" of development (i.e., the functional domains) will flow or unfold parallel to one another and that they will proceed along the same approximate course and at the same approximate rate. When a particular stream (or streams) varies from the expected path (e.g., motor function and functional

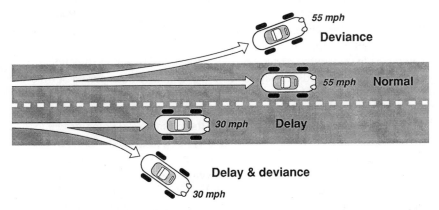

Figure 2.3. Three ways that development can depart from the expected path. First, *delay* (i.e., slower rate of development); second, *deviance* (i.e., abnormal quality of development); and third, *delay and deviance* (i.e., slower rate and abnormal quality of development combined).

mobility in the case of cerebral palsy), the term *dissociation* is applied (Capute & Accardo, 1996).

A particular stream of development may dissociate from the other streams in three ways. First, a stream may slow its rate of development in comparison with the other streams, which is called *delay*. Second, a stream may veer entirely from its expected course; this is called *deviance*. Establishing any developmental diagnosis involves identifying dissociation in the developmental process and further defining the delays and deviance associated with the particular child's developmental profile.

THE DIAGNOSIS OF CEREBRAL PALSY: MOTOR DEVELOPMENT AND FUNCTIONAL MOBILITY

The classical definition of cerebral palsy as presented in Chapter 1 can be incorporated into the terminology of this chapter: Cerebral palsy is a developmental disability that is first identified as a significant decrement in functional mobility during early childhood. This decrement is a result of an impairment of the brain's ability to regulate muscle tone and motor control; however, if the CNS impairment seems to worsen with time, this suggests that a progressive (i.e., degenerative) neurological condition, which supersedes the disability diagnosis because of its overriding functional and medical implications.

Once a professional involved in the diagnostic process of cerebral palsy is convinced that a progressive neurological condition is not in evidence, the next step is to define the presence of delayed motor development as well as the type of motor impairment associated with this delay.

Establishing Delay: Typical Motor Development

Typical motor development is the direct result of a carefully orchestrated and a relatively invariant series of maturational events in the developing brain. The basic structure of the brain is fully developed in the full-term infant; the neurons the infant will need for the rest of his or her life are already formed, as well. The brain in the full-term infant will continue to experience significant growth during the next several years; however, this growth is primarily a result of the expansion of white matter (i.e., glial) elements—which form the brain's infrastructure—supporting the billions of connections among neurons in different parts of the brain (Volpe, 1995). In the full-term infant, the infrastructure of the brain is not fully developed. Lower centers in the CNS (in particular, the brain stem and the spinal cord) that control vital functions and basic motor processes are more developed than higher brain centers (e.g., the cortex) that integrate sensory and motor processes and eventually come to dominate the control of motor function. Motor patterns in all newborns emanate primarily from the brain stem and the spinal cord and represent the scaffolding on which more complex motor patterns are later built.

Typical newborn infants have relatively lower muscle tone than older children, and they tend to hold their limbs in a partially flexed position. Deep tendon reflexes (e.g., the familiar knee-jerk response) are increased, which is a manifestation of the relative lack of inhibitory influences of higher brain centers over the reflex activity in the brain stem and the spinal cord. Other "release of inhibition" phenomena seen in typical newborns include clonus (i.e., rapid oscillation of a tendon reflex, which is sometimes mistaken for a tremor) and the Babinski response (i.e., when the outside edge of the foot is stroked, the big toe pulls upward and the other toes splay out).

Primitive Reflexes

The most characteristic feature of movement and motor control in newborns is the presence of complex, stereotypical movement patterns known as *primitive reflexes* (Capute, Accardo, & Vining, 1977). However, primitive reflexes are not truly "reflexes" in the same way that the knee-jerk response is a reflex. These reflexes represent complicated patterns of responses to a variety of sensory stimuli. Primitive reflexes are, in fact, conveniently classified according to the sensory modality that instigates a response (see Figure 2.4).

Cutaneous/Segmental Tactile stimuli to the skin or to mucous membranes elicit a variety of primitive reflex patterns. The most familiar of these are the rooting and the suckling responses that occur when a nipple or a similar object comes into contact with an infant's cheek, lips, or oral mucosa. Light pressure applied to the palms of the infant's hands and soles of the feet elicits the palmar and the plantar grasp responses. A favorite reflex response of pediatricians is the *Gallant response:* Stroking the skin on either side of an infant's spine causes him or her to curve his or her back toward the side being stroked.

Labyrinthine The labyrinthine apparatus (or semicircular canals) is a part of the inner ear and provides important sensory input to the brain in terms of the position of the head with respect to gravity (e.g., the dizziness induced by spinning in one direction for too long is caused by currents produced in the labyrinths). In the newborn at term, and more prominently in the preterm infant, the position of the head (i.e., face up versus face down) influences muscle tone throughout the body. In *supine* (i.e., face up), the back arches, the shoulders pull back or retract, and the legs extend. In *prone* (i.e., face down), the shoulders pull forward or protract and the knees pull up toward the chest as a result of flexion at the hips.

Proprioceptive Sensors located in muscles throughout the body monitor muscle activity and joint position and then return this information for processing to the brain and the spinal cord. *Proprioceptive stimuli,* originating in the muscles of the neck, have a particularly powerful influence on posture in newborns. The asymmetric tonic neck reflex (ATNR) response is seen when the head turns to one side or the other, and the arm and the leg extend to that side while the opposite side of the body flexes. The symmetric tonic neck reflex (STNR) is seen when

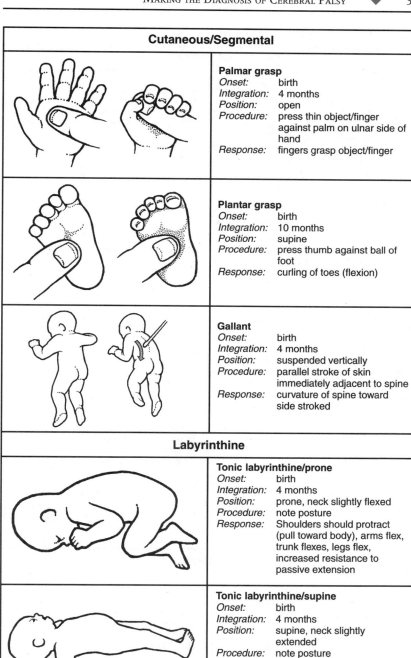

Cutaneous/Segmental	
	Palmar grasp *Onset:* birth *Integration:* 4 months *Position:* open *Procedure:* press thin object/finger against palm on ulnar side of hand *Response:* fingers grasp object/finger
	Plantar grasp *Onset:* birth *Integration:* 10 months *Position:* supine *Procedure:* press thumb against ball of foot *Response:* curling of toes (flexion)
	Gallant *Onset:* birth *Integration:* 4 months *Position:* suspended vertically *Procedure:* parallel stroke of skin immediately adjacent to spine *Response:* curvature of spine toward side stroked
Labyrinthine	
	Tonic labyrinthine/prone *Onset:* birth *Integration:* 4 months *Position:* prone, neck slightly flexed *Procedure:* note posture *Response:* Shoulders should protract (pull toward body), arms flex, trunk flexes, legs flex, increased resistance to passive extension
	Tonic labyrinthine/supine *Onset:* birth *Integration:* 4 months *Position:* supine, neck slightly extended *Procedure:* note posture *Response:* Shoulders retract (pull back), trunk extends/arches, legs extend, increase resistance to passive flexion

Figure 2.4. Primitive reflexes.

(continued)

Figure 2.4. (*continued*)

Proprioceptive/Tonic neck	
	Symmetric tonic neck *Onset:* birth *Integration:* 6 months *Position:* infant sitting or suspended prone *Procedure:* flex and extend neck *Response:* neck extended backward causes arms to extend and legs to flex, neck flexed forward causes arms to flex and legs to extend
	Asymmetric tonic neck *Onset:* birth *Integration:* 6 months *Position:* supine *Procedure:* passively or actively turn head to one side *Response:* arm and leg extend on side to which face is turned, other arm and leg flex
Multimodal/Noxious	
	Moro/startle *Onset:* birth *Integration:* 4 months *Position:* supine *Procedure:* allow neck to suddenly extend while supporting head *Response:* fast phase: extension and abduction of arms; slow phase: arms return to midline
Postural/Segmental	
	Segmental rolling *Emergence:* 5 months *Position:* supine *Procedure:* rotate head, observe response *Response:* body segments follow head rotation in sequence

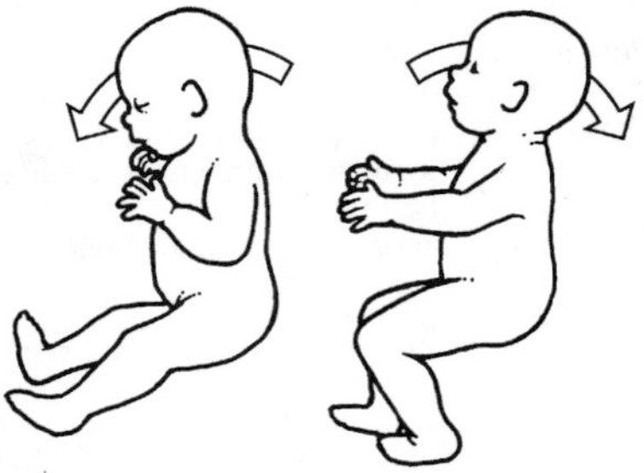

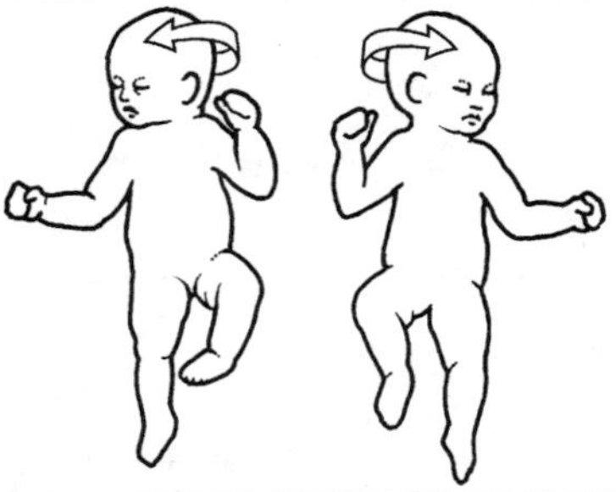

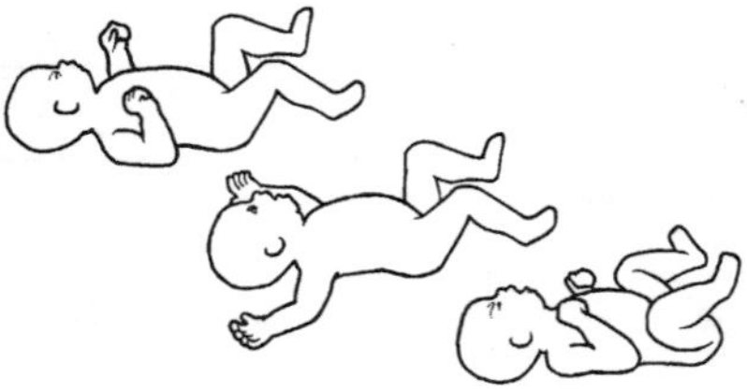

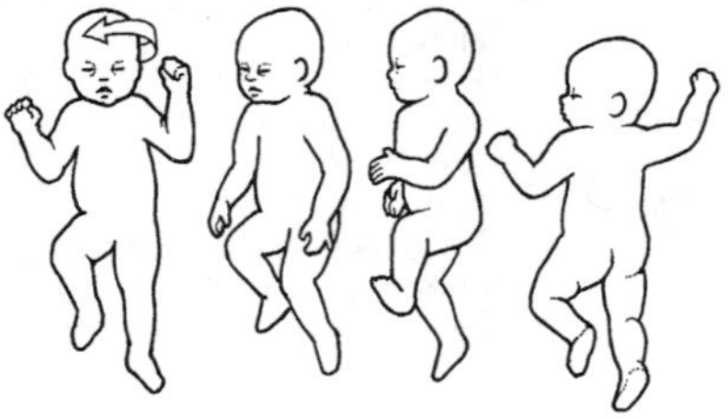

(continued)

Figure 2.4. (*continued*)

Postural/Antigravity

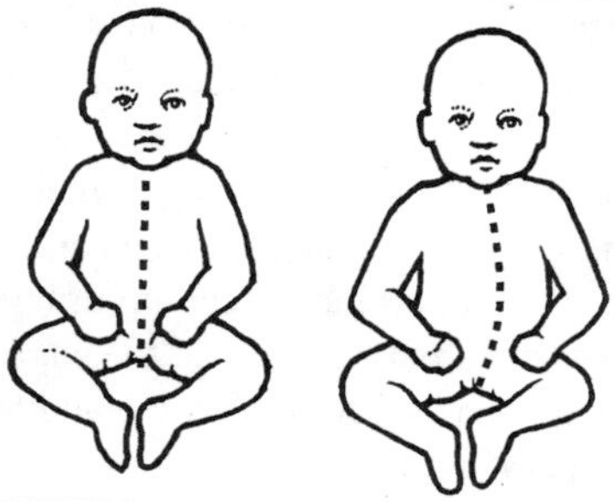

Head & trunk righting
Emergence: Head: 3 months; trunk: 5 months
Position: supine or suspended
Procedure: tilt upper body to one side
Response: head and trunk adjust to retain vertical posture

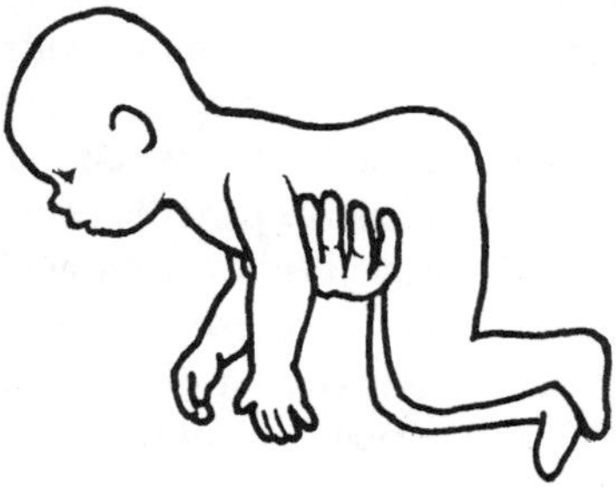

Landau
Emergence: 6 months
Position: suspended horizontal
Procedure: observe response
Response: neck and trunk extend, arms extend, legs partially flex

Protective/Antigravity

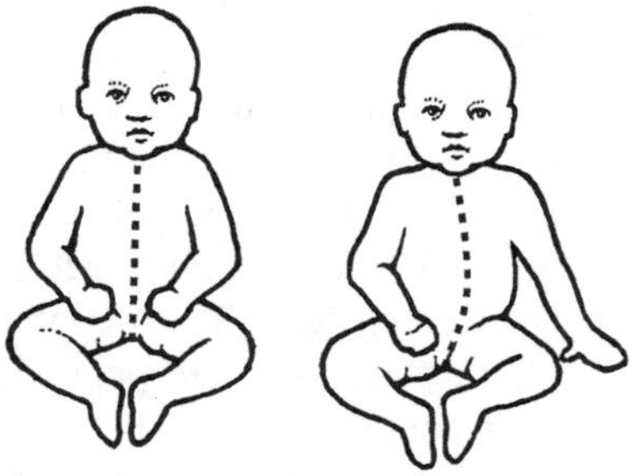

Lateral prop reaction
Emergence: 7 months
Position: sitting
Procedure: tilt to one side
Response: arm extends to support weight

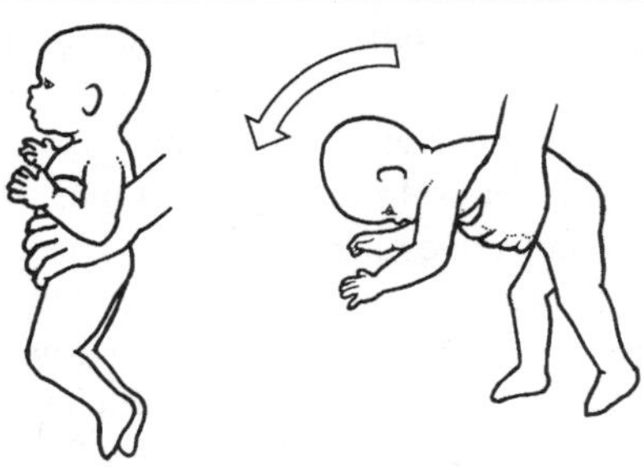

Parachute response
Emergence: 8 months
Position: suspended vertically
Procedure: tilt forward
Response: arms and legs extend to support weight

the head flexes and extends. When the neck flexes, the arms flex and the legs extend; when the neck extends, the arms extend and the legs flex. The STNR can be difficult to elicit in part because its responses overlap with the responses seen in the tonic labyrinthine reflexes. It helps to test the STNR with the child in a sitting position, which tends to minimize the influence of gravity on the labyrinths.

The positive support reaction (i.e., reflexive extension of the legs when the infant is held in a standing position and weight is put on his or her legs) and the stepping reflex (i.e., alternating steps taken when the infant's feet are dragged across a flat surface or the backs of his or her feet are dragged over the edge of a table) are primitive reflexes that probably have both proprioceptive and tactile components that elicit the characteristic response.

Multimodal/Noxious   Some primitive reflexes can be elicited through a variety of sensory modalities. The startle response (i.e., sudden convulsive movement of the entire body that is associated with facial grimace and flexion of the limbs) can be precipitated by a loud noise, a sudden movement, or an unexpected bump of the infant's bassinet. The Moro response partially overlaps with the startle response and has two components: 1) a rapid phase with sudden, wide extension of the arms, followed by 2) a slow phase during which the arms gather back toward the infant's trunk and midline. The Moro response is usually elicited by intentionally letting the infant's head extend suddenly; however, it is often elicited just as effectively by an accidental bump to the crib (as with the startle response).

The Emergence of Postural/Protective Reactions

By 1 year of age, the immature movement patterns of the infant are integrated into more complex patterns that directly reflect the increased control of higher CNS centers over lower CNS centers. This development is characterized by two mutually dependent phenomena: the emergence of postural/protective (i.e., automatic movement) reactions, and the increasing dominance of voluntary movement patterns (see section on "Postural/Segmental" responses in this chapter) over involuntary reflex responses (Capute et al., 1977).

Postural/protective reactions serve to properly position body segments (e.g., head, trunk, extremities) with respect to each other and with respect to gravity. In contrast to the primitive reflexes in which influence gradually recedes during the first year of life, the automatic movement reactions begin to emerge after birth and once established tend to persist in some form throughout life. Postural/protective reactions provide a protective function and are a necessary condition to the proper performance of voluntary movement. They may be categorized according to whether they involve movements of the head, the neck (i.e., postural), or the extremities (i.e., protective) or whether they are elicited in response to movements in other body parts (i.e., segmental) (see Figure 2.4).

Postural/Segmental When a newborn infant is laid down and rolled to one side, his or her head, trunk, and lower extremities tend to stay in line with each other (termed the *log roll*). In the early months after birth, a segmental rolling response emerges when movements in one body segment lead to successive movements in other body segments. For example, if the legs are turned over the hips, the trunk then turns, followed by the shoulders, and then the head. The reverse sequence is observed when the head is turned first.

Postural/Antigravity The newborn infant has no consistent head or trunk control when his or her body position changes with respect to gravity. The head righting reaction emerges within 2–3 months after birth and allows an infant to keep his or her head vertical even as the rest of the body changes positions. The head righting reaction is followed shortly by the emergence of the trunk righting reaction (i.e., when an infant is tipped in any direction, his or her back will curve in order to keep the trunk and the head relatively straight).

The Landau response becomes apparent approximately by 6 months of age. When an infant is suspended in a horizontal position (i.e., face down), the infant will lift his or her head and arch his or her back; younger infants cannot maintain the horizontal position and tend to "drape" over the examiner's hand.

Protective/Antigravity By 5 months of age, when an infant is tipped forward in a sitting position, the infant will reach his or her arms forward in order to catch him- or herself. This is called the *forward prop reaction. Lateral prop* (i.e., to the sides) and *backward prop reactions* become noticeable approximately at 6–8 months of age. The parachute response (i.e., arms and legs extending when the infant falls forward) emerges by approximately 10 months of age. The protective function of these reactions is self-evident and is a familiar (if unconscious) feature of adult motor responsiveness, highlighting the persistence of these patterns beyond infancy.

Pulling it All Together: The Emergence of Voluntary Movement Patterns

For the purposes of description, the development of motor skills is divided into either fine motor or gross motor components. *Fine motor development* involves refinements in the use of the hands; *gross motor development* involves the building of skills needed for locomotion. For both types of motor development, responses emerge in a neat progression that parallels maturational sequences in the CNS. These are the *vectors* of motor development during the first 12 months of life (see Figure 2.5). For fine motor development, prehensile activities are focused in the ulnar (i.e., fifth finger) side of the hand and gradually move toward the radial (i.e., first finger and thumb) side of the hand. For gross motor development, there is a cephalocaudal (i.e., top-to-bottom) and proximal-distal (i.e., body-center to body-peripheral) progression. In the early months after birth, head control precedes trunk and arm control, which precedes lower extremity control. Sphincter control emerges last around 18 months of age and signals a child's readiness to be toilet trained.

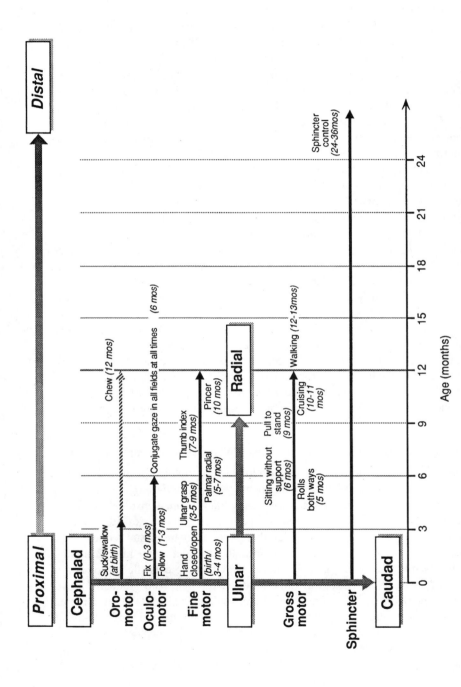

Figure 2.5. The "vectors" of infant motor development. Motor competence proceeds cephalocaudad (i.e., top-to-bottom), proximal-distal (i.e., body-center to body-peripheral), and ulnar-radial (i.e., fifth finger side of hand to thumb side of hand).

The successful integration of these emerging motor competencies into functional movement patterns requires that specific primitive motor patterns be subsumed by more mature, more flexible patterns. In addition, protective responses must be in place (i.e., in the case of gross motor development) to provide a "safety net" for future enthusiastic sensorimotor experiments. A graphic summary of these events is presented in Figure 2.6.

Functional Hand Use At birth, the palmar grasp response is dominant; and, as a result, the infant's hands remain clenched most of the time. By 4 months of age, this influence will recede, and the infant's hands will remain open most of the time. This progression sets the stage for the development of successively more mature grasp patterns, culminating in the pincer grasp, a key milestone in the development of functional hand use. The coordination of visual and motor responses provides for the emergence of visually directed reaching, another key milestone that can be recognized by 6–7 months of age. The development of prehensile (i.e., grasp) and ballistic (i.e., visually directed reaching) functions is often referred to as *manual dexterity*: a person's capacity to manipulate the world and to put his or her body at the service of the mind.

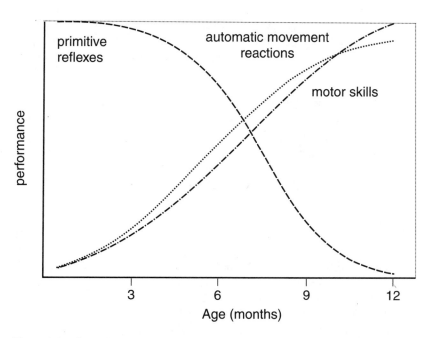

Figure 2.6. Changing patterns of motor response during the first year after birth. Infancy is characterized by the emergence of voluntary motor skills and postural/protective (i.e., automatic movement) reactions and the integration of primitive reflex patterns. (Adapted from Capute & Accardo, 1996.)

Rolling　Infants typically can roll both ways (i.e., front to back and back to front) by approximately 5 months of age. However, there are several prerequisites for this response. The ATNR must be significantly reduced; if it is not, the child will turn his or her head to begin a roll, and the arm and leg on the same side will extend and prevent the roll from starting. Sufficient head and trunk control are necessary in order to provide support for the rolling movement, and the segmental rolling response must have emerged, as well.

Sitting　Most infants can sit independently by 6 months of age. At this stage, the responses that are required for rolling are also needed. In addition, the STNR and labyrinthine responses must be integrated at this point (otherwise, movement of the head will result in postural changes that conflict with the sitting position). Head and trunk control must be well established, and the forward and lateral prop reactions must be available to catch the infant if he or she should fall forward or to the side (in the sitting position, the backward prop reaction can take a month or two longer to mature because the center of gravity is in front of the trunk).

Walking　The key milestone of walking, which every parent and professional worries about, is typically observed around 13 months of age. Any primitive reflex pattern involving the trunk or the extremities that continues to be dominant at this stage is likely to interfere with walking. Although remnants of the primitive patterns may still be observed, for the most part they are completely integrated by 13 months of age. The parachute response is another prerequisite to walking and, as previously described, serves as a protective function when the child inevitably falls in his or her early attempts at ambulation.

When Is a Delay Significant?

Many children do not begin sitting or walking when they are expected to, but this does not necessarily translate into their having a specific developmental problem. It is important to remember that developmental processes are best described in terms of rates rather than gaps. For instance, if a child begins to sit independently at 12 months of age instead of during the expected 6-month time frame, it would be appropriate to say that the child is 6 months delayed compared with his or her age-mates (i.e., a gap); it would also be appropriate to say that the child is developing at half the expected rate. This ratio is sometimes expressed as a developmental quotient: developmental age divided by chronological age. The important point to remember is that relying on rates of development allows for multiple observations over an extended period of time, which can help to establish a clear pattern of delay. At each point of development, standardized tests may be useful in helping to define the gap between observed and expected performance (see Chapters 12 and 13). For any particular milestone in development, a significant delay is usually defined with respect to a population norm (e.g., according to a frequently used screening test, 90% of children are walking by 15 months of age; thus, not walking by 15 months is defined as a significant delay for this particular milestone) (Frankenburg, Dodds, Archer, Shapiro, & Bresnick, 1992). Standardized tests attempt to aggregate categorically related milestones into groups for which composite scores can be derived. Performance is described in terms of standard deviations from the mean for a reference population (see Figure 2.7). A score that is 2 standard deviations below the mean is usually described as "significantly below average." However, the relationship between a child's true rate of development and the rate predicted by standardized tests is not precise. In general, the lower the predicted rate of development and the older the child, the more likely it is that the predicted rate will hold true over time. A child whose motor skills are developing at 25% of the expected rate is more likely to stay at this rate than a child who is developing at 75% of the expected rate. Standardized tests are therefore a useful and a necessary adjunct to the diagnostic process, but they should not be used in isolation to define significant motor delay or to determine the motor delay's implications.

Establishing Deviance in Motor Delay

Cerebral palsy is not the most common cause of significant motor delay. Significant motor delay is seen most often within the general context of developmental delay and leads to a diagnosis of mental retardation more often than it leads to a diagnosis of cerebral palsy (Batshaw, 1993). To establish the diagnosis of cerebral palsy—in addition to meeting the criteria previously

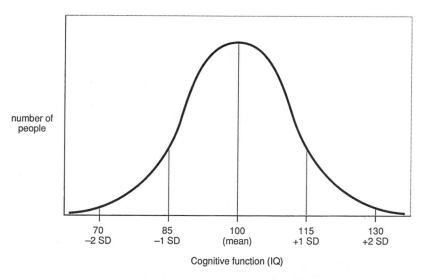

Figure 2.7.   Population distribution for an aggregate measure of cognitive function (IQ). Significantly abnormal scores are less than 70 (i.e., less than 2 standard deviations [*SD*] below the mean score of 100).

explained—a specific type of motor impairment must be present (i.e., the upper motor neuron syndrome).

The basis of motor control in the CNS consists of neuronal elements and anatomical structures at multiple levels from the muscle to the spinal cord to the brain (see Figure 2.8). It is important to remember that the final common pathway for all of these influences is the *alpha motor neurons (AMNs)* (Glenn & White, 1990). The AMNs reside in the spinal cord and are connected directly to muscle fibers via long extensions called *axons*. It is these axons that bundled together form a peripheral nerve. Impulses from several AMNs are the direct cause of muscle contraction. AMNs collectively are referred to as *lower motor neurons (LMNs)*. AMNs cannot spontaneously create nerve impulses; they can create nerve impulses only in response to stimuli from other neurons. There are three basic ways that AMNs can be stimulated. First, sensory nerve fibers that originate in the muscles can send signals back to the AMNs. For instance, in the stretch reflex, sensory nerves called *reflex afferents* fire in response to rapid

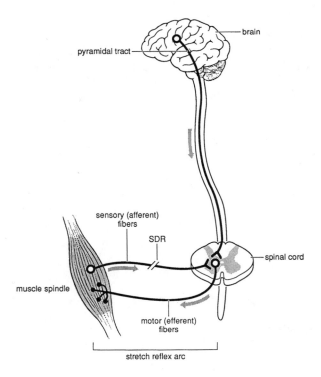

Figure 2.8. Levels of motor control in the CNS. The LMN (motor effect fibers) directly stimulates the muscle to contract. The LMN's output is modified by feedback from the muscle to the spinal cord transmitted via the reflex afferent; its output is also modified and controlled by UMNs ("pyramidal tract") that originate in the brain. The final output of the UMNs is influenced by other brain structures, including the basal ganglia and the cerebellum.

muscle stretch; this signal feeds back to the AMN, which is stimulated to fire, and this causes muscle contraction and counteracts the stretch. Second, other neurons in the spinal cord (i.e., interneurons) can influence the AMN to increase or decrease its rate of firing. Third, nerve fibers that originate in the brain can directly or indirectly influence AMN activity through interneurons. The nerve fibers that originate in the brain are known collectively as *upper motor neurons (UMNs)*. UMNs originate in the cortex and the brain stem and are a "final common pathway" for multiple influences from other parts of the brain's motor control system, most notably the basal ganglia and the cerebellum. Whereas the net or average influence of spinal interneurons is to cause an increase in the activity of the AMNs—resulting in increased muscle contraction and increased muscle tone—the net influence of UMNs is inhibitory (e.g., results in decreased muscle tone). Whenever there is a problem with UMN control of the LMN, there tends to be a relative increase in the activity of AMNs, and this activity results in what are known as *release from inhibition phenomena.*

The UMN syndrome is defined in terms of negative and positive signs and symptoms (Katz & Rymer, 1989). Positive symptoms are a direct result of the release of inhibition and include increased muscle tone, overactivity of reflexes, increased clonus, motor synergies (i.e., overactivity in one muscle group precipitating overactivity in another), and persistent primitive reflex patterns (i.e., because these patterns originate in the brain stem and the spinal cord, lack of control from higher centers via the UMNs results in pathological persistence of these reflexes). Negative symptoms are the deficits created by lack of UMN control (e.g., weakness, easy fatigability, poor dexterity, poor balance). Many of these negative symptoms are seen in primary muscle diseases (e.g., the muscular dystrophies) or in diseases of LMNs (e.g., a progressive, degenerating disease called *spinal muscular atrophy*), but these diseases are not associated with the positive symptoms described for the UMN syndrome. Primary muscle diseases are associated with low muscle tone, decreased or absent reflexes, and severe muscle atrophy and wasting.

Cerebral palsy is not the only example of the UMN syndrome. The same symptom complex is seen in adults who have had a stroke, in individuals with multiple sclerosis, and in individuals who have had a spinal cord injury. The major distinction is that cerebral palsy results from an injury to or a dysfunction of the brain that occurs during the period of rapid CNS development, whereas the other examples of the UMN syndrome occur during late childhood or during adulthood (or in the case of a spinal cord injury, do not involve injury to the brain).

Summary

The preceding sections have outlined the steps involved in making a diagnosis of cerebral palsy. The first step is based on the recognition that cerebral palsy is a developmental disability, and, as with other developmental disabilities, a diagnosis depends on the discovery of a break (or dissociation) in the profile of skills across functional and developmental domains. This break relates specifically to delayed and deviant motor skills and translates into impairments of functional mobility. Cerebral palsy is distinguished from other causes of motor delay by the presence of the signs and symptoms of the UMN syndrome; it is distinguished from other forms of the UMN syndrome by recognizing that damage or dysfunction has occurred in the developing (i.e., immature) brain rather than in the fully developed brain.

THE CLASSIFICATION OF CEREBRAL PALSY: MOTOR IMPAIRMENT SUBTYPES

Cerebral palsy is further classified according to the type of motor impairment that is evident. The UMN syndrome is actually a heterogeneous group of neurological entities with release of inhibition phenomena as its common denominator. As discussed in Chapter 1, three major subtypes of cerebral palsy are recognized: spastic cerebral palsy, dyskinetic cerebral palsy, and ataxic cerebral palsy. The spastic forms of cerebral palsy may be further categorized according to the distribution of the limbs involved. The dyskinetic types of cerebral palsy may be defined according to the presence of specific types of involuntary movements (i.e., athetoid versus dystonic). Assigning an appropriate subtype to a particular child can be problematic. It is notoriously difficult to obtain consistency among examiners in different settings or even to establish consistency among the same examiners in the same setting (Blair & Stanley, 1985). A consistent approach based on a series of logically connected questions and observations is needed to arrive at a rational methodology for dealing with this issue (see Figure 2.9). The following questions may help the clinician to begin this process.

Is it Cerebral Palsy?   Making the diagnosis of cerebral palsy has been the subject of this chapter to this point. The answer to the question is usually "yes" if there is significant motor delay, if there is evidence of UMN dysfunction (e.g., spasticity) first recognized in early childhood, and if the clinician can be reassured that the individual does not have a progressive metabolic or a neurodegenerative disorder. The presence of a known etiological risk factor for cerebral palsy (e.g., extreme prematurity) may increase the index of suspicion for the diagnosis, but it is not strictly necessary for making the diagnosis itself.

Does the Motor Impairment Involve the Whole Body?   In the young infant, it may be difficult to determine with confidence whether a motor impairment involves the whole body. In general, however, it should be possible to determine whether the motor impairment primarily involves the legs (i.e., diplegia), one side of the body (i.e., hemiplegia), or all of the extremities along with the trunk and the oral-motor apparatus (i.e., total body cerebral palsy). It is

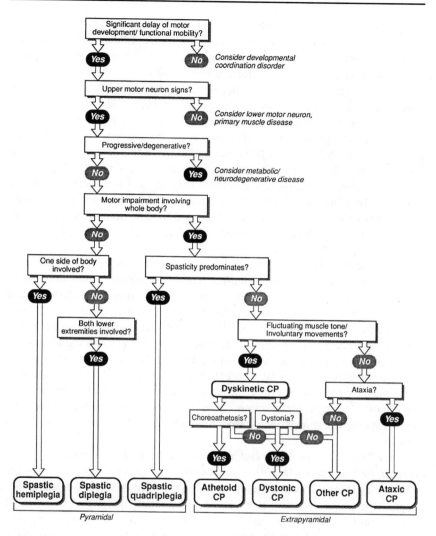

Figure 2.9. Evaluation of motor delay and classification of cerebral palsy subtype.

important to remember that if the impairment is confined to one part of the body, then it must, by definition, be one of the spastic forms of cerebral palsy. Although spasticity may involve the whole body, the dyskinetic and ataxic forms must, by definition, involve the whole body.

If the Motor Impairment Involves the Whole Body, then What Is the Predominant Muscle Tone Abnormality? The primary task is to determine whether spasticity is the dominant tonal abnormality. Specific features of the physical assessment can help at this point. Spasticity is usually defined as a velocity-dependent resistance to passive stretching of a muscle (i.e., the faster a muscle is stretched, the more resistance is encountered) and is usually associated with briskly overactive stretch reflexes (e.g., the knee-jerk response) and increased or sustained clonus. Another characteristic associated with spasticity is the clasp-knife response. When a spastic muscle is stretched past a certain length, there is a sudden release of resistance, which is recovered when the muscle is allowed to shorten again. Spasticity tends to involve the same muscle groups that are consistently identified over an extended period of time from one examination to the next and from one examiner to the next (e.g., if the left hamstring muscle is tight today, then it will be tight tomorrow). Because the same muscles have consistently increased tone, the same abnormal forces are applied across the same joints. This means that children with spastic forms of cerebral palsy have more problems with orthopedic deformities (e.g., contractures, hip dislocation) and develop these deformities at a younger age than children with other forms of cerebral palsy.

In contrast to spastic cerebral palsy, dyskinetic cerebral palsy is characterized by fluctuating tonal abnormalities. These fluctuations occur in terms of both location (i.e., different muscle groups are involved at different times) and muscle tone type (i.e., fluctuating between high muscle tone [i.e., rigidity] and low muscle tone [i.e., hypotonia]). When rigidity is evident, it can be distinguished from spasticity by less prominent stretch reflexes and clonus, by absence of velocity-dependent resistance to stretch, and by absence of the clasp-knife response. Rigidity is often characterized by active contraction of antagonistic muscles across the same joint (e.g., the biceps and the triceps across the elbow). Repeated stretching of rigid muscles can result in a gradual but persistent decrease in resistance to stretch, which is called *lead-pipe* or *candlewax rigidity.*

Are There Specific Abnormalities of Movement that Are Involuntary (Dyskinesia) or Voluntary (Ataxia)?   Although not always recognized, abnormal involuntary movements are one of the hallmarks of dyskinetic cerebral palsy. Rapid, jerking movements (i.e., chorea) are often combined with slow, writhing movements (i.e., athetosis) in athetoid cerebral palsy. Abnormal posturing centered in the trunk and the neck and extending to the extremities is observed in dystonic cerebral palsy. Ataxic cerebral palsy is characterized by abnormalities of movement that are observed after a voluntary action has been initiated.

THE TIMING OF DIAGNOSIS

The diagnosis of cerebral palsy prior to 2 years of age may be problematic for several reasons. According to one study, approximately 55% of children who are diagnosed with cerebral palsy prior to 1 year of age will no longer meet criteria for the diagnosis at 7 years of age (Nelson & Ellenberg, 1982). Children born prematurely are particularly likely to "outgrow" the early signs of cerebral palsy. This phenomenon has been called *transient dystonia of prematurity* (Drillien, 1972). Infants between 4 and 14 months of age may have increased muscle tone in their legs, which is associated with truncal hypotonia; this will generally resolve itself by 2 years of age. Overdiagnosis is more likely to occur among children of African descent who normally have higher muscle tone during infancy and achieve motor milestones earlier than do children of European descent (Super, 1976). In general, children with milder signs of motor impairment during infancy are more likely to demonstrate significant resolution of these signs by the preschool years. However, among children who do "outgrow" their cerebral palsy, there is an increased incidence of other neurodevelopmental problems (e.g., mental retardation, epilepsy, speech and language disorders, abnormal eye movements, small head size [i.e., microcephaly]) (Nelson & Ellenberg, 1982). Early abnormalities in muscle tone and motor control may therefore serve as a marker for other neurodevelopmental problems that become more evident in later years.

THE ETIOLOGY: DIAGNOSIS
OF THE CAUSE OF CEREBRAL PALSY

Given the heterogeneity of neurological conditions grouped under the rubric of cerebral palsy, it is not possible to create a diagnostic algorithm that would determine an etiology for every child with cerebral palsy. It is also important to consider the goals in pursuing an etiological diagnosis. In most cases, an etiological diagnosis does not result in a change in the recommendations for the child's care. It is important that the child's parents understand this before embarking on a course of extensive and expensive testing. A notable exception to this rule relates to the pursuit of inborn errors of metabolism and other neurodegenerative disorders. In some cases a specific treatment that could result in improved prognosis or even a cure may be indicated. Children who have a history of neurological deterioration—chronic or episodic—that excludes them by definition from a diagnosis of cerebral palsy are sometimes diagnosed as having "cerebral palsy" because of physical findings that are consistent with UMN dysfunction. When episodes of deterioration are associated with vomiting, changes in diet, or sudden weight loss (this may be difficult to distinguish from gastroesophageal reflux [GER]; see Chapter 11), concern regarding a possible metabolic disease should increase. If there is a high degree of suspicion, further evaluation by a metabolic specialist is recommended.

In cases in which a progressive neurological condition is not suspected, a review of the known causes of cerebral palsy will help direct the clinician along the most fruitful lines of investigation (see Chapter 1). Very often a diagnosis is suspected solely by investigating the child's history (e.g., premature birth, perinatal asphyxia associated with seizures in the immediate postnatal period). The single most helpful diagnostic test is magnetic resonance imaging (MRI), which provides detailed pictures of the brain anatomy and has a higher yield of positive findings in children with cerebral palsy than it does in children with other developmental disabilities (Barnes, 1992).

Another reason to pursue an etiological diagnosis of cerebral palsy is for the purposes of family and genetic counseling. A careful history and physical examination are required in order to raise suspicion about genetic disorders, and these should guide the selection of further laboratory data. A careful pregnancy history may suggest a specific prenatal etiology (e.g., infection). A family history should address questions regarding neurological, developmental, and psychiatric conditions and should also explore any history of recurrent fetal loss or prematurity. An infant who was small for gestational age or has a number of physical anomalies not attributable to the child's neurological condition is more likely to have a diagnosable genetic syndrome. A child with ataxic cerebral palsy also is more likely to have a diagnosable genetic syndrome (Hughes & Newton, 1992).

THE DIAGNOSIS OF ASSOCIATED IMPAIRMENTS AND DISABILITIES

Other impairments and disabilities that are associated with motor impairments and are characteristic of cerebral palsy are found frequently in children (see Chapter 1). These impairments and disabilities can be classified into three groups: sensory, cognitive, and physiological.

Sensory impairments in children with cerebral palsy are very common and easily can be overlooked in the clinician's zeal to address motor abnormalities. There is a high incidence of visual impairments, including myopia (i.e., nearsightedness), amblyopia (i.e., loss of vision related to disuse, often referred to as "lazy eye"), loss of vision in segments of the visual field (especially in children with hemiplegia), and cortical blindness (i.e., loss of vision caused by abnormalities of the brain rather than abnormalities of the eye or the optic nerve). Oculomotor disturbances (e.g., strabismus) are also common in children with cerebral palsy and predispose the development of amblyopia (Menacker, 1993). There is an increased incidence of hearing loss, particularly among former premature infants (Thiringer, Kankkuren, Liden, & Niklasson, 1984). Many children have somatosensory deficits (e.g., abnormalities of proprioception) (Molnar, 1992); however, somatosensory deficits are difficult to test for and to quantify, and the benefits of intervention strategies for these deficits are unclear. All children with cerebral palsy should have early and regular examinations by a pediatric ophthalmologist, and hearing should be tested by a licensed audiologist who has experience in the evaluation of children with developmental disabilities.

For many individuals with cerebral palsy, cognitive disabilities pose a greater obstacle than limitations of mobility in their effort to participate more freely in society. The identification of cognitive disabilities, such as mental retardation, learning disabilities, and developmental language disorders, may be promoted by involvement in early intervention programs. When a child enters school (or prior to the child entering school), detailed psychological testing should be obtained to help the education team delineate the child's relative strengths and weaknesses. This testing provides necessary information that can be useful in developing individualized education programs for children who will be enrolled in special education programs (see Chapter 19).

For the medical professional, the physiological impairments associated with cerebral palsy are of particular concern. Conceptually, these may be divided into impairments that are a direct manifestation of the CNS dysfunction, which gives rise to cerebral palsy, and impairments that are a secondary consequence of the primary disturbance in neuromotor function. For instance, spasticity may be seen as a primary manifestation of cerebral palsy in a particular child, whereas musculotendonous contracture is the long-term consequence of persistent hypertonicity and fiber shortening in particular muscle groups and is therefore considered to be a secondary impairment. In practice, it is often difficult to separate primary and secondary impairments. For example, GER—a common problem for many children with cerebral palsy—in part may be a result of neurologically based abnormalities in gastrointestinal motility; however, GER is clearly influenced by secondary factors such as increased intra-abdominal pressure related to spasticity of the abdominal musculature, constipation related to physical immobility and dietary factors, and abnormalities of position related to the physical characteristics of a particular child. For the pediatrician, awareness of the list of commonly associated problems of cerebral palsy is the first step toward developing a management strategy for the care of the child with cerebral palsy (see Chapters 4 and 11).

SUMMARY

Cerebral palsy is diagnosed according to a detailed analysis of a child's motor function and his or her development over an extended period of time. Significant delays in motor development are characterized by the pathological persistence of primitive reflex patterns and the delayed emergence of automatic movement reactions and voluntary motor control. Deviant motor function is manifest as "positive" and "negative" signs of UMN syndrome. The specific subtype of cerebral palsy is determined for a particular child by identifying the primary motor impairment that is in evidence. It is often difficult to make a definitive diagnosis of cerebral palsy prior to 2 years of age, particularly among children born prematurely.

It is not always possible to identify the etiology of cerebral palsy. It is important to distinguish between "true" cerebral palsy and neurodegenerative and metabolic conditions that mimic cerebral palsy. In cases in which a progressive neurological disorder is not suspected, a medical history and a physical examination will often suggest a specific etiological diagnosis. The most helpful adjunct to a medical history and a physical examination is MRI, which illustrates the anatomy of the brain in great detail. Specific clues in the medical history and the physical examination will also suggest whether genetic testing is warranted.

A number of developmental and medical problems are commonly associated with cerebral palsy. It is important to identify these problems because they may have as much of an impact on a child's life and function as the cerebral palsy itself.

REFERENCES

Barnes, P.D. (1992). Imaging of the central nervous system in pediatrics and adolescence. *Pediatric Clinics of North America, 39*(4), 743–776.
Batshaw, M.L. (1993). Developmental disabilities of childhood. *Pediatric Clinics of North America, 40*(3), 465–692.
Blair, E., & Stanley, F. (1985). Intraobserver agreement in the classification of cerebral palsy. *Developmental Medicine and Child Neurology, 25*, 615–622.
Capute, A.J., & Accardo, P.J. (Eds.). (1996). *Developmental disabilities in infancy and childhood.* (2nd ed., Vol. 2). Baltimore: Paul H. Brookes Publishing Co.
Capute, A.J., Accardo, P.J., & Vining, E.P.G. (1977). *Primitive reflex profile.* Baltimore: University Park Press.
Drillien, C.M. (1972). Abnormal neurologic signs in the first year of life in low-birthweight infants: Possible prognostic significance. *Developmental Medicine and Child Neurology, 14*, 575–584.
Frankenburg, W.K., Dodds, J., Archer, P., Shapiro, H., & Bresnick, B. (1992). The Denver II: A major revision and restandardization of the Denver Developmental Screening Test. *Pediatrics, 89*, 91–97.
Glenn, M.B., & White, J. (Eds.). (1990). *The practical management of spasticity in children and adults.* Philadelphia: Lea & Febiger.
Hughes, I., & Newton, R. (1992). Genetic aspects of cerebral palsy. *Developmental Medicine and Child Neurology, 34*, 80–86.
Katz, R.T., & Rymer, W.Z. (1989). Spastic hypertonia: Mechanisms and measurement. *Archives of Physical Medicine and Rehabilitation, 70*, 144–155.
Menacker, S.J. (1993). Visual function in children with developmental disabilities. *Pediatric Clinics of North America, 40*(3), 659–675.
Molnar, G.E. (Ed.). (1992). *Pediatric rehabilitation* (2nd ed.). Baltimore: Williams & Wilkins.
Nelson, K.B., & Ellenberg, J.H. (1982). Children who "outgrew" cerebral palsy. *Pediatrics, 69*(5), 529–536.
Super, C. (1976). Environmental effects on motor development: The case of African infant precocity. *Developmental Medicine and Child Neurology, 18*, 561–567.
Thiringer, K., Kankkuren, A., Liden, G., & Niklasson, A. (1984). Perinatal risk factor in the etiology of hearing loss. *Developmental Medicine and Child Neurology, 26*, 799–807.
Volpe, J. (1995). *Neurology of the newborn* (3rd ed.). Philadelphia: W.B. Saunders.

CHAPTER 3

Interdisciplinary Care of the Child with Cerebral Palsy

Louis Pellegrino and Gretchen Meyer

The concept of interdisciplinary care has come of age in the latter half of the 20th century. The concept emerged gradually among professionals in response to a collective recognition that no one person or one discipline had all of the requisite skills or perspectives to adequately address the complex issues surrounding the evolving nature of developmental disabilities. An increasing sensitivity in society as a whole to issues of developmental change and developmental disability has refocused discussions regarding interdisciplinary care on the concept of family-centered care. This shift represents a welcome, although somewhat belated, recognition that families are key participants in the process of establishing the priorities as well as the specific forms of care for individuals with developmental disabilities.

A series of legislative initiatives that have become widely known and often quoted emphasize that family-centered approaches to interdisciplinary care should take precedence over other aspects of interdisciplinary care (see Chapters 18 and 19). The challenge for the professional in the field of developmental disabilities is to operationalize this philosophy by creating a sound conceptual framework for implementation and modification of family-centered care.

HISTORICAL NOTES:
THE DEVELOPMENT OF THE TEAM APPROACH

The evolution of the concept of cerebral palsy is described in Chapter 1. Cerebral palsy was first conceptualized as a group of neurologically based disorders that had in common not only an early manifestation but also a nonprogressive course. Gradually, cerebral palsy was reconceptualized as a developmental disability, which is defined as a condition that arises in early childhood and, although it has a neurological basis, is defined and diagnosed in terms of functional characteristics rather than biological or etiological characteristics (see Chapter 2). For example, mental retardation, another developmental disability, has many biological causes; however, it is still defined by deficits in intellectual and adaptive functioning (Batshaw & Shapiro, 1997). Likewise, cerebral palsy as a developmental disability is defined and diagnosed according to deficits in functional mobility that are associated with specific impairments of motor function.

With the shift in emphasis from cerebral palsy as a neurological entity to cerebral palsy as a developmental disability has come a parallel development in the professional approach to the management of cerebral palsy. In the late 1800s, the model of health care that came to be known as the "medical model" first took shape. Prior to this time, symptoms of diseases were generally attributed either to moral or to character flaws in an individual or to extreme external circumstances. However, as knowledge of biological systems increased, diseases began to be attributed to specific biological agents or to physiological alterations in the human organism. This new approach turned out to be enormously successful in the management of many acute illnesses but continued to yield disappointing results for many chronic illnesses and disabilities. By the mid-20th century, the inadequacy of this approach for the management of cerebral palsy became apparent. An effort was made to draw on the recognition that a complex disability such as cerebral palsy has varied biological, cognitive, and psychosocial influences and may require the talents of professionals representing several disciplines in order to properly manage it (see section on "Variations in the Team Approach" in this chapter). Crothers, a child neurologist and founding member of the American Academy of Cerebral Palsy and Developmental Medicine, wrote, "Unless the interests of doctors are widened beyond mere physical care, it is reasonable to suggest that they may encourage docility instead of welcoming experiments in independence by the child" (Crothers & Paine, 1959, p. 256). Phelps (1941) and later Deaver (1956) also called for a shift in emphasis toward an all-encompassing program in which the facilitation of movement was accompanied by attention to cognitive skills and functional activities.

It was the acceptance of this broadened approach (sometimes called the "psychoeducational model" to provide a contrast to the former "medical model") that led to the evolution of the team process. In the 1960s, the advent of legislation for improved education and treatment of children with special needs provided a federal mandate for coordinated team services to include physicians, allied health professionals, educators, social workers, and parents. The university affiliated facilities were created in 1963 by the federal government. These institutions were established to encourage ongoing research in the field of developmental disabilities, to ensure appropriate training of team-based health care providers, and to promote the comprehensive delivery of health care services to individuals with disabilities (Farrell & Pimentel, 1996).

In 1975, the Education for All Handicapped Children Act (PL 94-142), defined the team process in which school-age children were to be evaluated and served in the school setting via individualized education programs (see Chapter 19). The Education of the Handicapped Act Amendments of 1986, PL 99-457, amended the original 1975 law to include services to preschool-age children. This law explicitly stated that services were to be team focused, comprehensive, interdisciplinary, and family centered (Blackman, Healy, & Ruppert, 1992).

In 1990, the Individuals with Disabilities Education Act (IDEA), PL 101-476, further expanded the mandated educational services to include infants and toddlers. IDEA was amended in 1991 (PL 102-119) and 1997 (PL 105-17) and now guarantees the delivery of comprehensive, coordinated services for all individuals with disabilities from birth to 21 years of age.

VARIATIONS IN THE TEAM APPROACH

Three types of collaborative professional teams have been developed to address the complex issues of children with developmental disabilities (see Figure 3.1). Multidisciplinary teams consist of several professionals who represent different disciplines. These professionals see consumers independent of one another; however, consumers are often seen at the same time and in the same place. This approach provides a type of "one-stop shopping" and creates an opportunity for collaboration among disciplines.

Interdisciplinary teams also are composed of professionals from several different disciplines, but they take collaboration one step further than multidisciplinary teams. Interdisciplinary care tends to be both problem and issue oriented, rather than strictly discipline oriented. Individual members of the interdisciplinary team come together to forge an integrated analysis of pertinent problems and issues, and they work together to arrive at a set of consensus recommendations based on that analysis. Under the best circumstances, interdisciplinary collaboration becomes better than the sum of its parts, providing results that could not have been predicted from the efforts of an individual discipline. The disadvantage of interdisciplinary care is that it is time and labor intensive. It takes a great deal of effort and patience for an effective and efficient interdisciplinary process to be established. The point of departure for an effective collaboration is mutual respect among team members, which is based

Team type	Schematic of model	Potential advantages	Potential disadvantages
Multidisciplinary Multiple disciplines available simultaneously; degree of collaboration variable	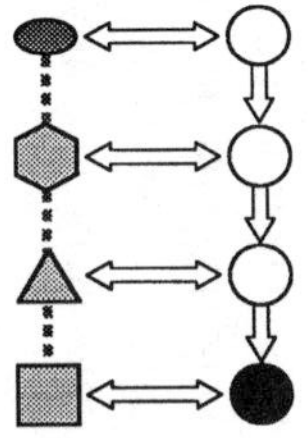	• "One-stop shopping" • Centralized data	• Conflicting recommendations • Insufficient synthesis of goals/objectives
Interdisciplinary Priority for establishing consensus of perceptions and recommendations	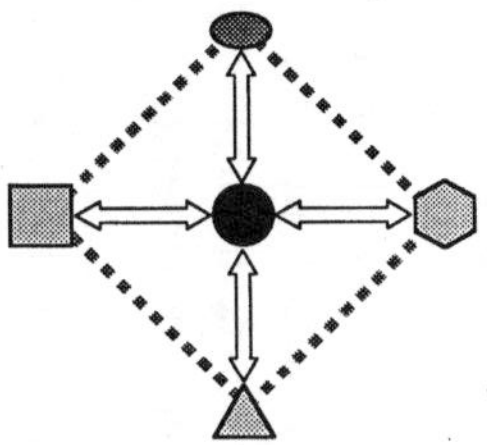	• Improved coordination of care • Consensus on goals/objectives	• Confusion regarding division of labor and responsibilities • Inefficiency resulting from need for collaboration
Transdisciplinary Individual professionals perform roles of several disciplines	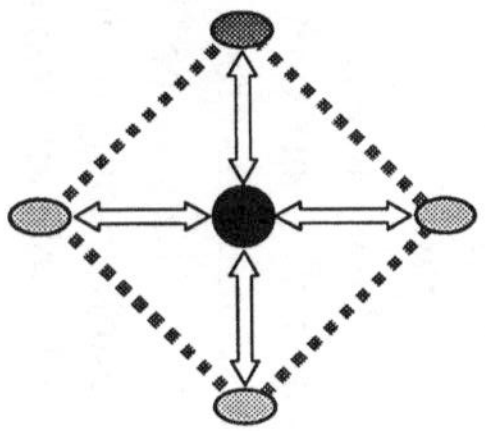	• Potential for improved efficiency with interchangeable roles	• Role confusion • Diffusion of responsibility

Figure 3.1. Types of professional teams. (Key: circle = child with disability; black oval = team leader; other shapes = other team members [different shapes symbolize different roles].)

58

on respect for one another and respect for one another's discipline. Although team members will vary in terms of training and experience, they must be viewed as equals in the collaborative process. An effective team also requires effective leadership. The specific person and discipline that provide that leadership are usually determined by the primary mission of the team and by the setting in which the collaboration occurs (e.g., school, hospital-based programs). Effective collaboration usually depends on effective service coordination. This means that one team member functions as the primary link between professionals and the family, and he or she works to bridge the priorities and concerns of the family with the priorities and concerns of the professional.

Finally, transdisciplinary teams are composed of professionals who represent different disciplines, at least in training, but whose roles become interchangeable in at least some aspect of collaborative care. An example of transdisciplinary care can be seen in educators and therapists who pursue similar goals and use similar methods in early intervention services for infants and young children. True transdisciplinary teams are rare. Collaboration tends to suffer from role diffusion and the inability to apply diverse points of view to a particular set of issues.

For children with cerebral palsy, the interdisciplinary model of collaborative care is the most favored. The disciplines typically involved in the interdisciplinary care of the child with cerebral palsy are listed in Table 3.1. Table 3.1 does not provide an all-inclusive list of disciplines that may be represented on an interdisciplinary team; any particular team will include only a subset of the disciplines cited. Larger teams involving more disciplines are more characteristic of large urban centers and are difficult to maintain without the support of federal, state, local, or private grants. Variations on the "gold standard" for interdisciplinary teams are therefore the rule rather than the exception. Regardless of the size of the team, the basic requirements of equal collaboration based on mutual respect, team leadership, and service coordination still apply.

FAMILY-CENTERED CARE
AND THE INTERDISCIPLINARY TEAM

To say that interdisciplinary care focuses on problems and issues is to say that interdisciplinary care is child centered. Determining what is "best" for the child is, therefore, the highest priority of interdisciplinary care. However, defining what is in the child's best interest is not always an easy task. This is particularly true when professional priorities come into conflict with family priorities. Emerging to address this issue has been the concept of family-centered care, which was first articulated in the late 1960s and was further defined and refined in 1987 (Shelton & Smith Stepanek, 1994). The key elements of family-centered care, as defined by the Association for the Care of Children's Health (sponsored by the Maternal and Child Health Bureau of the U.S. Department of Health and

Table 3.1. Professional discipines represented on teams for children with cerebral palsy

Disciplines usually represented

Physicians
    Pediatrics (e.g., general, neurodevelopmental)
    Orthopedic surgery
    Neurology
    Physical medicine and rehabilitation
Nursing
Social work
Physical therapy
Occupational therapy
Speech-language pathology
Orthotics

Disciplines often represented

Augmentative communication specialist
Psychology
Education
Neurosurgery
Nutrition/dietary
Dentistry

Disciplines occasionally represented

Vocational therapists/counselors
Art/music therapists
Recreational therapists
Service coordination
Urology
Genetics
Gastroenterology

Human Services) are presented in Table 3.2. The fundamental meaning of family-centered care is that family and cultural priorities take precedence over professional priorities when determining what is best for a particular child.

From the perspective of family-centered care, models of service delivery are seen in an evolutionary sequence that begins with professional-oriented services and ends with family-oriented services (Shelton & Smith Stepanek, 1994). The earliest stage is marked by professional-centered or system-centered models. In this stage, professional priorities determine the interventions that will be recommended and how they will be implemented. The next stage employs a family-allied model. In this stage, professionals allow family members to play a part in the decision-making process, but they still view families as agents of professional priorities. The next stage is a family-focused model, which creates

Table 3.2.   Elements of family-centered care

- Recognition that the family is the constant in a child's life
- Facilitation of family–professional collaboration at all levels of care
- Exchange of complete and unbiased information between professionals and family members
- Recognition of cultural diversity
- Recognition of different methods of coping
- Facilitation of family-to-family support
- Ensuring hospital, home, and community service and support systems that are flexible, accessible, and comprehensive
- Appreciation of families as families

Adapted from Shelton & Stepanek (1994).

a more equal partnership between families and professionals: Families are viewed as consumers; professionals are viewed as providers. The final stage features a family-centered model in which professionals become the agents of family priorities. In this stage, families determine the interventions that are appropriate based on their knowledge of their child and their own circumstances; professional advice is used only to augment the decision-making process. In family-centered models, families also determine the timing of interventions, which is based on the same considerations.

The assumption underlying family-centered care is that family priorities regarding what is best for the child will coincide with professional priorities. However, this may not always be the case. The most obvious example of this would be in instances of child abuse or neglect in which society mandates that professionals have a duty to circumvent family priorities for the child's best interest. In most cases, however, obvious neglect or abuse is not an issue. Family-centered care gives appropriate emphasis to the parental right to determine what is best for the child, regardless of professional opinions that might differ. The challenge for interdisciplinary care is to discover a way to take advantage of the family's expertise regarding their child and to integrate it with expertise that is both professional and discipline specific.

CEREBRAL PALSY AND THE LIFE CYCLE

Cerebral palsy is not static with respect to the human life cycle. As the child changes and grows, his or her attendant disability will change and grow as well. The dominant themes that mark the various stages of the human life cycle were described by Erikson (1985), a psychologist whose work represents a significant revision of the Freudian (Freud, 1897/1968) view of human development (see Table 3.3). Erikson's formulation emphasized the psychosocial context of human development. Every new stage builds on the one preceding it, and every

Table 3.3. Erikson's stages of the human life cycle

Stage	Age range	Primary task
Trust versus mistrust	Birth to 1 1/2 years	Establish a sense of basic trust that the world is on "your side."
Autonomy versus shame and doubt	1 1/2–3 years	Establish a sense of separateness from primary caregivers.
Initiative versus guilt	3–6 years	Establish a sense of independence in play and social interactions.
Industry versus inferiority	6–11 years	Establish a sense of competence and worthiness.
Identity versus role confusion	Adolescence	Establish a new sense of independence based on a renewed understanding of one's self-identity.
Intimacy versus isolation	Young adulthood	Establish a new sense of one's self as intimately connected with another person.
Generativity versus stagnation	Adulthood	Be productive and creative at work and at home; have a career, and raise a family.
Integrity versus despair	Old age	Establish a sense of completion to one's life as this relates to memories and current relationships.

stage comes to fruition through resolution of a central conflict. For example, the central tension during the toddler years is between an emerging sense of autonomy (i.e., self-defined action) and shame. Both autonomy and shame are emotional and psychological conditions that are defined with respect to other people, which for the toddler translates predominantly into interactions with his or her parents. The central tension that drives developmental change in the adolescent is the growing sense of identity, which is countered by the possibility of identity diffusion. This is the famous "identity crisis" for which Erikson is best known. Similar to the themes of the toddler years, the themes of adolescence are defined in terms of interpersonal relationships. The early consolidation of a sense of identity rests particularly in the balance that is struck between the values inculcated by the family and the values inculcated by the "outside world" (as represented by peers). Erikson's formulation is a reminder that development does not occur in a vacuum: It occurs within a context, and that context is other people.

The implications of a disability such as cerebral palsy are different at each stage of the human life cycle. For example, not being able to walk has very different implications for toddlers than it does for adolescents. For the toddler who is struggling to develop a sense of autonomy, impaired mobility may create a major hindrance to exploring the physical environment. For the adolescent, impairments of mobility may be less important than other issues (e.g., dysarthria [problems with the production of speech sounds], drooling due to oral-motor dysfunction) in working to establish a sense of identity. For interdisciplinary care to be effective, it must find a way to account for the developmental context of the disability. In order for family-centered care to be meaningful, it must adhere to a conceptual framework that can be used as a reference point when a child's best interests are unclear.

DEFINING A CONCEPTUAL FRAMEWORK
FOR FAMILY-CENTERED, INTERDISCIPLINARY CARE

In 1980, the World Health Organization (WHO) published the *International Classification of Impairments, Disabilities and Handicap,* which has become the point of departure for all subsequent discussions of the dimensions of disability. As the title implies, the report defines three key concepts: impairment, disability, and handicap. *Impairment* is defined as a fundamental structural, psychological, or physiological deficit (e.g., disordered motor control in cerebral palsy). *Disability* is defined as the functional deficit that a person experiences as a result of impairment (e.g., spasticity interfering with walking), and *handicap* is defined as the disadvantage a person with disability experiences in various societal settings as a result of that disability (e.g., people who cannot walk may be denied access to particular places).

A number of suggestions for modifying and refining the WHO model have been made since 1980. Most noteworthy among these recommendations is the model developed by the National Center for Medical Rehabilitation Research (NCMRR) (see Figure 3.2), which successfully integrates the WHO framework with other cogent models of disability (National Institutes of Health, 1993). The NCMRR construct defines five dimensions of disability. The WHO category of impairment is transformed in the NCMRR model into two categories: *pathophysiology* and *impairment* (the former emphasizing basic biological and psychological disturbances and the latter emphasizing the more generalized effects of these disturbances). For example, brain abnormalities resulting from adverse prenatal conditions (i.e., the pathophysiology) may be manifest as generalized abnormalities of muscle tone and motor control (i.e., the impairment). The WHO category of disability is then differentiated in the NCMRR model into functional limitations and disability. A *functional limitation* is a specific skill or set of related skills that cannot be executed and are often (but not always) a result of a preexisting impairment. *Disability* retains its original mean-

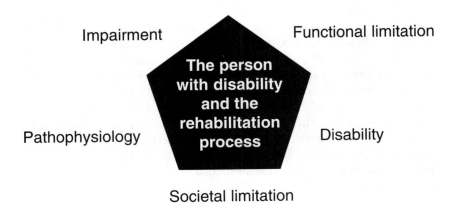

Impairment   Functional limitation

The person with disability and the rehabilitation process

Pathophysiology   Disability

Societal limitation

Figure 3.2. The NCMRR model of disability. The components of disability are shown arranged around a pentagon to emphasize the complex, rather than hierarchical, relationships among the components.

ing as the decrement in function that a person experiences as a consequence of his or her impairments and functional limitations (e.g., dysfunctional gait is a functional limitation that may result in impaired mobility, which is the disability experienced by the individual). Finally, the term *handicap* has been replaced in the NCMRR scheme by the term *societal limitation,* emphasizing the role of the environment and society in limiting the opportunities for growth and development. Environmental constraints, such as a lack of wheelchair ramps or "handicapped parking," are obvious examples of societal limitations. More subtle and more pervasive constraints are present within actual culture and limit opportunities for participation in the goods of society. The familiar metaphor of the "glass ceiling" in the workplace can be modified for people with disabilities as a series of "glass walls" that present barriers in every direction and often lack the transparency suggested by the image.

HABILITATION AND PARTICIPATION: PRIORITIZING GOALS FOR INTERDISCIPLINARY CARE

After reviewing the WHO and NCMRR models of the dimensions of disability, it should be clear that the field of developmental disabilities is semantically challenged and perhaps this is unavoidable. All of the major terms introduced in this chapter describe the dimensions of disability with respect to deficits or barriers (e.g., pathophysiology, impairment, functional limitation, disability, societal limitation, handicap). Although it is of no greater value to burden the lexicon with terminology that bows at every turn to political correctness, it is worth considering the current state of affairs more carefully and asking the question, "How can contemporary models of disability help to operationalize the priorities of family-centered, interdisciplinary care?"

We can begin by recognizing that deficits and barriers are mirror images of something in the human situation that is both desirable and affirming of the human person. To say that we wish to remediate deficits and remove barriers is true, but it falls short of the mark. To say that the goal of interdisciplinary care is to optimize development and to improve quality of life is admirable, but it leaves one wondering how these outcomes can be measured or even recognized.

We also must recognize that the term *rehabilitation,* which implies a return to some previous level of function, does not capture the full range of processes that family-centered, interdisciplinary care wishes to encompass for children with cerebral palsy and their families. The term *habilitation* has been used to describe the ongoing care and multiple medical, therapeutic, and educational interventions that children with developmental disabilities receive throughout their lives. If habilitation describes the collective activities that are the raison d'être of interdisciplinary care, then it must also attempt to characterize the overarching objective of that care.

One way to approach this issue is to define habilitation in terms of participation. The term *participation* broadly characterizes the core mechanism that operates at each stage of the human life cycle. As the child moves through each stage, he or she becomes further enmeshed in the structures of human society. With respect to participation, the child with disabilities is often like the child who is a member of a Little League baseball team who always sits on the bench. The child's parents may wonder if their child's lack of participation is a result of his or her inherently inferior athletic skills or if it is a result of the failure of the coach or the league to accommodate a wider range of skills because of an overemphasis on winning. In either scenario, the child is made to feel that he or she is not a part of the game and loses the opportunity to become a better player. This example refocuses the situation on society at large. Nothing characterizes disability in general so much as the loss of opportunities for participation in the goods of society. Working to enhance a person's ability to participate in settings and be engaged in relationships and activities appropriate to each stage of the life cycle does not guarantee an improved quality of life, but it is a concrete and potentially measurable way of increasing the probability that an improvement will occur.

In order for habilitation to be a successful venture, professionals must become as proficient in characterizing the child's real-life settings (i.e., environment) as they are at characterizing the specific aspects of the child's impairments, functional limitations, and disabilities. It is also necessary for professionals to draw on scientific perspectives that lie outside of the traditional domain of developmental disabilities. One potential source is found in the work of Bronfenbrenner, a Cornell psychologist. Bronfenbrenner (1979) defined *developmental change* as a property of settings as much as it is a property of individuals. The developmental setting is defined by the activities of the participants in that setting, by the roles that are assigned to participants by cultural standards, and by the relationships that exist as a consequence of these activities and roles. For example, the elementary school classroom is a developmental setting that is characterized by a set of educational activities (i.e., the curriculum), by the well-defined roles of the participants (i.e., student, teacher, or paraprofessional), and by the interpersonal relationships that are a consequence of these activities and roles.

In Bronfenbrenner's (1979) terminology, settings such as the elementary school classroom that are characterized by face-to-face interactions are called *microsystems* (see Figure 3.3). During infancy the child participates in primarily one microsystem, the home. As the child develops, he or she will begin to participate in an increasing number and variety of settings. The child will ultimately move regularly among several such settings, including home, school, and child care. From a developmental perspective, this "system of systems" eventually becomes more than the sum of its parts and is referred to as a *mesosystem*. Although other settings may exist and the child may not directly participate in them, they can still indirectly affect the child's development. These external settings are called *exosystems*. For example, the child's parent may work in an office that the child never visits or that the child may not even know

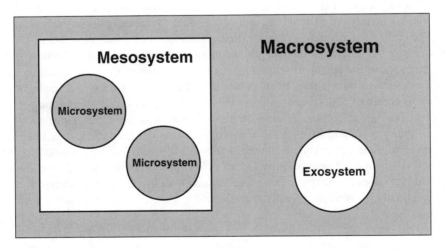

Figure 3.3. Bronfenbrenner's developmental settings. The relationships among the various types of settings are shown. Microsystems constitute the actual settings in which a child participates; a mesosystem is the collection of all such settings. Exosystems are settings to which a child does not belong but that nonetheless affect the child's development. The macrosystem is the cultural setting that determines the specific attributes (e.g., activities, roles, relationships) that constitute the microsystems within its domain. (Adapted from Bronfenbrenner, 1979.)

exists; however, the parent's being laid off or receiving a promotion can have a profound effect on the family and an indirect effect on the child's development. Finally, Bronfenbrenner defined *macrosystems* as the entire cultural standard or blueprint—encompassing microsystems, mesosystems, and exosystems—for all of the lower-order systems as they exist within a particular society. For example, classrooms vary greatly from one country and culture to the next; but, within a particular country, classrooms are fairly consistent and predictable with respect to the defining activities, roles, and relationships.

Bronfenbrenner's (1979) work has had surprising implications for professionals interested in designing interventions for children with disabilities. Therapeutic intervention is traditionally conceived as something that is done to a child to remediate a functional deficit that is a consequence of impairments and functional limitations. To return to a previous example, this would be like giving a Little League player who is stuck on the bench some remedial batting and fielding lessons. The idea is that practice (i.e., therapy) will result in improved participation and decreased time on the bench. If we think of the Little League team as a developmental setting, then Bronfenbrenner's formulation leads us to consider interventions that do not involve the child directly but rather focus on adjusting the activities, roles, and relationships within that setting. For example, a parental conference with the child's coach or with the Little League president may be necessary in order to adjust expectations and moderate competitive priorities in favor of inclusion and participation. Another possible reason for the child not participating in baseball is that the child cannot concentrate because of a problem at home. This would be an example of a circumstance in one setting influencing the ability to participate in another (i.e., the mesosystem effect). It is widely recognized that changes in the workplace since the 1970s have had a major effect on family life. The problems at home that are interfering with the child's ability to concentrate while playing baseball may be the result of parental concerns regarding a potential layoff (i.e., the exosystem effect). However, as Bronfrenbrenner would emphasize, it may be the whole idea of Little League that is flawed and discriminatory, and a change may be needed at the societal level in the form of changes in public policy (i.e., interventions at the level of the macrosystem).

Bronfenbrenner's (1979) formulation creates an enormous challenge for interdisciplinary care. When designing interventions for children, it is not sufficient to confine considerations exclusively to a child's functional characteristics. Consideration must be given to multiple aspects of the child's real-life settings and to the larger societal context in which these settings occur and derive their meaning. In addition, it cannot be assumed that the priorities of family-centered care automatically result in meaningful outcomes for the child with cerebral palsy until the ability to define the nature of meaningful outcomes has drastically improved.

THE ULTIMATE GOAL OF
FAMILY-CENTERED, INTERDISCIPLINARY CARE:
DEFINING AND CREATING MEANINGFUL OUTCOMES

The term *habilitation* is introduced in this chapter to describe the many activities that characterize the ongoing care of the child with a disability. It was posited that the overarching goal of habilitation was improved participation in real-life settings. With respect to the NCMRR model of disability, improved participation in the goods of society corresponds to minimizing societal limitations; with respect to the WHO model of disability, increased participation corresponds to minimizing or eliminating disadvantages or handicap. Bronfenbrenner's (1979) description of developmental settings and their societal context makes it possible to provide a more precise definition of habilitation:

> Habilitation is a comprehensive intervention strategy designed to facilitate adaptation to and participation in an increasing number and variety of settings in a particular society and culture. (Pellegrino, 1995, pp. 836–837)

Before any determination can be made regarding the potential benefits or risks of a particular intervention, habilitation must account for the specific circumstances of a child's life. In order for habilitation to be successful, interdisciplinary care must be family centered and family focused because it is family members who provide the critical information about the key settings in which the child lives. It is a common error among clinicians to determine a course of therapy or to recommend an intervention without sufficiently taking family priorities into account. For example, surgery is commonly recommended for a variety of orthopedic problems for children with cerebral palsy. The goals of surgery vary, but they typically include ameliorating an impairment to improve functional mobility, preventing or remediating pain, and improving positioning and personal hygiene. Many children undergo multiple surgical procedures and are away from home and absent from their schools and communities for extended periods of time. The underlying assumption in these instances is that surgery will usually prevent future limitations and enhance future participation in the goods of society, and these potential advantages for improved function outweigh or justify lost opportunities in the present. This is often but not always true. For some children, these short-term sacrifices accumulate until they represent a pattern of lost opportunities and the hope for the future never arrives.

Outcomes research in the field of developmental disabilities and cerebral palsy in particular has traditionally focused heavily on impairments and functional limitations. With the advent of functional outcome measures such as the Pediatric Evaluation of Disability Inventory (PEDI) (Haley, Coster, Ludlow, Haltiwanger, & Andrellas, 1992), the Gross Motor Function Measure (GMFM) (Russell et al., 1989), and the Pediatric Functional Independence Measure (WeeFIM) (Granger, Hamilton, & Kayton, 1989), progress in addressing outcomes at the level of disability has been made. The greatest challenge for the field is to define outcome measures that are contextually relevant. Efforts to characterize the specific, quantifiable aspects of participation in real-life settings are a necessary component of future research (see Chapter 5 for an attempt to apply these concepts to clinical decision making in the management of spasticity), and it is the NCMRR model of disability that provides a ready framework for discussion and progress in this endeavor.

SUMMARY

The team approach to cerebral palsy arose in response to the complex needs and issues that often attend this developmental disability. The coordinated efforts of professionals from several disciplines have been mandated through federal legislation, which targets the educational needs of children with disabilities. Although several types of coordinated teams exist, the most common type is the interdisciplinary team. The concept of family-centered care requires that interdisciplinary teams incorporate family members as key participants in the team process. When apparent conflicts exist between family or professional priorities and a child's "best interest," the team should revert to a set of principles that defines the dimensions of disability and provides an objective framework for assessing functional and psychosocial outcomes. These principles were originally set forth by the WHO in 1980 and were refined further by the NCMRR in 1993. Developmental theory informs interdisciplinary care by providing a life-cycle perspective of developmental disabilities and by drawing attention to environmental and social factors that influence functional outcomes and quality of life.

The team approach operates through the mechanism of habilitation, which aims to enhance participation in the benefits of society. Quantitative measures of functional outcome emphasize independence over participation: Improvements in the ability to accurately represent "enhanced participation" are needed to advance the cause of people with disabilities as well as the goals of interdisciplinary care.

REFERENCES

Batshaw, M.L., & Shapiro, B.K. (1997). Mental retardation. In M.L. Batshaw (Ed.), *Children with disabilities* (4th ed., pp. 325–348). Baltimore: Paul H. Brookes Publishing Co.

Blackman, J.A., Healy, A., & Ruppert, E.S. (1992). Participation by pediatricians in early intervention: Impetus from Public Law 99-457. *Pediatrics, 89,* 98–102.

Bronfenbrenner, U. (1979). *The ecology of human development: Experiments by nature and design.* Cambridge, MA: Harvard University Press.

Crothers, B., & Paine, D.S. (1959). *The natural history of cerebral palsy.* Cambridge, MA: Harvard University Press.

Deaver, G.G. (1956). Cerebral palsy: Methods of treating the neuromuscular disabilities. *Archives of Physical Medicine and Rehabilitation, 37,* 363–367.

Education for All Handicapped Children Act of 1975, PL 94-142, 20 U.S.C. §§ 1400 *et seq.*

Education of the Handicapped Act Amendments of 1986, PL 99-457, 20 U.S.C. §§ 1400 *et seq.*

Erikson, E.H. (1985). *Childhood and society.* New York: W.W. Norton.

Farrell, S.E., & Pimentel, A.E. (1996). Interdisciplinary team process in developmental disabilities. In A.J. Capute & P.J. Accardo (Eds.), *Developmental disabilities in infancy and childhood: Vol. 2. The spectrum of developmental disabilities* (2nd ed., pp. 91–109). Baltimore: Paul H. Brookes Publishing Co.

Freud, S. (1968). *Infantile cerebral palsy.* Coral Gables, FL: University of Miami Press. (Original work published 1897)

Granger, C.V., Hamilton, B.B., & Kayton, R. (1989). *Guide for the use of the Functional Independence Measure (WeeFIM) of the uniform data set for medical rehabilitation.* Buffalo: State University of New York, Research Foundation.

Haley, S.M., Coster, W.J., Ludlow, L.H., Haltiwanger, J.T., & Andrellas, P.J. (1992). *Pediatric Evaluation of Disability Inventory (PEDI).* Boston: New England Medical Center.

Individuals with Disabilities Education Act (IDEA) of 1990, PL 101-476, 20 U.S.C. §§ 1400 *et seq.*

Individuals with Disabilities Education Act Amendments of 1991, PL 102-119, 20 U.S.C. §§ 1400 *et seq.*

Individuals with Disabilities Education Act (IDEA) of 1997, PL 105-17, 20 U.S.C. §§ 1400 *et seq.*

National Institutes of Health. (1993). *Research plan for the National Center for Medical Rehabilitation Research.* (NIH Publication No. 93–3509). Bethesda, MD: Author.

Pellegrino, L. (1995). Cerebral palsy: A paradigm for developmental disabilities. *Developmental Medicine and Child Neurology, 37,* 834–839.

Phelps, W.M. (1941). The rehabilitation of cerebral palsy. *Southern Medical Journal, 34,* 770–776.

Russell, D.J., Rosenbaum, P.L., Cadman, D.T., Gowland, C., Hardy, S., & Jarvis, S. (1989). The Gross Motor Function Measure: Reliability, validity and responsiveness of an evaluative instrument. *Developmental Medicine and Child Neurology, 31,* 341–351.

Shelton, T.L., & Smith Stepanek, J. (1994). *Family-centered care for children needing specialized health and developmental services.* Bethesda, MD: Association for the Care of Children's Health.

World Health Organization. (1980). *International classification of impairments, disabilities and handicap.* Geneva, Switzerland: Author.

CHAPTER 4

Well-Child Care and Health Maintenance

Louis Pellegrino

The provision of well-child care for the child with cerebral palsy presents special challenges for families and professionals. In addition to the traditional emphasis on preventive care, well-child care for the child with cerebral palsy also must address a number of complex medical, developmental, and psychosocial issues. The interdisciplinary team approach (see Chapter 3), emphasizing the collaboration between family members and professionals, is an effective way of meeting the needs of the child who has a complex disability. Well-child care may be thought of as the aspect of interdisciplinary care that addresses the specific health care needs of the child and that provides the coordination and monitoring of other aspects of the child's care. Although the involvement of a large number of thoughtful and well-intentioned individuals in this caregiving process may create an opportunity for the provision of excellent care, it may also lead to confusion and miscommunication. Families are often bewildered and occasionally intimidated by the different and sometimes conflicting viewpoints of professionals. Families also may have difficulty integrating the recommendations of professionals into the realities of family life. A close partnership between family members and the primary care physician is needed to ensure that a child's overall best interests are being served. The primary care physician also plays an essential role in helping children and their families gain access to the various professionals involved in interdisciplinary care. Finally, the primary physician–primary caregiver partnership provides a "clearinghouse" for the recommendations generated by teams of professionals. This chapter discusses the key role of the primary care physician in the coordination of interdisciplinary care and reviews several of the special issues commonly encountered in the provision of well-child care for children with cerebral palsy.

CREATING APPROPRIATE EXPECTATIONS FOR WELL-CHILD CARE AND HEALTH MAINTENANCE

Since its inception as a medical specialty, pediatrics has always emphasized the importance of preventive health care for children. An obviously excellent example of this focus is the universal provision of immunizations for the prevention of certain infectious diseases. There also is a long tradition in pediatrics that emphasizes the importance of complete and adequate nutrition, particularly for infants, as the indispensable foundation for proper growth and good health. Finally, the sine qua non of pediatrics is the developmental perspective. The processes of growth and development transform every child into not one but several different patients, each following the other in sequence as the child grows and matures. The concept of *anticipatory guidance* (Hockelman, 1992) is founded on the principle that parents and professionals need to stay one or two steps ahead of children in order to provide the best preventive care. Families and professionals encounter their greatest challenges in attempting to anticipate the needs of the child with cerebral palsy. The point of departure for any discussion of well-child care for children with cerebral palsy must be the recognition that in most ways children with disabilities are not different from typically developing children in their needs for preventive care and anticipatory guidance. This assertion belies the fact that the priorities of preventive care and anticipatory guidance are frequently diluted and diffused by the presence of multiple medical issues and the involvement of multiple professionals. It becomes a goal of interdisciplinary care to refocus these priorities and to rediscover the basic elements of well-child care and health maintenance for children with cerebral palsy.

THE ROLES OF THE PRIMARY CARE PHYSICIAN AND THE CARE MANAGER

The primary care physician, often a pediatrician or a family-practice physician, has traditionally played the role of "case manager" with respect to health care for children with cerebral palsy; he or she has been the key person in the provision and the coordination of preventive care and anticipatory guidance. However, case managers, sometimes referred to as "care managers," have emerged in a variety of settings to provide additional coordination of care (Jacoby, Howard-Gleum, McGuire, & Hayashida, 1995). Care managers are typically better acquainted than most physicians with the various agencies and services that are available in a particular community and are therefore in a position to provide opportunities for and remove obstacles to the ongoing provision of care. The care manager is ideally an integral member of an interdisciplinary team that is organized around the habilitation goals and the medical needs of the child with cerebral palsy. A close collaboration among the care manager, the parents, and the primary physician forms a core group to monitor the child's process of habilitation over an extended period of time and ensures that the priorities of well-child care are not undermined.

CEREBRAL PALSY AND THE LIFE CYCLE

Cerebral palsy is in part defined as a disability that is a result of a nonprogressive neurological condition; however, this definition does not mean that the manifestations of the disability are static with respect to time. As the child with cerebral palsy grows and matures, so, in a sense, does the disability grow and mature. This is true not only of the physical and the obvious manifestations of the motor impairment but also of the important psychosocial implications of the disability at different stages of the life cycle (see Chapter 17). The anticipatory guidance provided to the 3-year-old child who does not walk must be very different from the guidance provided to the nonambulatory teenager. This is true not only because the younger child may have a better potential for ambulation but also because the implications for nonambulation are different at various ages. The priorities of adolescence are centered around the establishment of social identity and independence (Erikson, 1985). The implications of nonambulation in this context are clearly different from those in the preschool years, when freedom of mobility, in and of itself, is likely to be one of the child's main issues.

The medical problems associated with cerebral palsy also vary in importance at different stages of development. A particular issue in the provision of well-child care is the recognition of problems that yield better outcomes when identified and treated early (e.g., hearing loss, poor nutrition, hip dislocation; see sections on "Hearing and Vision" and "Growth and Nutrition" in this chapter). Professionals with expertise in the field of developmental disabilities and familiarity with the natural history of cerebral palsy have a special obligation to disseminate information regarding these opportunities for preventive care to families and to primary care physicians.

COMMON ISSUES IN THE PROVISION OF
WELL-CHILD CARE FOR CHILDREN WITH CEREBRAL PALSY

The diagnosis of cerebral palsy is discussed in detail in Chapter 2. The diagnosis is very often suspected early, particularly in children who had a difficult neonatal course; however, because of maturational issues, the diagnosis of cerebral palsy cannot be confirmed until the child is 2–3 years old (Nelson & Ellenberg, 1982). It is important to recognize that among children who have a suspected diagnosis of cerebral palsy that is not subsequently confirmed, there is an increased incidence of other neurodevelopmental problems (see Chapter 2).

It should not be assumed that children with significantly delayed motor development (e.g., a child who has not begun to walk by 18 months of age) will simply "outgrow" the problem. Although delayed motor development does not necessarily mean that a particular child has cerebral palsy, it may be an indication of other neurodevelopmental problems (e.g., mental retardation). Regardless of the situation, the appropriate response to recognizing significant motor delay is vigilance and in-depth analysis of the child's neurodevelopmental status. Parental concern regarding their child's development also should prompt further evaluation. Although parents may misinterpret the significance of developmental problems, they are, in general, excellent at recognizing and reporting motor delays (Glascoe & Dworkin, 1995). A good rule of thumb is that if either the parent or the primary care physician has concerns about a child's development (motor or otherwise), a referral to a professional with expertise in child development and neurodevelopmental disabilities should be made.

Making the Correct Diagnosis and
Explaining and Presenting the Diagnosis of Cerebral Palsy

The primary care physician is often involved in presenting the diagnosis of cerebral palsy to families. (This is especially true when the diagnosis is suspected early but cannot be confirmed for several months or years.) The manner in which the diagnosis is first presented to a child's caregivers has a critical impact on the family's subsequent ability to cope with the disability and its implications (Sharp, Strauss, & Lorch, 1992). How a family learns to cope with the diagnosis of a developmental disability may be as important to prognosis and to outcome as is the specific profile of impairments that characterizes the actual disability. The following suggestions on how to present the diagnosis of cerebral palsy may help to set the process of family coping and adaptation on a sound footing.

Set Aside Sufficient Time The diagnosis of cerebral palsy cannot be presented to a caregiver in a few minutes. Explanations that are hastily presented are a source of great distress for families as well as a fertile breeding ground for miscommunication, misunderstanding, anxiety, and litigation. What is said at the time of diagnosis leaves a permanent, vivid impression. A misspoken word or a misunderstood phrase may rankle in the parental psyche for years and may require heroic efforts to redress. An investment of 45 minutes or an hour at this critical juncture can save families great heartache and save professionals great amounts of wasted effort and backtracking in years to come.

Meet with More than One Caregiver Caregivers are typically overwhelmed by the news that their child has cerebral palsy, and, as a result, they often hear only a fraction of what is said at the time of the initial diagnosis. Having another caregiver present increases the likelihood that what is said will be heard and what is heard will be correctly understood. It is difficult for one parent to absorb and accurately convey the content and the implications of an entire meeting without creating further misunderstanding and confusion for the parent who was not present. In a sense, one parent is asked to carry the entire burden of the diagnosis. The process of coping and adaptation begins with conversation; thus, having two caregivers present at the time of the initial diagnosis gives the professional an opportunity to start family dialogue on the right track.

Meet without the Child Present Having the child present at the time of diagnosis often proves to be an overwhelming distraction. Caregivers and professionals need time in a quiet atmosphere of adult conversation to sort through the implications of the diagnosis. A separate meeting can be arranged after the initial diagnosis is presented to communicate with caregivers and the child together; this also can be a very useful way to follow up on questions that arise subsequently.

Engage in Dialogue Rather than Monologue Professionals are prone to expansive monologue when presenting a diagnosis. Very often once the words "cerebral palsy" are spoken, nothing else that is said by the professional is clearly heard or understood by the caregivers. It is helpful to stop frequently during the discussion to elicit feedback from the caregivers about what has been said. It is particularly important to ask the caregivers what they have heard in the past regarding cerebral palsy. Misconceptions abound and must be addressed before any meaningful discussion of the implications of the diagnosis for a particular child can occur. A good rule of thumb is to ask the caregivers many open-ended questions (e.g., "What have you heard about cerebral palsy?") and to spend at least half of the time listening and asking questions.

Do Not Be Gloomy The diagnosis of cerebral palsy is generally received by caregivers as bad news. Making constructive comments about a child's potential for progress and helping caregivers to understand what they can do to help their child grow and develop goes a long way toward establishing a sense of purpose and control, and this plants the seed for a healthy sense of optimism. Clinicians often feel that it is their duty to dissuade caregivers from entertaining any semblance of denial regarding their child's diagnosis or prognosis, and they can be overzealous in their efforts to make caregivers be "realistic" about their child's condition. Denial is an expected element in the process of coping (Kübler-Ross, 1969); and when it is handled with a sense of equanimity over an extended period of time, it can lead to a balanced view of the diagnosis and the disability.

Follow Up with a Telephone Call or Another Meeting   Regardless of how well the diagnosis of cerebral palsy is presented and explained, caregivers will always have questions that occur to them later, and typically they will experience some confusion and disorientation. A follow-up telephone call or a meeting with the caregiver within a week or two allows the professional to consolidate the progress made at the initial meeting.

Recognition of Associated Developmental Disabilities in the Child with Cerebral Palsy

Although the diagnosis of cerebral palsy per se relates to problems with motor control and functional mobility, children with cerebral palsy are much more likely than typically developing children to have concomitant cognitive deficits leading to a diagnosis of mental retardation, a learning disability, or a developmental language disorder (see Chapter 1). It is common for motor delays and cerebral palsy to be recognized earlier than cognitive delays. It also is common for problems with functional mobility to be overemphasized in relation to other issues in the design of early intervention strategies. Associated cognitive impairments may be drastically more important for prognosis than the cerebral palsy itself, particularly for the child with milder forms of motor impairment. In other words, disabilities in the areas of communication, socialization, and daily living skills are often more significant for function than deficits in mobility.

Hearing and Vision

A common issue in the provision of well-child care is recognizing deficits in hearing and in vision. Children with cerebral palsy have a high incidence of sensory deficits that have significant functional implications, and these may be overlooked in the clinician's enthusiasm to address more visible developmental and medical needs (see Chapters 1 and 2). Nearsightedness (i.e., myopia) or abnormalities of eye muscle control (e.g., strabismus) can lead to permanent secondary loss of vision in the most affected eye (i.e., "lazy eye" leading to amblyopia). Unrecognized hearing loss may interfere with language development, further complicating a child's disability profile. Parents and professionals alike are prone to overinterpreting visual-tracking and auditory-orienting behaviors as evidence of normal vision and hearing. Overrelying on such clinical impressions leads to missed diagnoses and lost opportunities for intervention (Coplan, 1987). It is, therefore, recommended that all children with significant neurodevelopment concerns undergo hearing and vision testing as soon as these concerns surface, ideally during infancy. Vision testing should be performed by an ophthalmologist with experience in both pediatrics and developmental disabilities. Hearing testing should be performed by a licensed audiologist in a soundproof environment. The types of audiological assessments available are listed in Table 4.1.

Table 4.1. Types of audiological tests

Test	Method	Advantages	Disadvantages
Brain stem auditory evoked response	Auditory stimulus applied to each ear while child is sedated; scalp electrodes measure response to stimulus	Establishes integrity of auditory pathway for each ear; child's cooperation is not necessary	Need for sedation; measures neuro-logical response rather than the true measure of hearing
Behavioral audiometry	Auditory stimulus provided in a sound-proof booth while child is awake; differential behavioral responses used to determine acuity	No sedation required; noninvasive, non-threatening; true measure of hearing	Differences between ears are not defined (only hearing for *best ear* is established); dependent on behavioral responses that are intact
Pure tone audiometry	Pure tones introduced to each ear via headphones; child indicates with gesture when sound is heard	Gold standard hearing test	Requires at least 3-year-old cognitive level and adequate motor control for responses

Growth and Nutrition

Multiple factors contribute to problems with growth and nutrition in children with cerebral palsy (Stallings, Charney, Davies, & Cronk, 1993b) (see Chapter 11). These factors can be divided broadly into nutritional and nonnutritional factors. There are many misconceptions regarding what constitutes appropriate growth for children with cerebral palsy. Parents often report that their children "have a good appetite" and that being underweight or "small" is a familial trait. Many parents of children who are nonambulatory worry that if their child gains weight, they will no longer be able to carry him or her. Professionals may assume that nonnutritional factors predominate in the growth deficits of children with cerebral palsy or that a child who is significantly below his or her typical weight on a growth chart is nevertheless "growing along his [or her] own curve." It also may be assumed that children with cerebral palsy "burn more calories" (i.e., have a higher than typical resting metabolic rate) as a result of spasticity or rigidity. But, in fact, because of decreased lean-body mass and relative immobility, most children with more severe cerebral palsy burn fewer calories than typically developing children their age (Fried & Pencharz, 1991; Taylor & Shelton, 1995).

Poor nutrition has been shown to be a significant factor in poor weight gain in children with cerebral palsy, particularly among children with more severe motor impairment types such as spastic quadriplegia (Stallings, Charney, Davies,

& Cronk, 1993a). In these children, measures of fat stores indicate chronic undernutrition in relation to insufficient caloric intake. Behavioral, neuromuscular, physiological, and environmental factors contribute synergistically to this poor caloric intake. Although these facts are well documented in medical literature, they are not widely appreciated. The state of knowledge in the medical community regarding the nutritional status of children with cerebral palsy is akin to the general knowledge that prevailed for children prior to the advent of nutritional science and pediatrics in the 19th and 20th centuries. It is incumbent on all primary care physicians who care for children with cerebral palsy to become more familiar with these issues and the methods for recognizing and ameliorating nutritional problems in these children.

Obesity also can be a significant problem for some children with cerebral palsy. Although it is a concern that is less common than undernutrition, obesity can have a significant impact on the health and the function of individual children. In some cases, obesity can even prevent or severely limit a child from walking who would otherwise be fully ambulatory. Some children with cerebral palsy may have significantly reduced caloric requirements as a result of inactivity, and they also may have a less-than-typical percentage of lean-body mass; under these conditions, intake of normal amounts of food can result in abnormal weight gain (Taylor & Shelton, 1995).

Gastroesophageal Reflux and Oral-Motor Dysfunction

A common issue in the provision of well-child care is recognizing how gastroesophageal reflux (GER) and oral-motor dysfunction contribute to poor nutritional status and to increased risk for aspiration in children with cerebral palsy. Children with cerebral palsy are prone to functional abnormalities of the gastrointestinal tract (i.e., mouth, pharynx, esophagus, stomach, and small and large intestines) that often have a significant effect on growth and nutrition on the one hand and on respiratory functioning on the other. In the normally functioning gastrointestinal tract, food and water pass in an orderly and well-coordinated sequence from the esophagus to the stomach and then to the intestines. GER represents a problem with the stomach contents backing up (i.e., refluxing) into the esophagus. GER actually is a common phenomenon and typically is present in newborns whose gastrointestinal systems have not fully matured (i.e., "spitting-up"). Most people experience GER in the form of episodic, self-limited bouts of heartburn. In many children with cerebral palsy, however, GER persists beyond early infancy and may be frequent (i.e., multiple daily episodes) and severe (i.e., extending to the upper esophagus, which sometimes results in vomiting) (Hebra & Hoffman, 1993).

There are two major potential consequences of severe chronic GER. First, because the lining of the esophagus is not designed to resist the acid contents of the stomach, GER results in irritation and inflammation, called *esophagitis*. Over an extended period of time, esophagitis may cause permanent scarring and abnormal motility of the esophagus. Esophagitis contributes to poor appetite, which results in decreased caloric intake and poor weight gain. Second, if GER is severe enough, stomach contents may reach the oral pharynx and be drawn from there into the trachea and lungs, resulting in *aspiration.* Multiple episodes of aspiration may eventually lead to chronic damage to the lungs and are a major factor in increasing morbidity and mortality in children with cerebral palsy.

Oral-motor dysfunction is described in detail in Chapters 11 and 14. A highly complex series of coordinated motor events is required for the many functions of the oral-motor apparatus, which include the generation of speech, the preparation and swallowing of liquids and solids, and the maintenance of the integrity of the airway. Problems with speech production and articulation related to oral-motor dysfunctions are referred to as *dysarthria.* Problems with typical swallowing may result in poor intake of food and water, which may contribute to problems with growth. Many children with significant oral-motor dysfunction have problems with drooling, which causes skin breakdown around the mouth and in extreme cases causes problems with dehydration as a result of excessive fluid loss. The main problem for most children with oral-motor dysfunction is the social stigma attached to drooling. Several intervention approaches to drooling have been employed and are summarized in Table 4.2 (Blasco & Allaire, 1992).

When oral-motor dysfunction leads to inadequate protection of the airway, aspiration of saliva and other contents of the mouth and the pharynx may occur. In many cases, identifying appropriate food textures (many children have difficulty swallowing thin liquids or chunky solids) for the individual child can help minimize the risk of this type of aspiration. When oral-motor problems are suspected, consultation with a speech-language pathologist or a feeding specialist should be scheduled. Radiological studies, such as a modified barium swallow (see Chapter 11), also may be conducted.

Constipation

Constipation is very common among children with cerebral palsy; however, the way in which it contributes to feeding problems and irritability is often underrecognized as well as undertreated. Constipation causes decreased appetite and contributes significantly to poor growth in some children. It also may contribute to irritability that may be attributed incorrectly to other causes. Untreated, chronic constipation can result in dramatic dilation of the intestine with permanent dysfunction and, in extreme cases, in bowel perforation requiring surgical intervention.

The goal of treatment is to establish daily bowel movements that are soft and well formed. Significant improvements in appetite can be seen in children who go from moving their bowels every other day to moving them once or twice daily. There are three phases of therapy. The *clean-out phase,* usually completed in 1–3 days, involves complete evacuation of the bowels. This is

Table 4.2.   Types of intervention for significant drooling

Intervention	Method	Advantages	Disadvantages
Behavioral techniques	Various "hands-on" methods using neurodevelop-mental techniques, behavioral modification, and biofeedback	Noninvasive, generally well tolerated	Time-intensive; problems with generalizing outside of therapy situation
Medications	Various medications, especially anti-cholinergic medications, which decrease salivary flow	Ease of administration	Problems with side effects and decreasing efficacy with time
Surgical interventions	Interruption of nerve supply to salivary glands; disruption of salivary glands or ducts	One-time procedure	Invasive; unclear long-term efficacy

Source: Blasco & Allaire (1992).

necessary before effective, long-term treatment can be initiated. The *equilibration phase* involves establishing daily bowel movements, usually with a combination of stool softeners, which improve the consistency of the stool, and laxatives, which promote bowel motility. During the *maintenance phase,* a combination of dietary measures (e.g., increased fiber and fluid in the child's diet) and medications is used to maintain daily bowel movements. The use of suppositories and enemas for long-term maintenance is avoided.

Dental Care

Ensuring adequate dental care for children with cerebral palsy is an important aspect of well-child care. Children with cerebral palsy are at greater risk for dental problems than are children without developmental disabilities for several reasons (Batshaw, Helpin, & Rosenberg, 1997). Abnormal oral-motor reflexes, such as the tonic bite reflex and the tongue-thrust reflex (see Chapters 11 and 14), may make it difficult for caregivers to provide adequate oral hygiene. Problems with swallowing may lead to retention of food particles in the oral cavity, thus promoting bacterial growth and contributing to tooth decay. The need to use anticonvulsants such as phenytoin (Dilantin) may result in overgrowth of the gums, which is known as *gingival hyperplasia.* Abnormal positioning of the jaw, the lips, and the tongue may promote malocclusion (i.e., any deviation from a physiologically acceptable contact of opposing dentitions). Abnormalities of the embryonic formation of tooth dentin have been associated with cerebral palsy and have been suggested as markers for adverse prenatal events leading to dentin abnormalities and cerebral palsy by parallel pathways (Bhat & Nelson, 1989). Poor dental health contributes to feeding difficulties and can result in significant pain and discomfort that may not be recognized. The components of good dental care include fluoride supplementation (often accomplished via fluoridation of public drinking water), good oral hygiene, moderation of simple sugars in diet, and regular professional dental care. In general, children with cerebral palsy should be monitored closely by a dentist with experience and interest in working with children with developmental disabilities. Parents should schedule their child's first dental appointment by 2 years of age or within 6 months of the appearance of the first tooth (Griffen & Goepferd, 1991).

Asthma/Reactive Airways Disease and Upper Airway Obstruction

Recognizing the variety of respiratory ailments common to children with cerebral palsy is another common issue in the provision of well-child care. Problems with aspiration related to oral-motor dysfunction and GER are discussed in this chapter in the section on "Gastroesophageal Reflux and Oral-Motor Dysfunction." Children with cerebral palsy also have an increased incidence of primary respiratory disorders. Asthma (i.e., reactive airways disease) is especially prevalent among children born prematurely (Batshaw & Bernbaum, 1997). Shortly after birth, many premature infants develop respiratory difficulties that are related to immaturity of the lungs (i.e., respiratory distress syndrome [RDS]). For many children, RDS resolves itself after a few days or a few weeks, but some children go on to exhibit signs of chronic lung disease with a persistent need for oxygen (i.e., bronchopulmonary dysplasia). As these children grow, they will often "outgrow" the need for oxygen as their pulmonary functioning improves, but there may remain persistent problems with wheezing and shortness of breath, especially during the winter months when viral diseases of the respiratory tract are prevalent. Among these respiratory ailments, respiratory syncytial virus infections are the most problematic and sometimes require hospital admission to provide careful monitoring, oxygen, and, occasionally, ventilatory support.

Upper airway obstruction refers to problems with maintaining airway patency above the level of the thoracic inlet (i.e., the base of the neck). A variety of structural and functional problems can contribute to upper airway obstruction (see Table 4.3). A particularly important issue related to upper airway obstruction is intermittent interruptions of normal breathing at night, which are known as *obstructive sleep apnea* (Kotagul, Gibbons, & Stith, 1994). An apneic episode is usually defined as a cessation of breathing for longer than 20 seconds. Position during sleep and decreased state of arousal may contribute to increased upper airway obstruction during sleep. Prolonged or repeated episodes of apnea may result in decreased oxygen delivery to all body tissues,

Table 4.3. Examples of conditions that cause upper airway obstruction

Nose and pharynx
- Allergy
- Choanal atresia (i.e., congenital narrowing of the nasal passage)
- Chronic sinus infection
- Craniofacial anomalies
- Enlarged nostrils/adenoids
- Large tongue
- Poor tongue and pharyngeal muscle tone

Larynx
- Congenital anomalies (e.g., webs)
- Laryngomalacia (i.e., laxity of laryngeal structure)
- Subglottic stenosis (i.e., narrowing caused by trauma)

Trachea and bronchi
- Bronchitis/asthma
- Congenital anomalies
- Tracheal stenosis bronchitis
- Tracheomalacia (i.e., laxity of tracheal structure)

Extrinsic compression
- Obesity (i.e., Pickwickian syndrome)
- Positioning (e.g., overextension, overflexion of the neck)

including the brain and the heart. Chronic oxygen deprivation of the heart may result in compensatory thickening of the right ventricle, which is one of the main pumping chambers of the heart. This is called *right ventricular hypertrophy* and can be detected by electrocardiogram. Right ventricular hypertrophy results in abnormally high blood pressures in the main blood vessels (i.e., pulmonary arteries) that supply venous blood to the lungs. This is a potentially life-threatening condition that is notoriously difficult to treat. It has been associated with episodes of sudden death in people with obstructive sleep apnea. Prevention of this condition remains the only truly effective intervention and is contingent on early identification.

If obstructive sleep apnea is suspected, consultation with a pediatric pulmonologist is necessary. A sleep study, which monitors how multiple aspects of respiratory function relate to various facets of sleep, is recommended in order to determine the character and the severity of apneic episodes and to provide parameters for therapeutic intervention. Although some children with obstructive sleep apnea may require only nighttime monitoring, others may require supplemental oxygen or a special ventilatory apparatus that provides continuous or intermittent pressure along with oxygen to help maintain patency of the airway.

The respiratory and the gastrointestinal problems described in this chapter often coexist in the same child and may interact to produce synergistic effects. For example, worsening asthma may cause fluctuations of pressure in the chest cavity (i.e., intrathoracic pressure), which effectively produces negative forces that draw stomach contents into the esophagus and exacerbates GER. Conversely, GER is thought to aggravate asthma via reflex stimulation of the parasympathetic nervous system, which when activated tends to cause constriction of small airways, thus worsening the symptoms of asthma (Grill, 1995). Aspiration of stomach contents related to GER also is more likely to occur in the context of worsening respiratory status. Another example relates to upper airway obstruction, which is often associated with poor oral-motor control and risk of aspiration via the upper airway. Respiratory and gastrointestinal dysfunction very often are closely related in the same child and must be evaluated and treated concurrently.

Hip Dislocation, Scoliosis, and Contractures

Early recognition of musculoskeletal problems and timely referral to an orthopedic specialist is a common issue in the provision of well-child care for children with cerebral palsy. A variety of interventions are available for the treatment of the various musculoskeletal problems associated with cerebral palsy. Although there is a great deal of debate among professionals regarding the interventions that are most effective for individual children, it is generally agreed that more conservative treatments introduced at an earlier age have a better chance of success than more invasive and complex procedures introduced at a later age.

Hip dislocation is an excellent example of this rule. *Hip dislocation* refers to a displacement of the head of the femur from its typical position in the hip socket (i.e., acetabulum). The term *hip subluxation* is applied when the head of the femur is only partially displaced (see Chapter 6). If subluxation is recognized early, physical therapy and positioning techniques (e.g., use of an abduction pillow [see Chapter 6]) may be effective in preventing or delaying frank dislocation. If surgery is needed at this stage, it may be possible to address the problem by releasing (i.e., dividing) or lengthening the hypertonic or contracted muscles around the hip joint that exert the unbalanced forces and promote dislocation. Once a hip is frankly dislocated and secondary changes occur to surrounding bone and soft tissues, this relatively simple surgery will no longer be effective and more complex surgery involving reconstruction of bony structures may be necessary. These complex procedures are not as likely to be effective as early muscle-tendon releases or lengthenings in preventing pain and functional limitations associated with hip dislocation (Scrutton, 1989). Children with greater degrees of motor impairment (e.g., spastic quadriplegia) are more likely to present signs of hip dislocation at an early age, sometimes as early as 2–3 years of age. In general, children should begin to see an orthopedic specialist as soon as the diagnosis of cerebral palsy has been recognized, and they should have X-rays to monitor the status of the hips at regular intervals.

Contractures and scoliosis are two other musculoskeletal problems associated with cerebral palsy. *Contractures* represent chronic shortening of spastic muscles, resulting in abnormal positioning of joints. *Scoliosis* refers to curvature of the spine caused by unbalanced muscular forces in the back and the pelvis. Both problems tend to worsen with time, and both tend to become more pronounced during periods of rapid linear growth (e.g., during the adolescent "growth spurt"). Worsening contractures can result in problems with positioning, with functional mobility, and with the provision of basic care; they can contribute to the development of hip dislocation (see the definition of hip dislocation presented previously). Worsening scoliosis, in addition to causing difficulties with positioning and mobility, also may result in a compromise of cardiorespiratory function via compression of vital internal structures (Kalen, Conklin, & Sherman, 1992). A wide variety of interventions are available for dealing with these problems and are discussed in several chapters of this book (see Chapters 5, 7, 10, and 12). In general, during physical examinations, problems with contractures and scoliosis are often more easily identified than are problems with hip dislocation. Therefore, the child who has received an appropriate early referral to an orthopedist for monitoring hip subluxation and dislocation should receive appropriate anticipatory guidance regarding contractures and scoliosis.

Spasticity

The appropriate application of available therapeutic modalities for the treatment of spasticity is a complex issue and is considered in detail in Chapter 5. When confronted with a child who has high muscle tone, it is tempting for the therapist to try medications with the hope of finding a quick solution to the problem. However, this rarely works. First, it can be difficult to distinguish spasticity from other forms of muscle hypertonia. Because most of the medications commonly used for increased muscle tone target spasticity, these medications would not be effective if spasticity were mistakenly diagnosed. Second, spasticity may not be the key factor contributing to the child's functional disability. Spasticity is only one of the components of the upper motor neuron syndrome (see Chapters 2 and 5) that contribute to the motor impairments seen in cerebral palsy. Third, all of the medications available for the treatment of spasticity have untoward side effects, particularly on cognition, and do not target specific muscle groups. Medications such as diazepam, which can be very helpful for the short-term treatment of muscle spasms (e.g., after orthopedic surgery [see Chapter 7]), are often ineffective for the chronic treatment of spasticity. Before medications for the treatment of spasticity are begun, it is best to carefully consider the goals of treatment and to review the other options available before proceeding.

Immunizations

Well-child care must consider how to provide adequate immunization against infectious diseases during childhood. The immunization schedule recommended by the American Academy of Pediatrics (AAP; 1997) is shown in Figure 4.1. In general, children with cerebral palsy should receive the same immunizations on the same schedule as typically developing children. Concerns have been raised regarding the safety of using the measles-mumps-rubella (MMR) vaccine and the diphtheria-tetanus-pertussis (DTP) vaccine with children who have cerebral palsy and other neurological disorders. The AAP (1997) recommended that all children, including those with neurological conditions, should receive the MMR vaccine (except in special circumstances with children who have known infection with the human immunodeficiency virus [HIV]). Although there is a slightly increased risk of seizures following MMR in children with known epilepsy or a family history of epilepsy, there is no evidence of serious acute or chronic sequelae from such seizures (AAP, 1997).

The use of the DTP vaccine, however, has generated more controversy. There have been concerns (followed by lawsuits) alleging that the pertussis component of the DTP vaccine either precipitates neurological damage, resulting in disorders such as infantile spasms (i.e., a severe form of epilepsy in

Type of immunization	Ages of administration					
Polio	2 months	4 months	6–18 months			4–6 years
Diphtheria, tetanus, pertussis	2 months	4 months	6 months	12–18 months	4–6 years	14–16 years (Td only); repeat every 10 years
Measles, mumps, rubella				12–15 months	4–6 years or 11–12 years	
Haemophilus influenza type B	2 months	4 months	6 months	12–15 months	4–6 years or 11–12 years	
Hepatitis B	2 months or 0–2 months	1–2 months or 2–4 months	6–18 months			
Varicella				12–18 months		

Figure 4.1. The American Academy of Pediatrics (AAP) immunization schedule.

infancy) and permanent neurological disability, or worsens neurological conditions that already exist. These concerns are weighed against acquiring clinical pertussis that results from a lack of immunization and can lead to seizures, pneumonia, apnea (i.e., discontinuities of breathing), encephalopathy (i.e., central nervous system [CNS] dysfunction/damage), and death. There is no scientific evidence that the DTP vaccine causes permanent brain damage, aggravates preexisting neurological conditions, or affects the prognosis of children with neurological disorders in any way (Gale et al., 1994). Because the DTP can cause brief, self-limited seizures in children who are prone to seizures (or in children who have a family history of epilepsy), the AAP (1997) has suggested that the DTP vaccine be deferred in specific cases in which DTP-related seizures might complicate the interpretation of seizures caused by other factors. (In a child with a suspected neurodegenerative condition, for example, increased seizure activity may be a marker for progression of the disease. However, DTP-related seizures could be misinterpreted in such a case as a worsening of the neurological condition.) The AAP (1997) also has recommended caution in giving the DTP if any of the following occur: 1) a convulsion within 3 days of receiving the vaccine; 2) persistent crying for more than 3 hours within 48 hours of receiving the vaccine; 3) shocklike state within 48 hours of receiving the vaccine; or 4) temperature of 40.5° C (104.9° F) or higher, unexplained by another cause, within 48 hours of receiving the vaccine. Otherwise, the AAP has recommended that all children with "static" neurological conditions (including cerebral palsy) receive the DTP vaccine on schedule.

Seizure Disorders

There is a high incidence of seizures and seizure disorders among children with cerebral palsy (see Chapter 1); recognizing and characterizing these correctly and obtaining adequate seizure control while minimizing medication side effects are important to the provision of well-child care. A *seizure* refers to an episode of abnormal, disorganized electrical activity in the brain that usually results in abnormal involuntary movements, sensations, or alterations of consciousness. A *convulsion* refers to the involuntary muscle activity that is often but not always associated with seizures.

Seizures are classified according to the extent of the involvement of the brain and according to the clinical manifestations, particularly if there are associated alterations of consciousness. A *generalized seizure* involves both sides of the brain and, when associated with convulsions, results in involuntary muscle contractions on both sides of the body. Generalized seizures are always associated with alterations of consciousness and are usually associated with a postictal-period (i.e., period after the interval of seizure activity) period of disorientation or sleepiness (an exception to this rule is an *absence seizure,* which is multiple episodes of very brief loss of consciousness with little or no involuntary muscle activity, followed by periods of complete lucidity). *Partial seizures* originate in one part or one side of the brain. They may be recognized as convulsions that affect only one side of the body. Partial seizures may also manifest as abnormal sensations (e.g., sensations of smell, which are called *olfactory seizures*), autonomic signs or symptoms (e.g., pallor, flushing, sweating, dilated pupils), or psychic symptoms (e.g., sensations of fear, disturbed sense of the passage of time, structured hallucinations). Partial seizures can be further classified as simple or complex—the latter if they are associated with alterations of consciousness, the former if they are not. *Seizure disorder, epilepsy,* and *epileptic syndrome* are synonymous terms that indicate a persistent pattern of seizure activity over an extended period of time for a particular child. A number of specific epileptic syndromes have been defined. For example, Lennox-Gastaut syndrome is a form of epilepsy that includes multiple seizure types in the same person (Lockman, 1994).

Not all seizures or all children with seizure disorders require medical therapy. For example, seizures associated with fever (i.e., febrile convulsions) may not require therapy (Freeman & Vining, 1992). When medications to treat seizures are recommended, it is generally true that "less is better." In other words, the lower the dose and the fewer the number of medications necessary to adequately control seizures, the better. All anticonvulsant medications have some risk of side effects, ranging from subtle effects on cognition to life-threatening bone marrow, pancreatic, or liver toxicity. Experience has shown that for most people, a specific range of blood levels for anticonvulsant drugs (termed *therapeutic range*) is associated with the best therapeutic effect and minimizes the risk of side effects. However, experienced physicians often will tailor dosing for a particular child, which results in blood levels that may be lower or higher than the typical therapeutic range.

Hydrocephalus

Pressure hydrocephalus is encountered with increased frequency in children with cerebral palsy, especially among those born prematurely (Liptak, 1997). It results from an obstruction to the free flow of cerebrospinal fluid (CSF), a clear liquid that surrounds the brain and fills its central cavities (i.e., ventricles). A ventriculo-peritoneal (VP) shunt is commonly used to treat pressure hydrocephalus by providing a safety valve for the egress of excess spinal fluid. A catheter, which creates a conduit from the ventricles to the surface of the scalp, is usually inserted. From there, a plastic tube is tunneled under the skin to the abdomen, which allows excess CSF to drain into the abdominal (i.e., peritoneal) cavity where the fluid is then reabsorbed (see Figure 4.2).

VP shunts are prone to mechanical problems, including clogged and disconnected tubing and malfunctioning valves. These problems may result in increased CSF pressure. Early clinical symptoms of increased CSF pressure include mild lethargy or irritability and vomiting. Later symptoms include profound lethargy or coma; protracted vomiting; high blood pressure; low heart rate; and

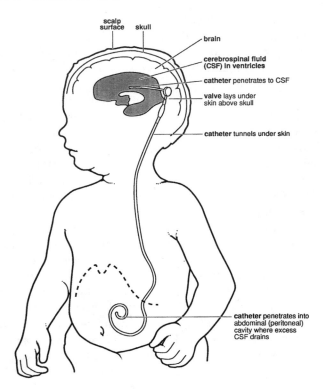

scalp surface   skull

brain

cerebrospinal fluid (CSF) in ventricles

catheter penetrates to CSF

valve lays under skin above skull

catheter tunnels under skin

catheter penetrates into abdominal (peritoneal) cavity where excess CSF drains

Figure 4.2.   Hydrocephalus and the ventriculo-peritoneal shunt. A catheter inserted through the scalp penetrates the skull and the brain in order to reach the brain ventricles, which contain the cerebrospinal fluid (CSF). When CSF pressure exceeds a predetermined value, excess fluid is shunted through a one-way valve to a catheter that has tunnels under the skin; these tunnels carry the CSF to the abdominal or the peritoneal cavity where it is deposited and reabsorbed.

eventual displacement of the brain from its normal position (i.e., herniation), which results in compromise of vital functions and death.

Because VP shunts represent a foreign material within the body, they also can serve as a nidus for bacterial growth, increasing the risk of meningitis (i.e., infection of the CSF and membranes covering the brain, which are called *meninges*) and encephalitis (i.e., infection of the brain itself). In addition to aggressive antibiotic therapy, it is usually necessary to remove the compromised shunt to allow for complete eradication of the infection.

Children with VP shunts are more vulnerable to latex allergies, a problem that is most often seen in individuals who require chronic urinary catheterization (e.g., many people with spina bifida). Latex is a synthetic material used in some household products and many medical and surgical products (e.g., the latex gloves used in the operating rooms of hospitals). Although VP shunts are not composed of latex, their presence apparently can provoke an immune reaction against latex-containing products. Exposure to these latex products, especially during invasive surgical procedures, can result in potentially life-threatening allergic reactions, known as *anaphylaxis*. Regardless of a child's history, it should be assumed that children with VP shunts or other permanent, indwelling catheters may have latex allergy and appropriate substitutes should be used in medical and surgical settings (Dormans, Templeton, Edmonds, Davidson, & Drummond, 1994).

Infant Colic, Irritability, and Cerebral Palsy

Overattribution of discomfort to colic (i.e., relating to the colon) or neurologically based irritability is a common issue in the provision of well-child care. Many children with cerebral palsy have problems with persistent irritability at different stages in their lives. If this irritability is especially pronounced during early infancy, it may be labeled "colic"; it also may be attributed to a neurologically based propensity to irritability. Brazelton (1973) developed a system for analyzing the behavioral characteristics of newborn infants. Some infants, especially those whose mothers abused drugs such as cocaine during pregnancy, have demonstrated a tendency to be easily overstimulated by visual, auditory, and tactile stimuli; these infants have demonstrated difficulty habituating to repeated or continuous stimuli (Mayes, Bornstein, Chawarska, & Granger, 1995). As these infants grow older, it is presumed that they will continue to demonstrate difficulties with self-regulation of behavioral and emotional states.

Because children with cerebral palsy have a "neurological condition," it is often assumed that irritability represents a primary manifestation of the condition. Although this may be true in a minority of cases, this is not true for the majority. It is best to assume that when a child with cerebral palsy is irritable, he or she has good reason. Many children with cerebral palsy experience gastrointestinal-related problems such as GER and constipation; when these problems go unrecognized and untreated, they can result in chronic irritability caused by chronic pain and discomfort. The basis for irritability in other children with cerebral palsy could be an undiagnosed hip dislocation, an incipient pressure ulcer, a urinary tract infection, or a dental disease. It also is possible that some children may be irritable as a result of lack of sleep caused by obstructive sleep apnea. The best approach to the child with cerebral palsy who is irritable is to carefully look for potentially treatable underlying causes of chronic pain and discomfort and to retain colic and neurologically based irritability and diagnoses of exclusion.

Skin Breakdown and Pressure Sores (Decubitus Ulcers)

Children with cerebral palsy are particularly vulnerable to developing pressure sores (i.e., decubitus ulcers). Prevention and early recognition of these ulcers and appropriate treatment are important components of well-child care provision. Decubitus ulcers are a result of the prolonged compromise of blood flow to an area of skin that is caused by persistent, unrelieved pressure. They usually occur over bony prominences, such as the lower back (i.e., sacrum), lower buttocks (i.e., ischium), and heels. Older children with severe cerebral palsy are especially at risk for developing skin breakdown and subsequent decubitus ulcers because of prolonged relative immobility. In addition, older children may have poor fat stores caused by chronic poor nutrition, which results in insufficient "padding" over bony prominences; these two factors contribute synergistically to the development of decubitus ulcers. Decubitus ulcers are graded according to severity (see Table 4.4). Preventive care for decubitus ulcers rests chiefly on the provision of appropriate positioning (e.g., a well-designed seating system), frequent repositioning for children who are not sufficiently mobile, and adequate nutrition to bolster fat stores. Decubitus ulcers are particularly problematic after surgery that requires prolonged follow-up casting (see Chapter 9); in this situation, it is essential to give extra attention to frequent repositioning and checks of skin integrity.

Pressure relief is the sine qua non of treatment for decubitus ulcers. For children with Grade 1–2 ulcers, gauze dressings and bio-occlusive dressings, which provide a protected, moist environment that is conducive to healing, are the mainstay of therapy. However, deeper, more severe ulcers require aggressive cleaning and debridement and, in some cases, prompt a hospital admission. The higher grade ulcers can be very difficult to treat and may require months or even years to resolve. Many of these cases require the involvement of a plastic surgeon; it is not uncommon for skin and skin/muscle grafts to be used in extreme cases.

Urinary Tract Disorders

Recognizing problems with lower urinary tract function and preventing damage to the upper urinary tract are key elements in the provision of well-child

Table 4.4.   Grading system for pressure (decubitus) ulcers

Grade 1
Redness of superficial skin layers
Grade 2
Ulcer extends into dermis (i.e., deep skin layer)
Grade 3
Extension into subcutaneous tissues but not into muscle
Grade 4
Extension through muscle to bone
Grade 5
Ulcer becomes continuous with joint spaces or body cavities (e.g., rectum, vagina)

Source: DeLisa & Gans (1993).

care. The urinary system is commonly divided into the upper tract (i.e., kidneys and ureters) and the lower tract (i.e., bladder, bladder neck, sphincter, and urethra) (see Figure 4.3). Urine that is produced at a fairly steady rate by the kidneys (typically 1–5 milliliters/kilogram/hour) flows through the ureters into the bladder. The bladder is composed of smooth muscle under the control of the parasympathetic nervous system (i.e., part of the autonomic nervous system), called the *detrusor muscle.* The bladder can expand significantly in order to store urine for short periods of time. In children, bladder capacity can be calculated by the formula (age x 25) + 25 milliliters. For example, a typical 5-year-old will have a bladder capacity of about 150 milliliters (Reid & Borzyskowski, 1993). By 2–3 years of age, children typically have achieved daytime urinary continence, which means that the sphincter muscle remains tonically contracted until sufficient bladder distention produces the urgency to void.

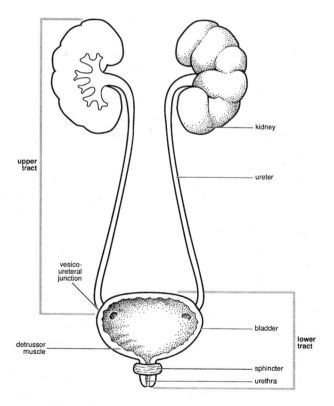

Figure 4.3. The human urinary tract. Urine is produced by the kidneys and flows freely through the ureters to the bladder, where it is then stored. The anatomical configuration of the vesicoureteral junction acts as a one-way valve, preventing reflux of urine back to the ureter and the kidney. Stimuli resulting in micturition (i.e., urination) lead to coordinated contraction of the bladder detrusor muscle and relaxation of the urinary sphincter, which leads to egress of urine through the urethra.

Children with cerebral palsy are at risk for several problems related to the urinary tract, including incontinence; urgency (i.e., abnormal sensation of the need to void); frequency (i.e., abnormally short intervals between voids); difficulty initiating void; urinary retention (i.e., residual urine in the bladder after a void); and urinary tract infection, which is called *cystitis* when involving the bladder and *pyelonephritis* when involving the kidney (Reid & Borzyskowski, 1993). Many children with cerebral palsy have hyperreflexia, or overactive contractions of the detrusor muscle, which is often associated with small bladder capacity and leads to problems with urgency, frequency, and incontinence. For some children, detrusor muscle contraction during voiding is out of sync with sphincter relaxation (i.e., detrusor-sphincter dysynergy): If the sphincter does not relax as the detrusor muscle contracts, bladder pressure increases and may overpower the protective mechanisms that prevent reflux of urine back into the ureters and the kidneys. When urine does back up, it is known as *vesicoureteral reflux (VUR)*. Prolonged or frequent episodes of VUR may lead to abnormal dilation of the ureters (i.e., hydroureter) and the kidneys (i.e., hydronephrosis). These conditions, as a result of reflux of bacteria from the bladder, can cause permanent kidney damage as well as make kidney infection more likely. Fortunately, this does not commonly occur in children with cerebral palsy, but careful monitoring for these conditions in a child with symptoms related to the urinary tract is warranted. If these symptoms should present themselves, a prompt referral to a urologist who is familiar with the problems of children with developmental disabilities is necessary. Some of the commonly used studies of the urinary tract are listed in Table 4.5.

The likelihood of discovering a urinary tract abnormality in children with cerebral palsy who do not have symptoms of a urinary disorder is small; routine screening tests or routine referral of such children to a urologist is not recommended (Brodak, Scherz, Packer, & Kaplan, 1994).

Sexuality and Health

Puberty is a difficult time for everyone, and it can be particularly challenging for people with disabilities. The situation can be further complicated for adolescents with cerebral palsy who have poor access to information about sex and sexuality (Blum, Resnick, Nelson, & St. Germaine, 1991). Preventing sexually transmitted diseases (STDs) and pregnancy as well as recognizing the importance of sexuality in people with disabilities are thus important issues in the provision of well-child care. Given the prevalence of STDs and most notably the prevalence of the HIV, which causes the acquired immunodeficiency syndrome (AIDS), this issue is of particular concern. Information regarding these issues should be disseminated among children and adolescents; however, this approach remains controversial. The fact remains that children with cerebral palsy are not learning about sexuality and health issues at home. In one study, 58.3% of adolescents with cerebral palsy reported receiving some sex education in school,

Table 4.5. Commonly used studies of the urinary tract

Study	Method	Use
Urinalysis	Chemical and microscopic examination of urine	Screens for infection and evidence of kidney or bladder dysfunction
Urine culture	Culture of urine to establish the presence of bacteria	Rules out urinary tract infection
Renal ultrasound	High-frequency sound waves are used to image the urinary tract	Rules out anatomical abnormalities of the urinary tract, especially the kidney
Renal scan	Nuclear medicine study	Provides information about the anatomy and functional integrity of the kidney
Voiding cystourethrogram	Radiographic studies in which dye is injected into bladder through catheter to provide contrast	Delineates the anatomy of the lower urinary tract; rules out reflux of urine from bladder to ureters
Urodynamic studies	Measures of bladder pressure and urinary volume over time	Provides information about bladder and sphincter function

whereas only 12% reported discussing sex-related issues in any way at home. The tendency of families to infantilize adolescents with cerebral palsy may contribute to this situation (Magill-Evans & Restall, 1991).

Among girls with cerebral palsy who have more severe cognitive impairments, regulation of menstruation may become an issue for the maintenance of personal hygiene. In this situation, oral contraceptives are sometimes recommended in order to regulate the menstrual cycle and to moderate menstrual flow. In selected cases, long-acting contraceptives (e.g., Depo-Provera) may be considered. When consideration is being given to such interventions, it is best to consult with an obstetrician/gynecologist. Regardless of specific issues and circumstances, all girls with cerebral palsy should receive regular gynecological care once they have reached menarche.

SUMMARY

A high degree of coordination of care is required to meet the often complex medical needs of the child with cerebral palsy. Primary care physicians continue to play the key role in this coordination, and care managers have emerged since the 1980s to supplement and augment the primary care physician's role.

As a developmental disability, cerebral palsy is a dynamic condition and its impact changes as the child grows and matures. Anticipatory guidance is an indispensable aspect of well-child care and health maintenance that allows professionals and families to increase the likelihood of optimal health throughout the child's life cycle. In addition to the health and developmental issues that apply to all children, specific problem areas exist for the child with cerebral palsy, and these problems require special attention in order to ensure that the child receives the best possible well-child care and health outcomes. Professionals with expertise in the care of children with cerebral palsy have a special obligation to disseminate information about these special health concerns to families and to the wider medical community.

REFERENCES

American Academy of Pediatrics (AAP), Committee on Infectious Diseases. (1997). *Red book.* Elk Grove Village, IL: Author.

Batshaw, M.L., & Bernbaum, J. (1997). Born too soon, born too small. In M.L. Batshaw (Ed.), *Children with disabilities* (4th ed., pp. 115–140). Baltimore: Paul H. Brookes Publishing Co.

Batshaw, M.L., Helpin, M.L., & Rosenberg, H.M. (1997). Dental care: Beyond brushing and flossing. In M.L. Batshaw (Ed.), *Children with disabilities* (4th ed., pp. 643–656). Baltimore: Paul H. Brookes Publishing Co.

Bhat, M., & Nelson, K.B. (1989). Developmental enamel defects in primary teeth in children with cerebral palsy, mental retardation, or hearing defects: A review. *Advances in Dental Research, 3*(2), 132–142.

Blasco, P.A., & Allaire, J.H. (1992). Drooling in the developmentally disabled: Management practices and recommendations. *Developmental Medicine and Child Neurology, 34*(10), 849–862.

Blum, R.W., Resnick, M.D., Nelson, R., & St. Germaine, A. (1991). Family and peer issues among adolescents with spina bifida and cerebral palsy. *Pediatrics, 88*(2), 280–285.

Brazelton, T.B. (Ed.). (1973). *Neonatal Behavioral Assessment Scale.* Philadelphia: J.B. Lippincott.

Brodak, P.P., Scherz, H.C., Packer, M.G., & Kaplan, G.W. (1994). Is urinary tract screening necessary for patients with cerebral palsy? *Journal of Urology, 152*(2), 1586–1587.

Coplan, J. (1987). Deafness: Ever heard of it? Delayed recognition of permanent hearing loss. *Pediatrics, 79*(2), 206–212.

DeLisa, J.A., & Gans, B.M. (Eds.). (1993). *Rehabilitation medicine.* Philadelphia: J.B. Lippincott.

Dormans, J.P., Templeton, J.J., Edmonds, C., Davidson, R.S., & Drummond, D.S. (1994). Intraoperative anaphylaxis due to exposure to latex (natural rubber) in children. *Journal of Bone and Joint Surgery (American Volume), 76*(11), 1688–1691.

Erikson, E.H. (1985). *Childhood and society.* New York: W.W. Norton.

Freeman, J.M., & Vining, E.P. (1992). Decision making and the child with febrile seizures. *Pediatrics in Review, 13*(8), 293–304.

Fried, M.D., & Pencharz, P.B. (1991). Energy and nutrient intakes of children with spastic quadriplegia. *Journal of Pediatrics, 119*(6), 947–949.

Gale, J.L., Thapa, P.R., Wassilak, S.G., Bobo, J.K., Mendelman, P.M., & Foy, H.M. (1994). Risk of serious acute neurological illness after immunization with diphtheria-tetanus-pertussis vaccine: A population-based case controlled study. *Journal of the American Medical Association, 271*(1), 37–41.

Glascoe, F.P., & Dworkin, P.H. (1995). The role of parents in the detection of developmental and behavioral problems. *Pediatrics, 95*(6), 829–836.

Griffen, A.L., & Goepferd, S.T. (1991). Preventative oral health care for the infant, child and adolescent. *Pediatric Clinics of North America, 38*(5), 1209–1226.

Grill, M.F. (1995). Respiratory manifestations of gastroesophageal reflux in children. *Journal of Asthma, 32*(3), 133–189.

Hebra, A., & Hoffman, M.A. (1993). Gastroesophageal reflux in children. *Pediatric Surgery, 40*(6), 1233–1251.

Hockelman, R. (Ed.). (1992). *Primary pediatric care* (2nd ed.). St. Louis: Mosby Yearbook.

Jacoby, A., Howard-Gleum, L., McGuire, C., & Hayashida, B. (1995). A CNS integrated health care delivery system model. *Nursing Management, 26*(11), 37–40.

Kalen, V., Conklin, M.M., & Sherman, F.C. (1992). Untreated scoliosis in severe cerebral palsy. *Journal of Pediatric Orthopaedics, 12*(3), 337–340.

Kotagul, S., Gibbons, V.P., & Stith, J.A. (1994). Sleep abnormalities in patients with severe cerebral palsy. *Developmental Medicine and Child Neurology, 36*(4), 304–311.

Kübler-Ross, E. (1969). *On death and dying.* New York: Macmillan.

Liptak, G.S. (1997). Neural tube defects. In M.L. Batshaw (Ed.), *Children with disabilities* (4th ed., pp. 519–543). Baltimore: Paul H. Brookes Publishing Co.

Lockman, L. (1994). Nonabsence generalized seizures. In K.F. Swaiman (Ed.), *Pediatric neurology: Principles and practice* (4th ed., p. 537). St. Louis: C.V. Mosby.

Magill-Evans, J.E., & Restall, G. (1991). Self-esteem of persons with cerebral palsy: From adolescence to adulthood. *American Journal of Occupational Therapy, 45,* 819–825.

Mayes, C., Bornstein, M.H., Chawarska, K., & Granger, R.H. (1995). Information processing and developmental assessment in 3 month old infants exposed prenatally to cocaine. *Pediatrics, 95*(4), 539–545.

Nelson, K.B., & Ellenberg, J.H. (1982). Children who "outgrew" cerebral palsy. *Pediatrics, 69*(5), 529–536.

Reid, C.J.D., & Borzyskowski, M. (1993). Lower urinary tract dysfunction in cerebral palsy. *Archives of Disease in Childhood, 68,* 739–742.

Scrutton, D. (1989). The early management of hips in cerebral palsy. *Developmental Medicine and Child Neurology, 31,* 108–116.

Sharp, M.C., Strauss, R.P., & Lorch, S.C. (1992). Communicating medical bad news: Parents' experiences and preferences. *Journal of Pediatrics, 121*(4), 539–546.

Stallings, V.A., Charney, E.B., Davies, J.C., & Cronk, C.E. (1993a). Nutrition-related growth failure of children with quadriplegic cerebral palsy. *Developmental Medicine and Child Neurology, 35,* 126–138.

Stallings, V.A., Charney, E.B., Davies, J.C., & Cronk, C.E. (1993b). Nutritional status and growth of children with diplegic or hemiplegic cerebral palsy. *Developmental Medicine and Child Neurology, 35,* 997–1006.

Taylor, S.B., & Shelton, J.E. (1995). Caloric requirements of a spastic immobile cerebral palsy patient: A case report. *Archives of Physical Medicine and Rehabilitation, 76*(3), 281–283.

SECTION II

Management of Impairments Related to Cerebral Palsy

CHAPTER 5

The Management of Spasticity

Stephanie Ried, Louis Pellegrino,
Shirley Albinson-Scull, and John P. Dormans

Spasticity is a specific type of motor impairment that characterizes several forms of cerebral palsy (see Chapter 1). Its management has been a subject of intense interest for many years among professionals who care for children with cerebral palsy. Renewed interest in spasticity has been fueled by the advent of several new treatment modalities that have greatly increased the range of choices for intervention available to the clinician. However, with greater choice has come greater confusion. The complex process of clinical decision making has become complicated not only by the availability of new treatments but also by the recognition that treatment should lead to demonstrable improvements in functional outcome. Creating a rational and reproducible approach to the management of spasticity requires the development of a clear framework as well as a common vocabulary for defining the dimensions of outcome. This chapter reviews what is known about the pathophysiology of spasticity, defines the range of interventions available for its management, considers models that are being used for clinical decision making, and presents an integrated model for the management of spasticity based on this information.

THE PATHOPHYSIOLOGY OF SPASTICITY

Spasticity may be defined as a motor disorder characterized by a velocity-dependent increase in tonic stretch reflexes (i.e., muscle tone) caused by hyperexcitability of the stretch reflex (Massagli, 1991). In addition, spasticity represents one of the positive signs that composes upper motor neuron (UMN) syndrome (see Chapter 2). Wright and Rang (1990) demonstrated that neurophysiological, biochemical, and structural abnormalities from the brain to the muscles contribute to spasticity in an animal model. In any discussion of spasticity, it is important to consider the role that spasticity may play in impeding or in facilitating the function of a given individual and to recognize that other components of UMN syndrome also may have a significant effect on motor skills. Other positive components of UMN syndrome that may affect motor skills include athetosis, primitive reflexes, rigidity, and dystonia; negative components include weakness, paralysis, and fatigue (Gans & Glenn, 1990).

Generally, it is believed that a loss of supraspinal inhibition linked to lesions in the central nervous system (CNS) is the underlying cause of cerebral palsy, and this leads to an increase in muscle tone and hyperactive reflexes (see Figure 5.1). Alpha motor neurons (AMNs) within the anterior horn of the spinal cord innervate striated muscle (i.e., extrafusal fibers). The activity of these AMNs is influenced and regulated to some extent by supraspinal pathways. In addition to innervating striated muscle, AMNs also innervate interneurons in the anterior horn (i.e., Renshaw cells), which helps to suppress repeated, rapid firing of the AMNs and, thus, acts to modulate muscle contraction via a negative feedback system. Renshaw cells also receive input from supraspinal regions, which allows lesions in the brain to decrease their inhibitory control on muscle contraction. Because Renshaw cells also are believed to play a role in inhibiting the stretch reflexes of antagonist muscles that otherwise would be active during voluntary contraction of the agonist, loss of these inhibitory influences contributes to the rhythmically repetitive stretch reflexes (i.e., clonus) that are seen in UMN lesions. In addition to providing an inhibitory influence, Renshaw cells tend to promote the activity of the motor neurons that are being driven sufficiently to overcome the inhibitory influence within their domain. This facilitates the activity of the most active members of a synergy group while inhibiting others (Whitlock, 1990). Studies of Renshaw cell function in spastic states provide evidence that the inhibitory function of Renshaw cells is decreased in spasticity while its facilitory effect is increased (Veale, Rees, & Mark, 1973).

Muscle spindles (i.e., intrafusal fibers) are structures that function as muscle stretch receptors within skeletal muscles. They provide the sensory component to the muscle stretch response and inform the nervous system of the length and rate of change in the length of the muscle. *Gamma motor neurons,* also found in the anterior horn of the spinal cord, provide the motor innervation for the muscle spindles. Highly sensitive receptors called *Golgi tendon organs,* which are located within muscle tendons, provide afferent feedback to the spinal cord and

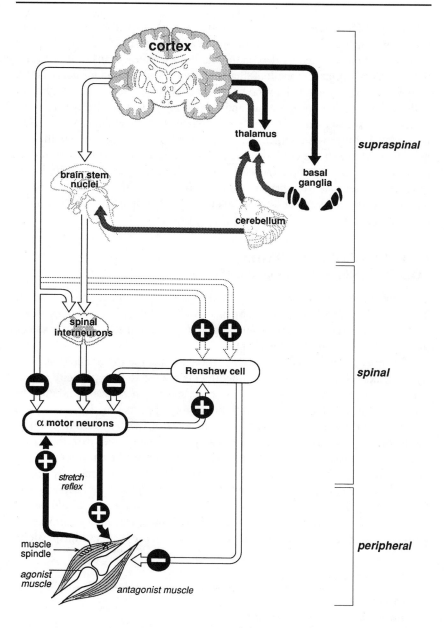

Figure 5.1. The motor system and spasticity. Multiple influences in the supraspinal (i.e., brain and brain stem) and spinal components of the nervous system affect the activity of the stretch reflex response. The net effect of supraspinal influences is to inhibit the stretch reflex response, either directly or indirectly, through spinal mechanisms (e.g., enhancing the inhibitory activity of Renshaw cells on alpha motor neurons). Brain damage or dysfunction may result in a net decrease in inhibition, resulting in overactivity of the stretch reflex response and clinical spasticity.

influence AMN activity through numerous connections within the spinal cord (i.e., polysynaptic pathways). Similarly, the activity of the Golgi tendon organ is controlled or inhibited by descending inhibitory interneurons. Nerve bodies in the cerebral cortex, cerebellum, thalamus, and basal ganglia influence AMN activity by sending axons into the brain stem and the spinal cord via multiple pathways, including corticospinal and corticobulbar (i.e., pathways from the cortex to the spinal cord and brain stem, respectively) and reticulospinal, vestibulospinal, and rubrospinal tracts (i.e., pathways from the brain stem to the spinal cord). Although the corticospinal tract is the main pathway for volitional motor control, a major function of the descending pathways is to restrain the lower motor neurons from producing uncontrolled primitive reflex-type activity. Thus, with damage to or dysfunction of the CNS, impairment of this inhibition can occur.

INTERVENTION STRATEGIES
FOR THE TREATMENT OF SPASTICITY

The decision to treat spasticity should always focus on functional goals (see Table 5.1 for a list of goals of treatment). A clinical decision-making process for identifying such goals and developing a rational treatment strategy based on those goals is discussed in this chapter.

In general, the choice of a specific modality for the treatment of spasticity is influenced by whether the impediments related to the spasticity are localized to a particular muscle group or are more generalized. It should be established whether spasticity contributes to or supports function in any way and whether the positive or negative components of UMN syndrome contribute to the targeted dysfunction. For example, marked lower extremity tone and extensor synergy pattern may facilitate the ability of an older child to perform a standing pivot transfer. Measures to decrease this tone may impair the child's ability to perform this transfer and result in increased dependence. In addition, pain or discomfort may exacerbate spasticity and should be addressed prior to instituting other interventions. Significant motor control problems (e.g., weakness) that might be unmasked with the decrease in spasticity

Table 5.1.   Goals of treatment

- Increase ease of care
- Prevent pressure ulcer, skin breakdown
- Relieve spasms or pain
- Limit progression of contractures, hip dislocation, and scoliosis
- Improve seating, positioning
- Improve motor performance
- Improve ability to perform activities of daily living

also should be considered. The evaluation should include thorough neurological, musculoskeletal, and general physical examinations as well as a careful nutritional assessment, some quantification of the spasticity, a measure of functional skills, and an assessment of quality of movement. In terms of good nutrition, there is usually more subcutaneous tissue; improved general health, comfort, and well-being also may play a role in decreasing spasticity (see Chapter 11). It is essential that a reliable sensory examination be completed whenever possible because limitations in these areas can have a significant impact on adjunctive modalities of treatment and response to that treatment. For example, tactile hypersensitivity may render a child unable to tolerate the foot plate of an inhibitive cast, and, as a result, a period of desensitization prior to initiating this treatment may be necessary. When significant impairment in proprioception is present in the child with cerebral palsy, it has the potential to be a major contributor to motor dysfunction once spasticity is reduced.

It becomes clear that multiple factors must be considered in reviewing the many issues associated with the evaluation and treatment of spasticity. In addition, a coordinated effort among family members and a cohesive team of professionals is essential in this process. The following sections review the various modalities available for the treatment of spasticity.

Oral Medications

When functional problems are related to more generalized spasticity, consideration may be given to oral medications as an adjunct to spasticity management (see subsequent section on "Intrathecal Medications"). Although a number of oral medications have been used to treat spasticity in children with cerebral palsy, none have been proven universally effective. The main problems with oral medications are

1. Variability of effectiveness among children
2. Cognitive side effects (the most common of which is sedation)
3. A narrow therapeutic window that excludes children when they or their families have demanding schedules that lead to subsequent decrease in dosing compliance
4. Systemic side effects

The most commonly used oral antispasticity medications are diazepam (Valium), dantrolene sodium (Dantrium), and baclofen (Lioresal). Many other medications have been reported as useful in the treatment of spasticity in other disorders (particularly in adults), including vigabatrin, clonidine, tizanidine, and idroclimide. There are, however, no studies as of 1997 that demonstrate the efficacy or safety of the use of these medications in the child with cerebral palsy.

Diazepam belongs to the benzodiazepine family of drugs. It exerts its antispasticity effect within the CNS by enhancing the presynaptic inhibitory effects of the inhibitory neurotransmitter gamma-aminobutyric acid (GABA). In addition to being the oldest antispasticity medication in widespread use (Whyte & Robinson, 1990), diazepam has been used extensively in controlling seizures in both adults and children. In general, this medication is not recommended for treating children with spastic diplegic cerebral palsy because of its CNS side effects, primarily sedation (Binder & Eng, 1989). Marsh (1965) reported that, as a result of relaxation, diazepam use in children with severe cerebral palsy with generalized spasticity leads to generalized improvement and elimination of startle response. However, no measures of spasticity were provided. Engle (1966) reported no significant effect of diazepam on spasticity in a double-blind study of children with cerebral palsy, which included both spastic and athetoid types. There was, however, behavioral improvement reported in the majority of the children irrespective of their type of cerebral palsy. In a 1993 double-blind, placebo-controlled study of clonazepam, Dahlin, Knutsson, and Nergardh used a dynamic dynamometer to document significant decreases in spasticity as indicated by resistance to passive movement. Clonazepam, similar to diazepam, is a benzodiazepine but with a slightly longer half-life. The majority of the children (ages 10–18 years old) in the Dahlin et al. (1993) study reported some degree of associated drowsiness or mild sedation. Other potential adverse effects of these benzodiazepines may include weakness, memory loss, ataxia, depression, or drug dependence.

Dantrolene sodium is unique among the oral medications commonly used to treat spasticity because its mode of action is within the muscle as opposed to within the CNS. Dantrolene inhibits the release of calcium from the sarcoplasmic reticulum (a storage area for calcium within muscle cells), thereby uncoupling electrical excitation from contraction in both extrafusal (i.e., muscle) and intrafusal (i.e., muscle spindle) fibers. It is uncertain to what extent the efficacy of its action is caused by the effect at the level of the muscle spindle. Studies evaluating the efficacy of dantrolene in treating spasticity in children with cerebral palsy have yielded some encouraging, yet mixed, results. Improvement in self-help skills, lower extremity scissoring tendency, and reflexes was demonstrated in a double-blind crossover study of 23 children with spastic cerebral palsy (Haslam, Walcher, Lietman, Kallman, & Mellits, 1974). Denhoff, Feldman, Smith, Litchman, and Holden (1975) evaluated the effects of dantrolene on neurological and orthopedic measurements, motor performance, and activities of daily living in children with spastic cerebral palsy. The latter study's results indicated only subtle improvements in activities of daily living; however, evaluations were subjective with low interobserver agreement. In an evaluation of 15 ambulatory children and adolescents with spastic cerebral palsy who were treated with dantrolene, improvements were demonstrated in both stride and step length, the ability to make small weight adjustments during balance testing, and the amount of vertical displacement of the center of gravity during gait (Ford, Bleck, Aptekar, Collins, & Sterick, 1976). Two thirds of the children also reported subjective improvement in gait and mobility, describing muscles as looser and walking as easier. Joynt and Leonard (1980) were unable to demonstrate significant changes in functional performance related to dantrolene use in children with cerebral palsy; however, physiological changes, including diminished muscle response to tibial stimulation, were reported.

The most serious potential adverse reaction to dantrolene is reversible hepatotoxicity; active liver disease is a contraindication to dantrolene use. Liver function should be assessed prior to initiating therapy and should be assessed periodically thereafter. Other potential adverse reactions to dantrolene include weakness, drowsiness, lethargy, fatigue, dizziness, nausea, and diarrhea. When these effects occur, they are usually transient and can be minimized by beginning with a small dose and gradually increasing it until an optimum regimen is achieved. Weakness can result from overshooting the optimum dose, which is the dose that provides the maximal benefit with the minimal adverse reactions.

Baclofen is a centrally acting GABA agonist that appears to reduce spasticity by acting primarily on inhibitory pathways within the spinal cord. Efficacy in the treatment of spasticity of spinal origin has been well documented. However, studies evaluating the use of oral baclofen in the management of spasticity of cerebral origin and particularly in children with cerebral palsy are limited. The pediatric studies that are available, including a double-blind crossover trial involving 20 children with cerebral palsy, document decreased spasticity with little change in adaptive or ambulation skills (Milla & Jackson, 1977; Molnar & Kathirithamby, 1979). Drowsiness, fatigue, and muscle weakness are common adverse effects; others include nausea, dizziness, intoxication, and paresthesias. Baclofen should be used with caution in children with impaired renal function. Hallucinations and seizures have been reported with abrupt cessation of baclofen usage; therefore, it is a medication that should be gradually weaned. In addition, there have been documented cases of extreme hyperthermia and increased spasticity associated with baclofen withdrawal during the weaning process (Mandac, Hurvitz, & Nelson, 1993). If individuals with gastrointestinal problems become unable to tolerate the medication orally, then complications associated with withdrawal may present a further problem because there is no parenteral form available.

Intrathecal Medications

The use of baclofen introduced directly into the spinal canal (i.e., continuous intrathecal baclofen infusion [CIBI]) has demonstrated efficacy in controlling severe spasticity. An externally programmable pump is implanted subcutaneously into the lateral abdominal wall and is attached to a catheter that tunnels under the skin and is connected to an intrathecal (i.e., within the spinal canal) catheter at the distal thoracic or lumbar spine (see Figure 5.2). The dose of a continuous infusion of baclofen is titrated to the desired clinical effect. Studies of CIBI use in children with cerebral palsy have shown significant improvement in the ability to

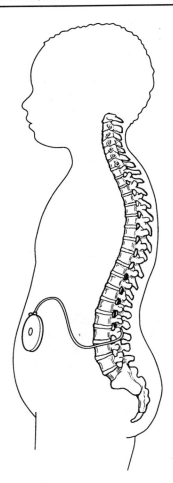

Figure 5.2. Continuous intrathecal baclofen infusion. Baclofen is injected through the skin into a reservoir, which is located within a surgically placed pump beneath the skin of the abdomen. The pump, which is about the size of a hockey puck, is programmable using a device placed against the skin and over the pump. Medication is continuously infused through a catheter that tunnels under the skin and is inserted directly into the spinal canal; baclofen mixes with the spinal fluid that bathes the spinal cord, thus directly affecting the spinal cord and resulting in a decrease in spasticity.

perform activities of daily living as well as demonstrated improvements in muscle tone, joint range, hamstring motion, and upper extremity function (Albright, 1991; Albright, Barron, Fasick, Polinko, & Janosky, 1993; Albright, Cervi, & Singletary, 1991). This treatment also has been found to be effective in managing dystonia. Transient side effects include urinary hesitancy and pedal edema, which responds to adjustments. Complications requiring surgical intervention include catheter-related problems, infection, and recurrent cerebrospinal fluid leaks. Seizures have been reported in adults following the administration of CIBI for the treatment of spasticity secondary to brain injury (Kofler, Kronenberg, Rifici, Saltuari, & Bauer, 1994). Other potential side effects include catheter migration, infection, subjective feelings of sensory or motor loss, loss of penile erections, and cystic myeloceles (Bennett, Tai, & Symonds, 1994; Meythaler, Steers, Haworth, Tuel, & Sesco, 1990). In general, long-term tolerance to CIBI has been good with devices that have been implanted for as long as 4 years (Albright et al., 1993; Massagli, 1991). There have been no studies to determine the long-term effects on the developing brain.

Chemoneurolysis

Chemoneurolysis is a nerve block that impairs conduction by destroying part of the nerve (Glenn, 1990). It can be used to treat more localized problems of spasticity without the systemic side effects that accompany oral medications. The procedure begins with the injection of a specific agent that chemically alters the nerve input to the target muscle(s), thereby significantly limiting the ability of the muscle to contract. This creates a window of opportunity in which an aggressive therapeutic program of casting, stretching, and exercise can be instituted to achieve improved position and joint range, increased strength of antagonist muscles, and clearer focus on specific functional goals. Chemoneurolysis can be performed at every level within the peripheral nervous system, from the nerve root as it exits the spinal cord to the motor end plate (i.e., terminal axon) within the muscle (Glenn, 1990). The site selected for injection has implications for the extent and duration of the effect achieved. In general, the more proximal (i.e., anatomically closer to the spinal cord) the injection, the greater the effect, both temporally and topographically. For example, chemoneurolysis of the sciatic nerve, which includes both the tibial and the peroneal nerves before it branches, will weaken not only the contractility of the muscles innervated by that nerve but also all of the distal muscles of the leg that are innervated by either the tibial or the peroneal nerves or their subsequent branches. This effect, in addition to being more widely distributed, also is of longer duration. In contrast, a more localized effect can be achieved (e.g., on the gastrocnemius muscle innervated by the tibial nerve) by intramuscular injection directly into that muscle. This is called a *motor point block* and results in neurolysis involving only the motor branches within the target muscle. The most commonly used agents for injection at the level of the nerve are phenol, alcohol, and local anesthetics such as lidocaine, procaine, and bupivacaine. The local anesthetics reversibly block conduction without causing actual structural damage to the nerve. This temporary effect, lasting from less than an hour to several hours, depends on the agent and aids in evaluating the potential impact on function of a longer lasting nerve block. Bupivacaine has been used at the root level to assist in candidate selection for selective dorsal rhizotomy (see discussion on dorsal rhizotomy in this section).

Phenol (i.e., carbolic acid) denatures protein in the myelin sheath of the nerve or terminal axon and is capable of destroying axons of all sizes. There is a large body of literature on the neurolytic action of phenol (Felsenthal, 1974; Fischer, Cress, Haines, Panin, & Paul, 1970; Fusfeld, 1968; Garland, Lucie, & Walters, 1982; Iggo & Walsh, 1959; Nathan & Sears, 1960). This effect is reversible as the nerve regenerates and may need to be repeated over time. Duration of effect is highly variable and usually ranges from 3 to 6 months (deLateur, 1972). Because it is important that the phenol be injected in close proximity to the nerve or the motor end plate, observing the strength of the muscle contraction and the amount of current required to achieve that contraction through electrical stimulation is very helpful in locating the optimum site for injection. This procedure may be difficult in young children or those with developmental delays because they have very little tolerance for the "shocks" that accompany nerve stimulation, the needle used to inject the agent, or the burning sensation that often accompanies phenol infusion. For this reason, sedation or general anesthesia may be necessary in order to perform this procedure on young children. The procedure is usually tolerated well by older children and adolescents with the use of either topical or subcutaneous local anesthesia. Side effects of motor point blocks are usually limited to local discomfort or bruising at the injection site. Injection of mixed nerves, however, may be complicated by dysaesthetic pain. Alcohol has a similar method of action on nerves but is not widely used.

In the early 1990s, botulinum toxin use was introduced as a treatment for spasticity in children with cerebral palsy. The effect on muscle function is similar to that of phenol; however, the mechanism of action differs. Whereas phenol actually denatures the protein in the peripheral nerve, botulinum toxin is a protein polypeptide chain that irreversibly binds to the cholinergic terminal in the neuromuscular junction and inhibits the release of the acetylcholine necessary for muscle contraction. This agent has a natural affinity for the neuromuscular junction and must be given intramuscularly. Although this is the same toxin responsible for botulism poisoning, the dosages used for this purpose are minute—a whole order of magnitude lower—in comparison to that required for systemic effects. The injection is given with a very small needle, requires a much smaller volume than when using phenol, and is essentially painless. Even in young children, it usually can be accomplished in the clinic with the use of conscious sedation. In older children, a topical anesthetic agent and distraction may be used. Topical anesthetic not only minimizes the discomfort for the child and his or her parents but also obviates the need for general anesthesia, which significantly decreases the cost of the procedure. However, this savings is partially offset by the very high cost of the botulinum toxin (greater than $300 per 100 units, using 8–10 units per kilogram). In a 1994 study (Cosgrove, Corry, & Graham) of botulinum toxin used to treat children with cerebral palsy and lower extremity dynamic contractures, muscle tone was decreased for 2–4 months with concomitant improvement in gait on gait analysis, some of which persisted after tonal effects of the botulinum toxin had worn off. In a placebo-controlled study of children with spastic diplegic cerebral palsy who underwent gastrocnemius injection with botulinum toxin for their spasticity, improved gait pattern also was documented (Sutherland, Kenton, Wyatt, & Chambers, 1996). Using a randomized, placebo-controlled study design, Corry, Cosgrove, Walsh, McClean, and Graham (1994) reported decreased tone and improved upper extremity function in children with spastic hemiplegic cerebral palsy who were treated with upper extremity botulinum toxin injection. Average duration of the effect is 2–3 months; however, the procedure can be repeated. It is important to remember that with repeated injections, botulinum toxin antibodies may develop and, as a result, render the injection ineffective. Reports suggest that this development of resistance is related to the use of higher doses of botulinum toxin and higher total cumulative dose (Borodic, Johnson, Goodnough, & Schantz, 1996; Jankovic & Schwartz, 1995). Although there are eight subtypes, only one immunotype (i.e., botulinum toxin type A) is available commercially as of 1997. With the introduction of other immunotypes, it is likely that development of antibodies will be much less of an issue because the immunotypes used could be rotated for subsequent injections. In addition, the required dose may be lower if electrical localization of the motor end plates is used. Although the majority of studies in the literature relating to the efficacy of botulinum toxin do not use motor end plate localization techniques for injections, there is evidence to suggest that an increased efficacy of botulinum toxin injection with lower dosing can be achieved by injecting the toxin nearer to the motor end plates (Shaari & Sanders, 1993). As a result of limited experience, the impact of botulinum toxin use on long-term functional outcome remains uncertain.

Casting

The concept of "tone-reducing" or "inhibitive" casting was introduced in the 1970s and is based on the premise that casting in a functional, tone-inhibiting posture, combined with therapy, increases joint range and facilitates improved quality of movement (Law et al., 1991). Although the mechanism that is responsible for this occurrence is unclear, both biomechanical and neurophysiological explanations have been offered. It has been postulated that casting in a correct position alters the positions of muscles and joints with resultant decrease in soft tissue contractures caused by changes of muscle length in the presence of spasticity (Tardieu, Tardieu, Colbeau-Justin, & Lespargot, 1982). This biomechanical explanation suggests that the change in these shortened spastic muscles is a result of a decrease in anatomical length rather than any neurophysiological impact; it also suggests that cast application in a lengthened position should stretch the connective tissue elements and actually add sarcomeres to the muscle fiber (Grossman, Sahrmann, & Rose, 1982). The neuro-physiological interpretation of the effects of inhibitive casting stresses an impact of the casting on the spasticity and abnormal reflexes (Sussman & Cusick, 1979). The theory is that inhibitive casting, by providing constant pressure, warmth, and protection, has the effect of attenuating sensory feedback that would ordinarily tend to aggravate spasticity (Feldman, 1990; Sussman & Cusick, 1979). Although tone may be decreased while the cast is worn, rebound spasticity may be a problem once the cast is removed. Casts may be "bivalved" (i.e., split lengthwise) at removal and may continue to be worn periodically throughout the day or at night in order to reduce tone, to facilitate learning new motor patterns and functional skills, or to maintain range of motion that may have been gained while the cast was being worn continuously. Another alternative is to fabricate a tone-reducing orthotic. A discussion of the techniques of fabrication and the types of cast and orthotics is beyond the scope of this chapter and is covered elsewhere (Feldman, 1990; see Chapter 16).

The biomechanics of muscle length forms the theoretical foundation for traditional serial casting in which gains in range of motion achieved by casting are incorporated into each subsequent cast until maximum increase in joint range is achieved. Serial casting is an important addition to therapy because it decreases joint contracture and improves range of motion, especially following chemoneurolysis and botulinum toxin injection targeting specific muscles. A common example of serial casting use is in the child with spastic diplegia who has marked gastrocnemius tone, heel cord shortening, or toe walking. Following injection of the gastrocnemius muscle with phenol or botulinum toxin, a series of casts is applied, with changes occurring almost weekly. Each new cast positions the foot in greater dorsiflexion, until the desired joint angle is achieved, which is then maintained by use of an ankle-foot orthotic (see Chapter 16). Appropriate monitoring during cast use is essential to prevent skin breakdown and circulatory complications. When used in this way, casting is a valuable adjunct to therapy and improves functional mobility of children with cerebral palsy. Casting is especially effective when used in younger children who have not yet developed chronic, irreversible contractures of joint capsules. Efficient use of the new movements made available by serial casting must be emphasized in follow-up physical therapy.

Neurosurgical Interventions

Selective dorsal rhizotomy (SDR) is a neurosurgical method for reducing spasticity by sectioning a portion of the sensory nerve roots, which are typically restricted to the lumbosacral plexus (i.e., the nerves that innervate the lower extremities). The procedure uses electromyographic (EMG) readings to help identify which subdivisions of the nerve roots (called "rootlets") are carrying "abnormal" information back to the AMN, thus contributing to increased hyperactivity of the stretch reflex response, and ultimately causing increased spasticity (see Chapter 10 for a detailed discussion). Following SDR, 6 months to a year of intensive rehabilitation is required for motor retraining and addressing the loss of muscle strength experienced by many children.

The ideal candidate for SDR is the near-ambulatory or ambulatory, preschool-age child with spastic diplegia, whose resting muscle tone interferes with his or her quality of gait. Arguments have been presented that the improved motor function following SDR is related more to the intensity of physical therapy provided than the procedure. Randomized, controlled clinical trials have yielded conflicting conclusions (McLaughlin et al., 1994; Steinbok, Reiner, Beauchamp, et al., 1997). SDR may also benefit children with spastic quadriplegia whose spasticity interferes with the provision of care or with positioning (e.g., seating). Older children with fixed contractures would be less likely to benefit from this procedure.

Outcome studies of SDR have used videography to show improved gait characteristics such as joint alignment, stride length, and speed (Vaughan, Berman, & Peacock, 1991; Vaughan, Berman, Staudt, & Peacock, 1988). However, the procedure does not change the timing of various muscle groups as they fire during the gait sequence (Cahan, Adams, Beeler, & Perry, 1989; Giuliano, 1991). Although complications are few, they may include leakage of cerebrospinal fluid, incontinence, lower extremity sensory loss, weakness, or scoliosis.

Other neurosurgical procedures include phenol rhizotomy, which lasts from only 6 months to 2 years, or intrathecal baclofen pumps (see section on "Intrathecal Medications" in this chapter). Cerebellar and dorsal spinal cord stimulators also have been used for spasticity reduction, but these procedures have fallen out of favor as a result of inconsistent benefit and problems with complications.

Orthopedic Interventions

In general, orthopedic interventions do not directly address spasticity; instead, they deal with the secondary complications of spasticity, such as contracture of the muscle–tendon unit, hip subluxation and dislocation, and scoliosis. Spasticity often limits range of motion and encourages fixed postures and a poverty of movement patterns, thereby resulting in secondary changes in the muscle and tendon. (Typical examples would include hip flexion contractures and limitations of hip abduction, straight leg raising [caused by hamstring contracture], and ankle dorsiflexion [caused by gastrocnemius contracture].) Orthopedic interventions such as tenotomy or tendon lengthening also may improve range of motion, and, as a result, joint alignment and functional mobility may be improved (see Chapter 7).

For example, tendo-Achilles lengthenings may be selected for children who cannot achieve a plantigrade (i.e., flat) foot position during the midstance phase of gait (see Chapter 8). This intervention deals primarily with the secondary effects of spasticity (e.g., contracture) rather than the primary impairment itself.

Tone is reduced postoperatively as a result of the lengthened muscle being less responsive to passive stretch, but spasticity per se is not addressed directly.

Improvement in gait characteristics can be measured using a gait laboratory with EMG input to select the appropriate strategy and to measure the outcome (see Chapter 8). Muscle transfer techniques may be used to achieve more typical balance around a joint; for example, the posterior tibialis muscle may be split and transferred laterally to balance a varus (i.e., bent inward) foot deformity by creating an eversion force (see Chapter 7).

When deciding on the appropriate intervention for a particular child with cerebral palsy, it is important to determine whether the deformities are fixed and a result of contracture or dynamic and a result of tone. An interdisciplinary model for clinical decision making is presented in the next section. This algorithm provides a rational approach for choosing treatment options and taking into consideration these and other factors that are important in increasing the likelihood of a desirable outcome.

THE DIMENSIONS OF CLINICAL DECISION MAKING

Since 1986, two prominent approaches to clinical decision making have provided the framework and guidelines for improving care for children with cerebral palsy. Both approaches are designed to assist clinicians with diagnosing, evaluating, and treating the complex nature of this disorder.

The Hypothesis-Oriented Algorithm for Clinicians

Rothstein and Echternach (1986) proposed a standardized approach to clinical decision making regarding therapeutic interventions. This model, called the Hypothesis-Oriented Algorithm for Clinicians (HOAC), is based on the following premises:

1. Clinical decision making should assume a problem-oriented approach.
2. Evaluation and treatment functions should be clearly distinguished.
3. Problem statements based on the primary concern of caregivers should yield a set of goals for intervention and a series of hypotheses regarding cause and effect; this should occur early in the decision-making process.
4. Treatment planning should be based on the most probable hypothesis.
5. Periodic review of progress toward goals should allow for the refinement of treatment strategies and tactics as well as the hypothesis.

Although the HOAC was originally formulated with the individual clinician in mind, it is easily adapted to the requirements of interdisciplinary collaboration. For the purposes of this discussion, a simplified version of the HOAC is presented in Figure 5.3. The clinical process represented by the HOAC is divided into two phases: 1) an initial evaluation and treatment phase and 2) a review phase.

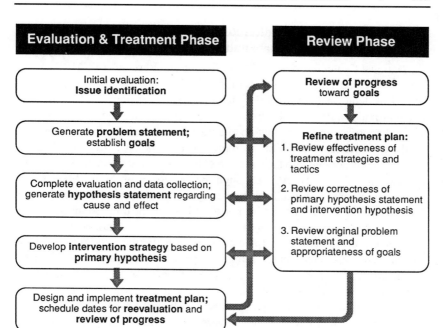

Figure 5.3. Simplified algorithm for clinical decision making based on the Hypothesis-Oriented Algorithm for Clinicians.

During the evaluation and treatment phase, the first step in the process is *issue identification.* A child's caregivers are the main source of information at this juncture. The clinician establishes a dialogue with caregivers that yields a *problem statement* and establishes *goals for intervention,* which are based on the primary issues identified. Following the completion of further evaluation and data collection, which may involve several clinicians representing several professional disciplines, a set of *hypothesis statements* are generated that attempts to provide a cause-and-effect explanation for the primary issues as explicated in the problem statement. The most probable hypothesis (i.e., *primary hypothesis*) is selected and from it an *intervention strategy* is derived. The intervention strategy forms the basis for developing a *treatment plan.*

During the review phase, progress toward goals is considered. Discrepancies between expected and unexpected outcomes are evaluated during this phase. Discrepancies may be a result of problems with the treatment plan itself, or they may reflect inaccuracies in the problem statement, primary hypothesis, or intervention hypothesis. Previously defined goals may have become inappropriate or unrealistic by this point. The process of review provides an analysis that allows for periodic refinement of the treatment plan by applying successive iterations of the HOAC.

The National Center for Medical Rehabilitation Research Model of Disability and Rehabilitation in Clinical Decision Making

The National Center for Medical Rehabilitation and Research (NCMRR) model of disability and rehabilitation (National Institutes of Health, 1993) was reviewed in detail in Chapter 3. By defining the dimensions of disability, the model provides a framework for the more general application of a hypothesis-oriented approach to the evaluation and the treatment of spasticity. In particular, the dimensions of disability as represented in the NCMRR model can be explicitly incorporated into the structure of the problem statements and hypotheses generated by the HOAC. Although the categories of the NCMRR model are best represented graphically along the edges of a polygon as shown in Chapter 3 (which emphasizes the complex interrelatedness of the dimensions of disability), it is more convenient to the HOAC to represent the model in a vertical arrangement of domains (see Table 5.2). For a particular child, three clinical "epochs" are considered, representing past, present, and future status. For each epoch, observations are recorded at each level of the NCMRR model. The child's current status is immediately available to the clinician via direct observation and examination. The child's past status (i.e., history) is made available primarily through interviews with caregivers. The child's future status is an extrapolation made by the clinician at each level of disability regarding possible favorable outcomes versus possible unfavorable outcomes.

The HOAC draws on the NCMRR model to extract its problem statements, goals, and hypotheses. A problem statement is derived from the identification of the aspect of the child's current status that is of greatest concern to the caregiver as well as a review of the child's history that led to the current state of affairs. Goals flow from the problem statement and anticipate potential favorable and unfavorable outcomes. Hypothesis statements regarding cause and effect attempt to explain the problem statement. The intervention hypothesis proposes how the previously identified goals for intervention can be met.

The NCMRR model also informs the review process. After the treatment plan has been formulated, progress toward goals in reference to the levels of disability can be assessed on a spectrum from most favorable to most unfavorable outcomes (as previously defined). The subsequent case study provides a specific example of how this review process can be applied in practice.

Case Study

Christopher is 3 years, 10 months. He has cerebral palsy in spastic diplegic distribution. He is the second twin born at 31 weeks' gestation

(continued)

Table 5.2. Epochs of the National Center for Medical Rehabilitation and Research model

Dimension	Past	Present	Future
Societal limitation	History of access to societal settings compared with typically developing age-mates	Current access to societal settings (e.g., home, school, work)	Improved versus decreased access to societal settings
Disability	Development of mobility/history decrement in mobility	Current mobility status (methods of locomotion, transfers, need for assistance)	Improved mobility versus decreased mobility (increased or decreased independence)
Functional limitation	Development of skills/history of loss or plateau in skills	Assessment of specific skills underlying mobility	Development of new skills versus loss of skills
Impairment	Evolution of impairments	Assessment of neuromotor, musculoskeletal status (spasticity per se, range of motion, strength, etc.)	Remediation of impairment versus worsening of impairments or development of new (secondary) impairments
Pathophysiology	Review of diagnoses	Current diagnoses	Unchanged diagnoses versus new diagnoses

115

Case Study–continued

with a birth weight of 4 pounds, 3 ounces. He required ventilatory support for 4 days and required oxygen by nasal cannula for 1 week. He also was treated for jaundice with phototherapy. He was discharged home on an apnea monitor with no further episodes of respiratory compromise.

Christopher attends a specialized preschool in his community where he receives regular physical, occupational, and speech-language therapy. His receptive language is better than his expressive language, which is limited to single words that are difficult to understand, and his pointing. He has received an augmentative communication device that was custom programmed, but he has not yet initiated training with this device. His history is significant for bilateral strabismus surgery at the age of 18 months.

Christopher travels in a custom-designed and fitted wheelchair that he can self-propel for household distances. He is unable to transfer without being lifted. He can balance in short-sitting position with both hands propping for 30 seconds; however, he cannot free his hands or reach outside of his base of support. His left leg tends to scissor in sitting; his hips and knees extend. He cannot balance independently in long-sitting position, and he also shows posterior tilting of the pelvis and scissoring in this stance. He can roll from supine (i.e., face upward) to prone (i.e., face downward) and back, but he is not able to assume a sitting position from prone. He can commando crawl (i.e., crawl on his belly) 15 feet, but he is unable to assume quadruped or "creep" (i.e., crawl on all fours) as a result of extensor patterns of the lower extremities. When placed in the parallel bars, Christopher attempts to walk forward 10 feet with contact guard. His legs scissor and cross the midline; his stride length is only a few inches. His attempts to walk are not functional. He also is unable to stand alone against a support or cruise.

Christopher's muscle tone was examined; his Ashworth scores (Bohannon & Smith, 1987) (see Chapter 12) were recorded as 4 in the hip and knee extensors; and 5 in adductors and plantar flexors. Hamstring tone was present and graded 3. Passive range of motion was difficult to examine as a result of the high muscle tone. Restrictions were present in hip extension (15 degrees), hip abduction (25 degrees), popliteal angles (40 degrees), and dorsiflexion of ankles to neutral. Hip films revealed partial subluxation with lateral migration of the head of the femur of 30%.

(continued)

Case Study–continued

In summary, Christopher's impairments included spasticity in a scissoring pattern in both legs, decreased range of motion in both legs, poor sitting balance, and lack of selective motor control. Although Christopher could assist nicely when asked to move from squat to stand, some weakness of antigravity muscles was suspected.

The family was very interested in improving Christopher's mobility, and they especially wanted Christopher to walk. Using the NCMRR model as a guide, Table 5.3 summarizes the dimensions of disability as they related to the stated parental concerns. The family's primary focus was on the level of disability (i.e., Christopher's inability to walk). Further questioning revealed that the family saw the inability to walk as a limiting factor in expanding both Christopher's educational goals and his participation in the school setting (i.e., societal limitations). Although it is less of a concern now, the family thinks that Christopher's inability to walk also limited family outings in the past. A careful assessment by the clinicians involved reveals that lower extremity spasticity (i.e., an impairment) has a significant impact on motor performance (i.e., functional limitation), and this is a major contributing factor in Christopher's inability to walk. It is known that the cause (i.e., pathophysiology) of Christopher's spasticity is cerebral palsy related to periventricular leukomalacia (see Chapter 1). Because the underlying neurological abnormality cannot be changed, interventions will focus on other levels of the NCMRR model.

Using the HOAC as a guide, the issue identified is impaired mobility. The problem statement is that impaired mobility related to problems with motor performance is preventing Christopher from fully participating both at school and at home. Several hypothesis statements are possible. For example, one hypothesis might be that the scissoring pattern was caused by a fixed contracture rather than spasticity; management of this contracture then would focus on orthopedic interventions. In this case, the primary hypothesis was that generalized lower extremity spasticity was interfering with functional mobility. In choosing an intervention strategy, it was desirable to find a therapy that would decrease spasticity in multiple muscle groups in the lower extremities and have a long-lasting effect. The three main options were, therefore, oral medications, intrathecal medications, or selective dorsal rhizotomy. The family was concerned about Christopher taking medications for long periods of time; the clinicians were concerned about sedating and other side effects. CIBI also

(continued)

Table 5.3. Dimensions of disability in relation to parental concerns

Dimension	Past	Before intervention	After intervention
Societal limitation	• Family activities limited by difficulty accommodating transportation	• Educational goals limited by physical restrictions imposed by decreased mobility	• Expanded goals of individual education plan possible
Disability	• Nonambulatory • Requires wheelchair for most distances • Dependent for transfers	• Nonambulatory • Requires wheelchair for most distances • Dependent for transfers	• Walk with walker after 6 months for household distances • Transfer sitting to standing
Functional limitation	• Roll supine to prone by 1° years • Commando crawl by 3 years	• Roll supine to prone • Commando crawl • Cannot maintain or assume sitting position • Cannot maintain or pull to stand	• No change in rolling or crawling • Maintain sitting position • Maintain standing position • Slow, unstable gait, apraxia unmasked
Impairment	• Lower extremity spasticity by 1 year of age • Development of lower extremity contractures, hip subluxation by 3° years of age	• Hip, knee extensors (Ashworth score: 4) • Hamstrings (Ashworth score: 3) • Hip adductors and ankle plantar flexors (Ashworth score: 5) • Decreased range of motion at hips, knees, and ankles	• Hip, knee extensors and hip adductors (Ashworth score: 3) • Hamstrings (Ashworth score: 2) • Ankle plantar flexors (Ashworth score: 4) • Significantly improved range of motion at hips, knees; mild improvement at ankles • Quadriceps weakness more notable
Pathophysiology	• Periventricular leukomalacia; cerebral palsy; spastic diplegia	• Periventricular leukomalacia; cerebral palsy; spastic diplegia	• No new diagnoses

118

Case Study–continued

was considered, but the procedure was not available close to the family's home, and they were unable to make frequent trips to the distant site that offered the procedure. Selective dorsal rhizotomy was believed to be the best option under the circumstances. A treatment plan was developed that included intensive, long-term, postoperative rehabilitation. There was a high degree of confidence among the clinicians involved that the family was sufficiently cohesive and motivated to "stay the course."

Following the selective dorsal rhizotomy, Christopher learned to walk for household distances with a reverse walker while wearing ankle-foot orthoses. He also was able to short-sit with his hands free for play and was able to transfer from sitting to standing. He did not learn to creep or high kneel within the first 6 postoperative months. His walking was slow and required close supervision and verbal cues. He sometimes collapsed suddenly while walking (the rhizotomy unmasked some underlying weakness of the quadriceps), and he cannot yet ascend or descend stairs.

One problem that was not recognized prior to the surgery was an apparent motor apraxia. Throughout his rehabilitation, Christopher had difficulty planning new movement sequences; for example, he was very slow to learn to ride an adapted tricycle. The speech-language pathologist also believed that apraxia was the cause of Christopher's poor expressive language ability.

As with many children undergoing rhizotomy, Christopher's range of motion improved at all joints. His only residual restriction is his popliteal angle, which now measures 25 degrees. It is possible that he may require lengthening of the hamstrings at some time in the future. Furthermore, he will need to be monitored for possible subluxation. In general, Christopher's family was happy with the outcome of his surgery. They believed that he was more independent at home, and his teachers and therapists reported that he was able to participate in more activities at school, although this had not yet resulted in expanded goals on his individualized education program.

OUTCOME MEASURES AND CLINICAL DECISION MAKING

In the literature for the treatment of spasticity in cerebral palsy, there has been a tendency to apply quantitative measures of spasticity with little or no attention given to recording, much less measuring, more contextually relevant aspects of outcome. It is widely recognized that available outcome measures, especially for children with disabilities, are inadequate to task. Some of the available measures are summarized in Table 5.4 and are arranged according to

Table 5.4. Outcome measure versus dimension of disability

NCMRR dimension	Measure	Comment
Societal limitation	Parent/teacher interview	Disability measures include components of societal limitation
Disability	Gross Motor Function Measure (GMFM) (Russell et al., 1989) Pediatric Evaluation of Disability Inventory (PEDI) (Coster & Haley, 1992) Functional Independence Measure for Children (WeeFIM) (Msall, DiGaudio, & Duffy, 1993)	Measures are reviewed in more detail in Chapters 12 and 13
Functional limitation	Gait analysis (see Chapter 8)	Results vary among centers
Impairment	Modified Ashworth scale (Bohannon & Smith, 1987) Range of motion Direct (mechanical) measures of spasticity	Most commonly used measures in research literature
Pathophysiology	Neuroimaging; genetic/ metabolic testing	Limited clinical utility for planning interventions for spasticity

their relationship with the dimensions of disability. As greater consistency is obtained in the application of clinical decision-making paradigms, a greater "market" for outcome measures with better validity and applicability will be created.

SUMMARY

The management of spasticity is a complex process that is best accomplished with a close collaboration between professionals and family members. The NCMRR model of disability provides a rational framework for identifying the goals of intervention. Although interventions targeting spasticity focus on the impairment level of the model, outcomes must be addressed and monitored at all levels. It is rarely advisable to treat spasticity for spasticity's sake alone.

A number of specific intervention strategies are available for the treatment of spasticity. These treatments can be classified according to whether their effects are local or general and according to whether the effects they produce are short, intermediate, or long term. Given the variety of choices and clinical circumstances encountered, it is important to invoke a logical, consistent decision-making strategy such as the HOAC to provide methods and outcomes that are reproducible and capable of being monitored.

REFERENCES

Albright, A.L. (1991). In reply [Letters to the editor]. *Journal of the American Medical Association, 266,* 66.

Albright, A.L., Barron, W.B., Fasick, M.P., Polinko, P., & Janosky, J. (1993). Continuous intrathecal baclofen infusion for spasticity of cerebral origin. *Journal of the American Medical Association, 270,* 2475–2477.

Albright, A.L., Cervi, A., & Singletary, J. (1991). Intrathecal baclofen for spasticity in cerebral palsy. *Journal of the American Medical Association, 265,* 1418–1422.

Bennett, M.I., Tai, Y.M., & Symonds, J.M. (1994). Staphylococcal meningitis following synchromed intrathecal pump implant: A case report. *Pain, 56,* 243–244.

Binder, H., & Eng, G.D. (1989). Rehabilitation management of children with spastic diplegic cerebral palsy. *Archives of Physical Medicine and Rehabilitation, 70,* 481–489.

Bohannon, R.W., & Smith, M.B. (1987). Interrater reliability of a modified Ashworth scale of muscle spasticity. *Physical Therapy, 67,* 206–207.

Borodic, G., Johnson, E., Goodnough, M., & Schantz, E. (1996). Botulinum toxin therapy, immunologic resistance, and problems with available materials. *Neurology, 46,* 26–29.

Cahan, L.D., Adams, J.M., Beeler, L., & Perry, J. (1989). Clinical electrophysiologic and kinesiologic observations in selective dorsal rhizotomy in cerebral palsy. *Neurosurgery: State of the Art Reviews, 4*(2), 477–484.

Corry, I.S., Cosgrove, A.P., Walsh, E.G., McClean, D., & Graham, H.K. (1994). Botulinum toxin A in the hemiplegic upper limb: A double blind trial. *Developmental Medicine and Child Neurology, 11*(11, Suppl. 70).

Cosgrove, A.P., Corry, I.S., & Graham, H.K. (1994). Botulinum toxin in the management of the lower limb in cerebral palsy. *Developmental Medicine and Child Neurology, 36,* 386–396.

Coster, W.J., & Haley, S.M. (1992). Conceptualization and measurement of disablement in infants and young children. *Infants and Young Children, 4*(4), 11–12.

Dahlin, M., Knutsson, E., & Nergardh, A. (1993). Treatment of spasticity in children with low dose benzodiazepine. *Journal of Neurological Sciences, 117,* 54–60.

deLateur, B.J. (1972). A new technique of intramuscular phenol neurolysis. *Archives of Physical Medicine and Rehabilitation, 53,* 179–185.

Denhoff, E., Feldman, S., Smith, M.G., Litchman, H., & Holden, W. (1975). Treatment of spastic cerebral-palsied children with sodium dantrolene. *Developmental Medicine and Child Neurology, 12,* 736–742.

Engle, H.A. (1966). The effect of diazepam (Valium) in children with cerebral palsy: A double blind study. *Developmental Medicine and Child Neurology, 8,* 661–667.

Feldman, P.A. (1990). Upper extremity casting and splinting. In M.B. Glenn & J. Whyte (Eds.), *The practical management of spasticity in children and adults* (pp. 149–166). Philadelphia: Lea & Febiger.

Felsenthal, G. (1974). Pharmacology of phenol in peripheral nerve blocks: A review. *Archives of Physical Medicine and Rehabilitation, 55,* 13–16.

Fischer, E., Cress, R.H., Haines, G., Panin, N., & Paul, B.J. (1970). Evoked nerve conduction after nerve block by chemical means. *American Journal of Physical Medicine, 49,* 333–347.

Ford, F., Bleck, E.E., Aptekar, R.G., Collins, F.J., & Sterick, D. (1976). Efficacy of dantrolene sodium in the treatment of spastic cerebral palsy. *Developmental Medicine and Child Neurology, 18,* 770–783.

Fusfeld, R.D. (1968). Electromyographic findings after phenol block. *Archives of Physical Medicine and Rehabilitation, 49,* 217–220.

Gans, B.M., & Glenn, M.B. (1990). Introduction. In M.B. Glenn & J. Whyte (Eds.), *The practical management of spasticity in children and adults* (pp. 1–7). Philadelphia: Lea & Febiger.

Garland, D.E., Lucie, R.S., & Walters, R.L. (1982). Current uses of open phenol nerve block for adult acquired spasticity. *Clinical Orthopaedics, 165,* 217–222.

Giuliani, C.A. (1991). Dorsal rhizotomy for children with cerebral palsy: Support for concepts of motor control. *Physical Therapy, 71*(3), 248–259.

Glenn, M.B. (1990). Nerve blocks. In M.B. Glenn & J. Whyte (Eds.), *The practical management of spasticity in children and adults* (pp. 227–258). Philadelphia: Lea & Febiger.

Grossman, M.R., Sahrmann, S.A., & Rose, S.J. (1982). Review of length-associated changes in muscle. *Physical Therapy, 62,* 1799–1808.

Haslam, R.H.A., Walcher, J.R., Lietman, P.S., Kallman, C.H., & Mellits, E.D. (1974). Dantrolene sodium in children with spasticity. *Archives of Physical Medicine and Rehabilitation, 55,* 384–388.

Iggo, A., & Walsh, E.G. (1959). Selective block of small fibers in the spinal roots by phenol. *Journal of Physiology, 146,* 701–708.

Jankovic, J., & Schwartz, K. (1995). Response and immunoresistance to botulinum toxin injections. *Neurology, 45,* 1743–1746.

Joynt, R.L., & Leonard, J.A. (1980). Dantrolene sodium suspension in treatment of spastic cerebral palsy. *Developmental Medicine and Child Neurology, 22,* 755–767.

Kofler, M., Kronenberg, M.F., Rifici, C., Saltuari, L., & Bauer, G. (1994). Epileptic seizures associated with intrathecal baclofen application. *Neurology, 44,* 25–27.

Law, M., Cadman, D., Rosenbaum, P., Walter, S., Russell, D., & DeMatter, C. (1991). Neurodevelopmental therapy and upper-extremity inhibitive casting for children with cerebral palsy. *Developmental Medicine and Child Neurology, 33,* 379–387.

Mandac, B.R., Hurvitz, E.A., & Nelson, V.S. (1993). Hyperthermia associated with baclofen withdrawal and increased spasticity. *Archives of Physical Medicine and Rehabilitation, 74,* 96–97.

Marsh, H.O. (1965). Diazepam in incapacitated cerebral-palsied children. *Journal of the American Medical Association, 191,* 797–800.

Massagli, T.L. (1991). Spasticity and its management in children. *Physical Medicine and Rehabilitation Clinics of North America, 2*(4), 867–889.

McLaughlin, J.F., Bjornson, K.R., Astley, S.J., Hays, R.M., Hofflinger, S.A., Armantrout, E.A., et al. (1994). The role of selective dorsal rhizotomy in cerebral palsy: Critical evaluation of a prospective clinical series. *Developmental Medicine and Child Neurology, 36,* 755–769.

Meythaler, J.M., Steers, W.D., Haworth, C.S., Tuel, S.M., & Sesco, D.V. (1990). Limitations and complications in the use of intrathecal baclofen. *Archives of Physical Medicine and Rehabilitation, 71,* 771.

Milla, P.J., & Jackson, A.D. (1977). Controlled trial of baclofen in children with cerebral palsy. *Journal of Internal Medicine Research, 5,* 398–404.

Molnar, G.E., & Kathirithamby, R. (1979). Lioresal in the treatment of cerebral palsy. *Archives of Physical Medicine and Rehabilitation, 60,* 540.

Msall, M.E., DiGaudio, K.M., & Duffy, L.C. (1993). Use of functional assessment on children with developmental disabilities. *Physical Medicine and Rehabilitation Clinics of North America, 4*(3), 517–527.

Nathan, P.W., & Sears, T.A. (1960). Effects of phenol on nervous conduction. *Journal of Physiology, 150,* 565–580.

National Institutes of Health. (1993). *Research plan for the National Center for Medical Rehabilitation and Research.* Bethesda, MD: Author.

Rothstein, J.M., & Echternach, J.L. (1986). Hypothesis-oriented algorithm for clinicians: A method for evaluation and treatment planning. *Physical Therapy, 66*(9), 1388–1394.

Russell, D.J., Rosenbaum, P.L., Cadman, D.T., Gowland, C., Hardy, S., & Jarvis, S. (1989). The Gross Motor Function Measure: A means to evaluate the effects of physical therapy. *Developmental Medicine and Child Neurology, 31,* 341–352.

Shaari, C.M., & Sanders, I. (1993). Quantifying how location and dose of botulinum toxin injections affect muscle paralysis. *Muscle & Nerve, 16,* 964.

Steinbok, P., Reiner, A.M., Beauchamp, R., Armstrong, R.W., & Cochrane, D.D. (1997). A randomized clinical trial to compare selective posterior rhizotomy plus physiotherapy with physiotherapy alone in children with spastic diplegic cerebral palsy. *Developmental Medicine and Child Neurology, 39,* 178–184.

Sussman, M.D., & Cusick, B. (1979). Preliminary report: The role of short leg tone-reducing casts as an adjunct to physical therapy for patients with cerebral palsy. *Johns Hopkins Medical Journal, 145,* 112–114.

Sutherland, D.H., Kenton, K.R., Wyatt, M.P., & Chambers, H.G. (1996). Injection of botulinum A toxin into the gastrocnemius muscle of patients with cerebral palsy: A 3-dimensional motion analysis study. *Gait and Posture, 4,* 269–279.

Tardieu, G., Tardieu, C., Colbeau-Justin, P., & Lespargot, A. (1982). Muscle hypoextensibility in children with cerebral palsy: II. Therapeutic implications. *Archives of Physical Medicine and Rehabilitation, 63,* 103–107.

Vaughan, C.L., Berman, B., & Peacock, W.J. (1991). Cerebral palsy and rhizotomy: A 3-year follow-up evaluation with gait analysis. *Journal of Neurosurgery, 74,* 178–184.

Vaughan, C.L., Berman, B., Staudt, L.A., & Peacock, W.J. (1988). Gait analysis of cerebral palsy children before and after rhizotomy. *Pediatric Neuroscience, 14,* 297–300.

Veale, J.L., Rees, S., & Mark, R.F. (1973). Renshaw cell activity in normal and spastic man. In J.E. Desmedt (Ed.), *Human reflexes, pathophysiology of motor systems, methodology of human reflexes: Vol. 3. New developments in electromyography and clinical neurophysiology* (pp. 523–538).

Whitlock, J.A. (1990). Neurophysiology of spasticity. In M.B. Glenn & J. Whyte (Eds.), *The Practical management of spasticity in children and adults.* Philadelphia: Lea & Febiger.

Wright, J., & Rang, M. (1990). The spastic mouse and the search for an animal model of spasticity in human beings. *Clinical Orthopaedics and Related Research, 253,* 12–19.

Whyte, J., & Robinson, K.M. (1990). Pharmacologic management. In M.B. Glenn & J. Whyte (Eds.), *The practical management of spasticity in children and adults* (pp. 201–226). Philadelphia: Lea & Febiger.

CHAPTER 6

Musculoskeletal Impairments

Introduction to the Orthopedics of Cerebral Palsy

John P. Dormans and Lawson A. Copley

This chapter reviews and discusses abnormalities, or disorders, of the musculo-skeletal system in children with cerebral palsy and concentrates on the early detection of orthopedic abnormalities and the basics of orthopedic intervention. The structure of a bone and its growth are illustrated in Figure 6.1. Terminology used for describing the musculoskeletal system is defined in Figure 6.2.

HISTORY TAKING

Obtaining the history for a child with cerebral palsy is usually a straightforward process and is discussed elsewhere in this book. Obtaining the "orthopedic" portion of the history, however, is mostly related to the child's past interventions, function, and comfort. Older, less-involved children are often able to supply much of this information, especially regarding function and comfort. The child's immediate family is the most common source for obtaining the orthopedic history;

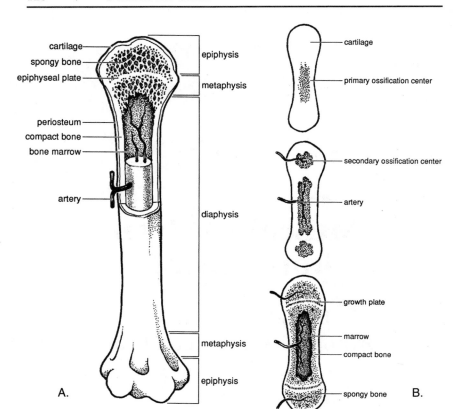

Figure 6.1. A) The structure of a typical long bone, the humerus. New bone arises from the epiphyseal plate, and the arm lengthens. The upper portion of the bone is the metaphysis, and the shaft is called the diaphysis. The bone marrow, which produces blood cells, lies in the center of the shaft. Surrounding the bone is a fibrous sheath, the periosteum. The bone facing the joint space is covered by articular cartilage. B) The long bone starts off as a mass of cartilage in fetal life. Gradually, the center is invaded by osteoblasts. These cells lay down minerals that form bone. The ossification centers spread and the bone enlarges. After birth, further bone growth occurs from the epiphyseal plate. (From Dormans, J.P. & Batshaw, M.L. [1997]. Muscles, bones, and nerves: The body's framework. In M.L. Batshaw [Ed.], *Children with disabilities* [4th ed., p. 318]. Baltimore: Paul H. Brookes Publishing Co.; reprinted by permission.)

however, background information might also be obtained from the child's relatives, therapists, nursing personnel, or teachers. Input from these other individuals is often helpful and can influence decision making for the child; if input from these individuals is unavailable, the child's history should be solicited (if these individuals are unable to attend the initial appointment, notes from an outside therapist can be particularly helpful). For "new patients," previous medical records and radiographs also can be very helpful and the child's family or

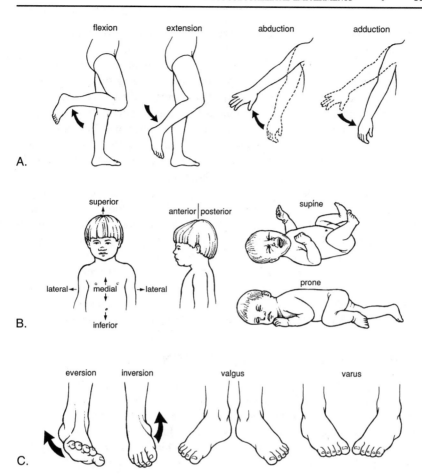

Figure 6.2. Various types of movements and postures. A) Flexion refers to the bending of a body part at a joint. Extension, the opposite of flexion, refers to the straightening of a body part at a joint. Abduction is the moving of a body part away from the midline, or middle segment, of the body; adduction is the movement toward the midline. The midline is also called the median plane. B) The outer parts of the body are the lateral sections. Anterior refers to the front of the body surface, whereas posterior refers to the back part (e.g., the chest is anterior, the back is posterior). The word *superior* means up or above; *inferior* means down or below (e.g., the head is superior to the shoulders, whereas the feet are inferior). For the extremities, *proximal* means toward the center of the body and *distal* means away from the center of the body (e.g., the hands are distal, the shoulders are proximal). *Supine* refers to lying on one's back facing upward; *prone* refers to lying on one's stomach facing downward. C) A foot is everted when the sole faces outward, or away from the midline and inverted when the sole faces inward. Valgus denotes a deformity in which the angulation of the distal body part is away from the midline of the body (talipes valgus, when the heel is turned outward from the midline of the leg); a varus deformity is the opposite. (From Dormans, J.P. & Batshaw, M.L. [1997]. Muscles, bones, and nerves: The body's framework. In M.L. Batshaw [Ed.], *Children with disabilities* [4th ed., p. 317]. Baltimore: Paul H. Brookes Publishing Co.; reprinted by permission.)

caregivers should be asked to provide these items prior to the first appointment. At some institutions, the caregivers fill out a "new patient" information sheet, which is useful in collecting the child's initial medical and social information.

The time when the child's orthopedic history is being obtained also is a good time to observe the child and his or her interaction with the environment and other individuals. If the child is ambulatory, this is a good time to observe him or her walking; if the child is nonambulatory, other mobility skills (e.g., rolling, pulling to kneel or stand) may be observed. A soft floor mat can facilitate this process. The child's sitting skills also can be observed at this time. In addition, the child's interactions with his or her family are noted.

As children get older, it is helpful to classify their ambulatory status. *Community ambulators* are able to walk both indoors and outdoors during most of their activities. Wheelchairs, if used, are needed only for long distances. *Household ambulators* are able to walk short distances on level ground within the home and are able to use wheelchairs for most outside activities. *Exercise ambulators* walk only during therapy sessions; they require wheelchairs for all other activities. *Nonambulators* are completely dependent on caregivers and adaptive equipment (especially wheelchairs) for mobility. Knowledge of the ambulatory status is important in establishing realistic therapeutic goals.

THE MUSCULOSKELETAL EXAMINATION

The musculoskeletal examination is an especially important component of the physical assessment of the child with cerebral palsy. The examiner needs to be familiar with the techniques of the musculoskeletal examination. This examination process should proceed in a systematic fashion, looking for signs of contractures (i.e., tight muscle tendon groups), hip subluxation (i.e., the hip coming partially out of the hip socket), scoliosis (i.e., curvature of the spine), and gait disturbances in children who can ambulate. The child should be relaxed and comfortable, and he or she should be undressed yet still covered when appropriate to avoid embarrassment or becoming cold.

Gait Observation

For ambulatory patients, the musculoskeletal examination should begin and end with gait observation. (This is discussed in more detail in Chapter 8.) It is frequently helpful to watch a child walk into the examination room because gait is more likely to be spontaneous and representative of usual gait if the child does not know that he or she is being observed. The child's parents also can be helpful in providing subjective evaluation of their child's gait pattern. After the static examination, it also is useful to have the child walk outside of the examination room. This activity is best observed in a private, long hallway with the child wearing gym shorts or a bathing suit.

Hip

After gait evaluation (when appropriate), the hip examination is usually performed. However, with an infant, hip examination may precede other examination when the infant is relaxed or sleeping (this ensures that the subtle signs of hip subluxation or instability will not be missed if the infant becomes excited by other parts of the examination). As previously discussed, with time, spasticity can lead to contractures. At the hip, the hip adductors and the flexors often are more involved than are the abductors and the extensors. With time, these contractures may contribute to the development of hip subluxation and dislocation (Moreau, Drummond, Rogala, Ashworth, & Porter, 1979). Hip pathology may be classified as *hip at risk, hip subluxation,* or *hip dislocation.* A hip at risk is defined as one in which abduction is limited to less than 45 degrees or one in which asymmetries of abduction exist on the clinical examination (see Figure 6.3). Hip subluxation describes the situation in which the femoral head has migrated partially out of the acetabulum. Although hip subluxation and dislocation can be detected clinically, they are best defined radiographically (see Figure 6.4). Hip dislocation is present when all contact is lost between the femoral head and the acetabulum. Hip dislocation may occur as early as 18 months of age, and most hips dislocate (if they are going to dislocate) by 6 years of age (Banks & Green, 1960).

During the hip examination, the child rests supine (i.e., face upward) on the examination table, and the hips are flexed to 90 degrees while abduction is performed slowly until spasticity is overcome (see Figure 6.3). Abduction also can be examined with the hips in extension. Limitation of abduction, asymmetries of abduction, or thigh shortening are all clues of underlying hip subluxation or dislocation. Asymmetry of hip abduction caused by unilateral hip subluxation needs to be distinguished from asymmetries of abduction caused by asymmetric contracture. The latter situation is often the case with the child who has a hemiplegic pattern of cerebral palsy or with the child who has a diplegia superimposed on a hemiplegic pattern. If there is any indication of hip pathology, a simulated standing anteroposterior hip radiograph may be useful in establishing the diagnosis and in characterizing the pathology (see Figure 6.4). Reimer's migration percentage (see Figure 6.5) is used to quantify the amount of hip subluxation. Using a radiograph, it measures the percentage of the epiphysis that lies lateral to Perkin's line.

Hip flexion contracture is quantitated using the Thomas test or the Staheli test. The Thomas test (see Figure 6.6A) is performed with the child lying supine on the examination table and the examiner flexing the child's contralateral hip. If there is no hip flexion contracture, then the opposite hip completely extends. If there is a hip flexion contracture, however, then there will be a limitation of hip extension on the nonflexed side. The amount of hip flexion contracture is quantitated as the amount of hip flexion on the side being tested. The Staheli test (see Figure 6.6B) is more accurate but can be difficult to perform on larger

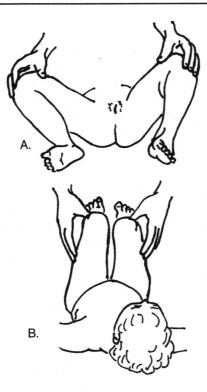

Figure 6.3. Asymmetries of abduction. A) The child is placed supine on the examination table. The hips and knees are flexed. With the child relaxed, the thighs are abducted slowly and gently. Asymmetries of abduction are noted. Any asymmetry of abduction can be an indication of underlying hip subluxation or dislocation. In this picture, there is decreased abduction on the left thigh. B) Femoral shortening can also be a sign of hip subluxation or dislocation. With the child lying supine, the hips are flexed to 90 degrees. Any shortening of one femur (the right in this case) can be indicative of underlying hip pathology.

children (Staheli, 1977). With this test, the child lies prone (i.e., face downward) on the examination table with his or her hips and legs extending off the end of the table. The examiner flexes the child's opposite hip to 90 degrees while gradually extending the hip being tested. The degree of hip flexion contracture is quantitated as the degrees short of full extension.

Rotational Assessment of the Lower Extremities

In typically developing children and adults, there is a rotation of the femur (i.e., thigh bone) between the hip and the knee joints such that the axis of the most upper part of the femur, or the femoral neck, is rotated forward (i.e., anteverted) compared with the axis of the knee joint; this is referred to as *femoral anteversion.* The child who does not have cerebral palsy typically has approximately

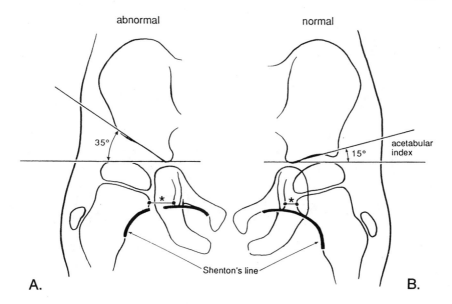

Figure 6.4. Radiographic features of hip subluxation as seen on a standing or a simulated standing anteroposterior pelvis radiograph. A) The normal radiographic appearance is represented by this child's left hip. B) The right hip shows radiographic signs of subluxation as well as an increased acetabular index (35% rather than the normal 15%) that is indicative of acetabular dysplasia. In addition, there is a break in Shenton's line, which indicates a right hip subluxation (see break in solid black line in the right hip). The amount of right hip subluxation can be quantified by measuring the teardrop distance (as indicated by *) that is increased on the right as compared with that on the left.

15–20 degrees of femoral anteversion. The child with cerebral palsy has abnormal amounts of femoral rotation that may affect his or her gait or the process of hip subluxation and/or dislocation. In children with cerebral palsy, this approximation may be abnormally increased or occasionally decreased; and this may contribute to the development of hip subluxation, hip dislocation, or gait rotational abnormalities. The prone rotation test can be useful in quantifying the amount of femoral anteversion (see Figure 6.7A).

In addition, tibial rotation should be assessed. With this test, the child lies prone on the examination table and the examiner notes the axis of the child's foot with the axis of his or her femur (see Figure 6.7B). This thigh–foot angle can be diagnosed as either internal, contributing to intoeing, or external, contributing to outtoeing. Using the information obtained from these tests, the examiner can create a rotational profile for the child; this can be compared with the child's gait to determine the cause and the location of rotational abnormalities.

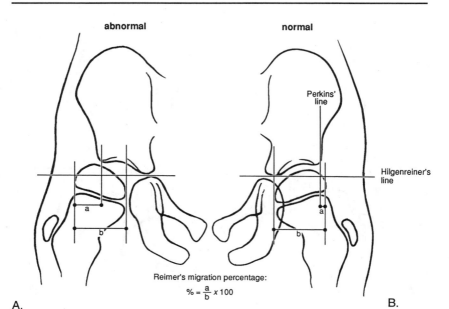

abnormal   normal

Perkins' line

Hilgenreiner's line

Reimer's migration percentage:

$$\% = \frac{a}{b} \times 100$$

A.   B.

Figure 6.5. Reimer's migration percentage. A) In this figure, the right hip is subluxated 50%. B) The typical radiographic relationships are demonstrated on this child's left hip (i.e., migration percentage of 15%).

Knee

In ambulatory children with cerebral palsy, hamstring contracture may lead to reduced stride length or crouched gait. In nonambulatory children with cerebral palsy, hamstring contracture may lead to lumbar kyphosis (i.e., reverse curvature of the lumbar spine such that the lower spine curves out or away from the midline of the body) during sitting, which is sometimes referred to as "sacral sitting." Although hamstring contracture may be detected by observing decreased straight leg raising, it can best be quantitated by measuring the popliteal angle (Bleck, 1987; see Figure 6.8). With the child lying in a supine position on the examination table, the examiner flexes the child's hip and knee of the extremity being evaluated until they reach 90 degrees. The opposite extremity is held in extension while the child's knee is gradually extended; once spasticity, if present, is overcome, the degrees of extension (from full extension) is measured and referred to as the *popliteal angle.* In order to eliminate any confusion as to the reference for the degree measurement, the popliteal angle is communicated as "X degrees from full extension." The typically developing child is approximately 15–20 degrees from full extension.

As a result of a preexisting hamstring contracture, contractures of the knee capsule and the cruciate ligaments may occur (usually in older children) with

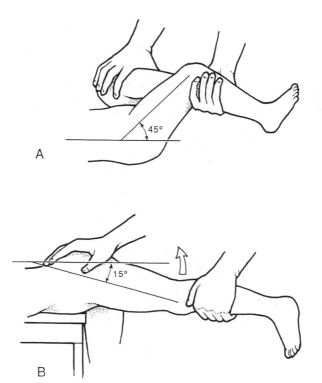

Figure 6.6. Tests for iliopsoas tightness. A) The Thomas test. In the typically developing child, full extension of the right hip is possible. In the child with iliopsoas tightness, less than full extension is achieved and is quantified using the angle that the femur forms with the examination table (this child's femur is 45 degrees from full extension). B) The Staheli test. The amount of iliopsoas contracture is quantified by evaluating the angle formed by the axis of the femur and the axis of the examination table (this child's femur is 15 degrees from full extension).

time. Hamstring spasticity and contracture can be differentiated from contracture of the deep structures of the knee (i.e., knee capsule and cruciate ligaments). With the child's hip extended in order to relax the hamstrings, any inability to fully extend the knee is a function of contracture of the deep posterior soft tissues of the knee (i.e., knee capsule and cruciate ligaments). This is particularly important in preoperative planning. If a fixed knee flexion contracture is present, no amount of hamstring lengthening will overcome the contracture of the deep structures of the knee joint.

If the ambulatory child with cerebral palsy experiences a contracted rectus femoris muscle—one of the quadriceps muscles (i.e., group of four knee extensor muscles)—the child may exhibit a stiff-legged gait with decreased knee flexion during the swing phase of gait (Gage, Perry, Hicks, Koop, & Werntz,

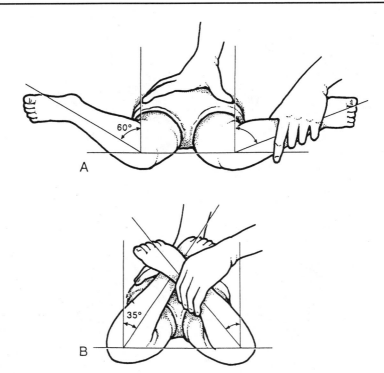

Figure 6.7. Assessing femoral anteversion. With the child lying prone and his or her hips extended, the knees are flexed to 90 degrees and the amount of A) internal and B) external rotation of the hips is assessed. An increased amount of internal rotation of the thighs can be consistent with an increased femoral anteversion. The average amount of rotation for a typical child is shown in this figure.

1987; Perry, 1987). Although rectus femoris contracture may be detected by the Ely test, it is best quantitated by the sidelying knee flexion test. The Ely test is performed with the child lying prone on the examination table while the examiner slowly flexes the child's knee on one side of his or her body (see Figure 6.9A). If there is a rectus femoris contracture, then the child's pelvis slowly rises off the examination table as the knee is flexed (see Figure 6.9B). This reaction is the result of the rectus femoris crossing both the hip and the knee joint. With knee flexion, the rectus femoris is placed on stretch and contracture causes the hip flexion. In addition to testing contracture, the Ely test also can examine the rectus muscle for spasticity. However, there is a problem with the Ely test because the quadriceps stretch has been shown to elicit a reflexive iliopsoas firing that may also cause hip flexion.

The sidelying knee flexion test is performed with the child lying on his or her side (see Figure 6.9C). As the examiner extends both of the child's hips, he or she gradually flexes the knee on the side being tested as far as the child can

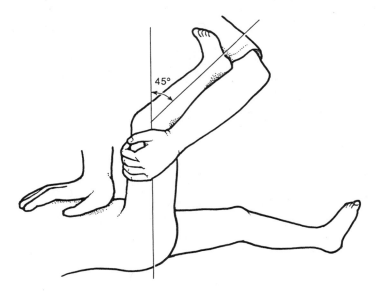

Figure 6.8. The popliteal angle.

comfortably tolerate. The amount of fixed rectus femoris contracture is referred to as "X degrees from full flexion."

Ankle and Foot

Achilles tendon contracture is manifested in a child as an equinus (i.e., tiptoe) gait or a deformity and is quantified by measuring the amount of dorsiflexion (i.e., how far the child's ankle passively can be extended beyond neutral) with the child's knee fully extended and flexed (see Figure 6.10). Children without cerebral palsy typically are able to dorsiflex their ankle 30–40 degrees beyond neutral with their knee extended. Children with cerebral palsy may have significant contractures in their flexion, and these are referred to as "an X-degree plantar flexion contracture."

Spine

Scoliosis (i.e., abnormal curvature of the spine in the frontal plane) is most common in nonambulatory children with more severe involvement (Lonstein & Akbarnia, 1983). The nonambulatory child's spine is best evaluated from behind with him or her sitting on the examination table (see Figure 6.11A). Any signs of scoliosis, such as asymmetries of the spine, the shoulders, the trunk, or the pelvis, are visible in this position. The child is then observed while bending forward (see Figures 6.11B and 6.11C). Any paraspinous elevations (i.e., evidence of lumbar spine involvement) or rib elevations (i.e., evidence of thoracic spine involvement) are carefully checked for at this time. The scoliometer can

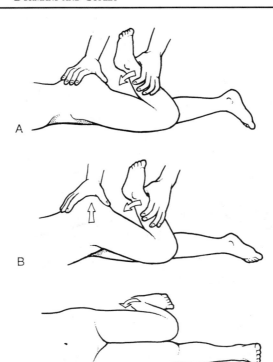

Figure 6.9. The Ely test. A) With the child lying prone and his or her hips extended, the knee on one side is flexed. B) If there is rectus femoris tightness, as the knee is flexed the hip also will flex, and this causes the child's pelvis to rise off the examination table. C) Rectus femoris tightness also can be quantified with the sidelying knee flexion test.

be used to quantitate thoracic rib or paraspinal elevation (see Figure 6.11D). Sitting balance and pelvic obliquity (i.e., abnormal inclination of the pelvis in the frontal plane), if present, are also noted. The flexibility of the spine also is assessed at this time. In the ambulatory child, scoliosis is best detected by observing the child's back while he or she is standing; contracture and/or limb length discrepancy, if present, can contribute to spinal asymmetries.

Pelvis

Pelvic obliquity is evaluated while the child is sitting in order to detect abnormal inclination of the pelvis, which is caused by asymmetrical pressure on one ischial tuberosity. Pelvic obliquity is correlated with the presence of scoliosis and/or hip dislocation (Cooperman, Bartucci, Dietrick, & Millar, 1987). Obliquity may be rigid or flexible and can be evaluated with lateral bending. The skin also is evaluated at this time for any signs of pressure sores.

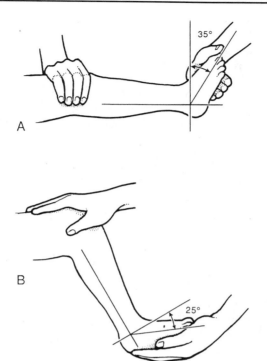

Figure 6.10.   Measuring the amount of dorsiflexion. A) Soleus and gastrocnemius contracture is evaluated by quantitating the maximum amount of ankle dorsiflexion with the knee extended. In this case, a 35-degree plantar flexion contracture is noted. B) Assessing the amount of contracture with the knee flexed versus the amount of contracture with the knee extended may help to differentiate how much contracture is caused by the gastrocnemius muscle as opposed to being caused by the soleus muscle. The gastrocnemius muscle crosses both the knee and the ankle joint. If the amount of plantar flexion contracture is greater with the knee extended than it is with the knee flexed, this indicates that the gastrocnemius is the primary offender (as shown in this case).

Upper Extremity Examination

Upper extremity examination includes inspecting for deformities, testing of range of motion, detecting contractures, and assessing functional use (Skoff & Woodbury, 1985; see Chapter 13).

Leg Length Discrepancy

Leg length discrepancy is not a common feature of children with cerebral palsy; however, it may occur as a result of contracture, hip dislocation, or previous surgery. Leg length discrepancy in the ambulatory child is best evaluated by palpating the iliac crests while he or she is standing (see Figure 6.12). Any shift of the pelvis may indicate a leg length discrepancy. The use of blocks can help

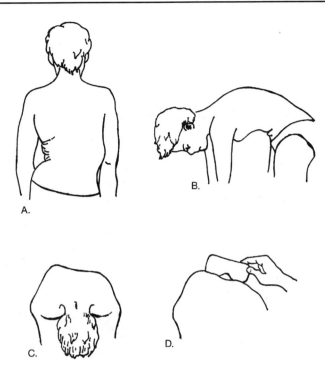

Figure 6.11. Physical examination for scoliosis. A) With the child sitting, any asymmetries of the shoulders, trunk, or pelvis usually are indicative of scoliosis. With forward bending, B) any thoracic rib elevation or C) lumbar paravertebral elevation can be noted. D) The scoliometer can be used to quantitate rib or paravertebral elevations.

quantitate the amount of leg length discrepancy. Contractures of the lower extremity, if asymmetric, can influence the detection and the quantification of leg length discrepancy (i.e., "apparent leg length discrepancy"), which occurs most often in children with hemiplegic cerebral palsy. The leg length discrepancy also may contribute to the appearance of scoliosis. If the scoliosis is nonstructural and is related to the leg length discrepancy, then the appropriate height block placed under the child's short leg should correct the problem.

Strength Testing

Strength is an important factor for both ambulatory and nonambulatory children with cerebral palsy. For the nonambulatory child, strength is an important factor that may affect transferring, powering a wheelchair, and other activities of daily living. For the ambulatory child, strength or lack thereof is critical in determining the quality of his or her gait. Assessment of strength is an essential component in surgical decision making. It is important to realize that spasticity

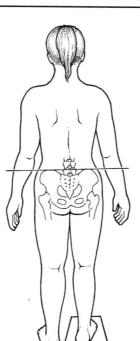

Figure 6.12. Physical examination for leg length discrepancy. The iliac crests are palpated from behind while the child is standing upright. The amount of leg length discrepancy is quantitated by placing blocks under the short leg until the pelvis is level.

may substitute for or augment strength, and, if taken away, functional limitations may result.

Gait

Most gait analysis is conducted with simple observation in the clinical setting (see Chapter 8 for discussion of formal gait laboratory analysis). In order to compare the static examination with the functional examination, gait is reevaluated after conducting all of the tests discussed in this chapter. The examiner should look for gait velocity, stride length, scissoring, and limping. It is important to check to see if the child has a heel strike or if he or she walks on tiptoes. It also is important to note any signs of knee crouch, incoordination, arm swing, abnormal hip flexion or extension, and intoeing or outtoeing.

Typical gait problems for the child with diplegic cerebral palsy include scissoring with increased hip flexion, knee flexion (i.e., *crouch*), and a tiptoe equinus gait (i.e., no heel strike). An associated feature of these problems is decreased knee flexion during the swing phase of gait (see Chapter 8).

Formal gait laboratory analysis can be particularly helpful in evaluating ambulatory children who are candidates for orthoses or for surgical correction of lower extremity abnormalities. Gait laboratory analysis is especially useful in evaluating children with foot and ankle deformities, in preparing for tendon transfers, in evaluating complex vocational problems, in evaluating cospasticity of the quadriceps and hamstrings, in considering rectus femoris surgery, and in evaluating children with atypical patterns of gait (postsurgical or otherwise) (Gage et al., 1987; Perry, 1987; Perry & Hoffer, 1977).

RADIOGRAPHS

The orthopedic assessment of cerebral palsy frequently involves radiographic studies. Radiographic evaluation is valuable for detecting scoliosis, hip subluxation and dislocation, and other extremity disorders (e.g., foot deformities). In nonambulatory children with cerebral palsy, for example, routine radiographic evaluation of the hips (in combination with physical examination) can help detect early subluxation and early hip dislocation (Rang, 1990). This type of care management is particularly common for nonambulatory children. The radiographic landmarks used in the evaluation of hip subluxation and dislocation are shown in Figures 6.4 and 6.5. In addition, radiographic evaluation of the spine at an early stage may be helpful to detect scoliosis.

SUMMARY

Children with cerebral palsy are a diverse group of individuals. There are many variables that will have an impact on their orthopedic care, including age, type and severity of involvement, functional abilities, previous treatment, and access to new treatment. The overall goal of orthopedic management is the detection of specific orthopedic problems at an early stage so that simple and more effective treatment options may be instituted. It is hoped that these children will have early evaluation and access to services that may prevent or lessen the impact of problems related to cerebral palsy. With continued efforts and research, it is hoped that new and better ways will be found to improve the care and thus the quality of life of children with cerebral palsy.

REFERENCES

Banks, H.H., & Green, W.T. (1960). Adductor myotomy and obturator neurectomy for the correction of adduction contracture of the hip in cerebral palsy. *Journal of Bone and Joint Surgery (American Vol.), 42A,* 111–126.

Bleck, E.E. (1987). *Orthopaedic management of cerebral palsy* (2nd ed.). Philadelphia: J.B. Lippincott.

Cooperman, D.R., Bartucci, E., Dietrick, E., & Millar, E.A. (1987). Hip dislocation in spastic cerebral palsy: Long-term consequences. *Journal of Pediatric Orthopedics, 7,* 268–276.

Dormans, J.P. & Batshaw, M.L. (1997). Muscles, bones, and nerves: The body's framework. In M.L. Batshaw (Ed.), *Children with disabilities* (4th ed., pp. 315–334). Baltimore: Paul H. Brookes Publishing Co.

Gage, J.R., Perry, J., Hicks, R.R., Koop, S., & Werntz, J.R. (1987). Rectus femoris transfer to improve knee function in children with cerebral palsy. *Developmental Medicine and Child Neurology, 29,* 159–166.

Lonstein, J.E., & Akbarnia, A. (1983). Operative treatment of spinal deformities in patients with cerebral palsy or mental retardation. *Journal of Bone and Joint Surgery (American Vol.), 65,* 43–55.

Moreau, M., Drummond, D.S., Rogala, E., Ashworth, A., & Porter, T. (1979). Natural history of the dislocated hip in spastic cerebral palsy. *Developmental Medicine and Child Neurology, 21,* 749–753.

Perry, J. (1987). Distal rectus femoris transfer. *Developmental Medicine and Child Neurology, 29,* 153–158.

Perry, J., & Hoffer, M.M. (1977). Preoperative and postoperative dynamic EMG as an aid in planning tendon transfers in children with cerebral palsy. *Journal of Bone and Joint Surgery (American Vol.), 59,* 531–537.

Rang, M. (1990). Cerebral palsy. In R.T. Morrissy (Ed.), *Pediatric orthopaedics* (pp. 465–506). Philadelphia: J.B. Lippincott.

Skoff, H., & Woodbury, D.F. (1985). Current concepts review: Management of the upper extremity in cerebral palsy. *Journal of Bone and Joint Surgery (American Vol.), 67,* 500–503.

Staheli, L.T. (1977). The Prone Hip Extension Test: A method of measuring hip flexion deformity. *Clinical Orthopaedics and Related Research, 123,* 12–15.

CHAPTER 7

Orthopedic
Approaches to Treatment

John P. Dormans and Lawson A. Copley

Many children with cerebral palsy have significant problems of the musculo-skeletal system that cause impaired mobility or that are related to contractures. Most of these problems are evaluated, treated, or tracked by an orthopedic surgeon and/or a physical therapist. These musculoskeletal problems are often a central concern of the child's family and caregivers. In many health care environments, the orthopedic surgeon sees children with cerebral palsy more often than other medical specialists and, therefore, has the opportunity to have a positive influence on the overall management of these children's care. Many children require surgical intervention in order to manage their underlying musculoskeletal problems. These procedures can range from relatively simple preventive interventions to more complex and invasive procedures. With this in mind, an introduction to the musculoskeletal aspects of care of children with cerebral palsy is presented in this chapter.

As discussed previously, contracture resulting from spasticity is the underlying feature in cerebral palsy that most commonly leads to surgery. In general, with time, spasticity leads to contractures of muscle and tendon groups. Without treatment, the other soft tissues surrounding the joints (i.e., ligaments and capsule) also become contracted and eventually present a further obstacle to restoring the natural motion of the joint. Ultimately, the joint itself can become damaged by the continued presence of spasticity and joint contracture. Therefore, the role of the orthopedic surgeon is to identify those individuals at risk for these more serious sequelae of spasticity and to intervene with effective treatment before more severe damage occurs.

In the past, preventive surgeries such as soft-tissue lengthening procedures to prevent progressive hip dislocation or to improve gait have been the mainstay of orthopedic intervention. However, as of 1998, the focus of orthopedic research for children with cerebral palsy is on assessing the outcomes of the various procedures that are used in treating the underlying musculoskeletal disorders. Long-term follow-up data regarding a variety of surgical treatments are being compared with the outcomes when no intervention is used. With this information, physicians are becoming better aware of the efficacy of given procedures based on the natural history of the particular deformity, its response to treatment, and the deformity's overall impact on the child and his or her family. This chapter discusses the orthopedic treatment of cerebral palsy and concentrates on the early detection of orthopedic abnormalities and the basics of orthopedic surgery.

ORTHOPEDIC INTERVENTION

Although no satisfactory treatment exists for the underlying central nervous system disorder in cerebral palsy, support, preventive interventions, and overall optimization of musculoskeletal system function can frequently improve the quality of life of the child who has this condition. Musculoskeletal intervention is chosen according to the type of cerebral palsy, the severity of involvement, the particular child's needs and expectations, the expectations of the child's family, the functional limitations of the child, and the experience and judgment of the child's therapists and surgeons. Treatment of musculoskeletal problems begins with educating the child and his or her family. Once the diagnosis of cerebral palsy is made, other appropriate subspecialists and individuals with experience in caring for children with cerebral palsy need to be introduced into the management of the child's care. The child's family is instructed, supported, and educated in the diagnosis, prognosis, and treatment that the child will receive in the future. If necessary, intervention may include some combination of occupational and physical therapies, orthoses (i.e., braces), or other adaptive equipment and surgery.

Because the problems that children with cerebral palsy may encounter can be complex and may require long-term comprehensive care, the orthopedic surgeon must develop an overall plan of management with which to evaluate and treat the wide variety of children who will need assistance in the future. From this more generalized perspective, the surgeon may then individualize treatment based on the particular needs of each child. The primary concern is to help the child achieve his or her maximum potential when performing daily activities and to prevent the sequelae of progressive deformity.

There are four common scenarios that occur with regard to orthopedic surgical intervention. Most often, the child is seen and evaluated by the orthopedic surgeon and no surgical intervention is planned. In this scenario, the child continues with his or her therapy and/or splinting programs and is scheduled for a follow-up evaluation. When indicated, surgical intervention is planned in conjunction with the therapy team and executed with a detailed postoperative, interdisciplinary plan. Some children are referred for other interventions, such as rhizotomy or motor point blocks (see Chapters 5 and 10). Occasionally, two separate modalities are recommended for the same child in the same surgical setting (e.g., rhizotomy with tendon Achilles lengthening).

CLASSIFICATION IN RELATION TO TREATMENT

As part of the general framework in managing children with cerebral palsy, the orthopedic surgeon must be able to classify the type and the severity of cerebral palsy affecting the child (see Chapter 1). This classification will offer some insight into the likelihood that the child will gain the ability to walk. It also will provide some indication as to the type of deformity that may develop in a child with a particular "type" of cerebral palsy as well as provide a framework for its treatment. For example, nearly all children with hemiplegia (i.e., paralysis of one side of the body) will eventually walk; this often will occur at the same time of development (between 12 and 18 months of age) or slightly later as it would in typically developing children. Many children with hemiplegia require Achilles tendon lengthening at approximately 4–8 years of age; at this age or a few years later, some children also may require tendon transfers at the ankle (i.e., moving part of a tendon to a different portion of the foot to improve a muscle imbalance) or hamstring lengthening. Some children benefit from upper limb surgery between the ages of 10 and 12 years. Most children with diplegia (i.e., both legs more severely affected than the arms) have delayed developmental milestones; walking generally develops by 4 years of age, 3 years later than the typically developing child. Most children with diplegia will need hip, knee, and ankle soft-tissue lengthening procedures—with or without rotational osteotomies for intoeing (i.e., surgically dividing the bone and correcting a rotational abnormality)—when they start walking or shortly thereafter. Children who have total involvement (i.e., involvement of arms, legs, cranial nerves, and intelligence) have global functional impairments, which lead to significant delays of developmental milestones. As a rule of thumb, most children who have total involvement are unable to sit independently or walk. Only 10% of children with total body spastic cerebral palsy will begin to walk by 7 years of age (Tachdjian, 1990). By 3 or 4 years of age, children who have total involvement generally need preventive hip balancing procedures if radiographs and/or physical examination shows that their hips are at risk for subluxation. If scoliosis develops and interferes with seating, total contact seating and/or spinal fusion may be necessary.

Another important factor in surgical decision making is whether a child has potential for ambulation. Although this potential is most often obvious and easy to predict, it occasionally can be more difficult to assess. The presence or the absence of certain primitive reflexes can be used to predict ambulatory potential. Bleck (1987) found that by 12 months of age the persistence of certain primitive reflexes or the absence of certain postural reflexes can predict ambulation. However, Rang (1990) found that a child's inability to sit by 4 years of age is often a poor prognostic sign for walking. The potential for ambulation in children with cerebral palsy may influence the treatment team's decision making in addressing specific combinations of musculoskeletal problems.

Beyond classification, a general frame of management involves consideration of the natural, chronological progression of the effects of cerebral palsy on the child. In general, there are several age groupings in which a particular emphasis of management occurs. During the first 4 years of life, the primary modalities of treatment will involve physical therapy (PT) and the use of orthotics. Between 4 and 6 years of age, surgery often is necessary in order to correct progressive deformity and to assist in improving function. During the next 12 years, the focus is on the education and the psychosocial development of the child (Rang, 1990). It is important to remember that this does not suggest that other areas of focus are not important during these age groupings; these are broad generalizations for the major areas of focus in treating children with cerebral palsy during these ages.

One of the reasons that surgery is often postponed until the child reaches 4 years of age or older is related to the rapid growth of the musculoskeletal system. By 4 years of age, a child's muscles will double their birth length; by the time the child reaches adulthood, his or her muscles will have doubled in length again. Muscle lengthenings in children younger than 4 years of age will frequently need lengthening again at a later stage. Furthermore, because of the developmental delay in children who have diplegia or total involvement, gait patterns, which may affect surgical planning, may not have developed prior to 4 years of age (Gage, Fabian, & Hicks, 1984).

The orthopedic surgeon should assess a child several times before recommending surgery. Serial physical examinations may help to provide a more complete picture of the severity of involvement, the degree of musculoskeletal contractures, and the existing gait patterns of the child. Emergency orthopedic procedures are not a part of the management of children with cerebral palsy. It is best to be careful with decision making in regard to surgery. Surgery should ideally be done by a surgeon who has experience and training in caring for children with cerebral palsy (Rang, 1990; Tachdjian, 1990).

Surgeries should be grouped together to enable as many significant problems to be addressed at once. In the past, the difficulty for children with cerebral palsy has been that surgeries were done individually—one after the other—and with multiple hospitalizations and long extended periods of casting and rehabilitation in between. Rang (1990), who has been a pioneer in developing and teaching better ways of caring for children with cerebral palsy, has referred to this phenomenon as the *birthday syndrome*. Figure 7.1 shows what *should not* be done in planning surgeries and rehabilitation for children with cerebral palsy; the child in the figure had multiple contractures, all of which *should have* been addressed surgically at one time. First, the child had a tendo Achilles lengthening (see Figure 7.1A). After this surgery, the child's hamstrings and hip flexors were still tight and he subsequently assumed a crouch position as a result of these unopposed contractures (see Figure 7.1B). The next

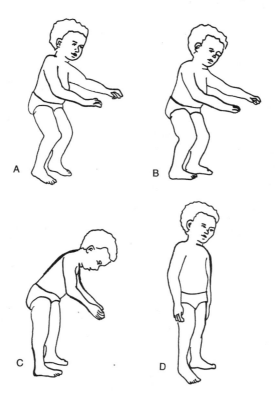

Figure 7.1. Rang's "birthday syndrome." A) A boy who has diplegia with contractures of tendo Achilles, hamstrings, and hip flexors; B) as a result of the child's hamstrings and hip flexors being tight after tendon Achilles lengthening, the child assumed a crouch position; C) following hamstring lengthening and subsequent rehabilitation, the child was left with unaddressed illiopsis contracture; D) after a third operation to address illiopsis, the child stood erect.

year—on the child's birthday—the child had a hamstring lengthening and subsequent rehabilitation that left him with an unaddressed iliopsoas contracture
and caused him to lean forward and to the left through the hip joints (see Figure
7.1C). The child then underwent a third operation to address the tight iliopsoas,
which required yet another rehabilitation (see Figure 7.1D). In the meantime,
the child had missed school, had been hospitalized, and had missed the opportunity to live a more typical childhood. Ideally, all contractures should be addressed surgically at one time. The concept of linkage should be taken into
account, and there should be an effort to minimize repeated surgical endeavors
as well as an effort to enable the child to live as typical a childhood as possible.

Every treatment endeavor should have a realistic goal. Both short- and long-
term goals should be set within a comprehensive program of child caregiving.
Once surgery is accomplished, the plan should include a quick return to the
previous level of activity. After surgery, continued non–weight bearing and immobilization are undesirable and may produce functioning limitations that are
worse than those present before the operation.

Principles of Surgical Correction of Contracture

Because children with cerebral palsy often have abnormal and asymmetrical
tone (i.e., spasticity), muscle–tendon contractures often develop. The surgical
methods for addressing these contractures are illustrated in Figure 7.2 and include Z lengthening, intramuscular lengthening, and recession. In Z lengthening, the contracted tendon is longitudinally split in half and is allowed to slide
into a lengthened position before being surgically repaired. In intramuscular
lengthening, the tendinous portion of the muscle–tendon junction is divided
and the musculotendinous unit stretches through muscle. In recession, the tendinous insertion is released from its insertion and is transferred to a more proximal portion of the bone of insertion or to the capsule of the joint.

SPECIFIC ABNORMALITIES

Children with cerebral palsy often encounter a variety of muscoloskeletal abnormalities. The spectrum ranges from hip subluxation or dislocation and pelvic obliquity to knee abnormalities (e.g., flexion deformity, extension deformity)
and genu recurvatum.

Hip Subluxation or Dislocation

In nonambulatory children with cerebral palsy, contractures of the hip are one
of the most commonly encountered musculoskeletal abnormalities of the lower
extremities (Hoffer, 1986). These contractures can lead to progressive hip subluxation (i.e., partial dislocation) or dislocation.

In terms of the treatment of hip abnormalities, the old adage "an ounce of
prevention is worth a pound of cure" is particularly true. For instance, the

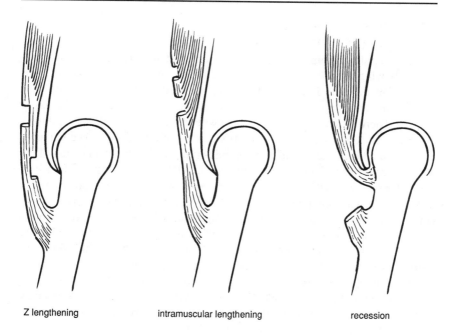

Z lengthening   intramuscular lengthening   recession

Figure 7.2. Three general ways of addressing tendon contracture. In Z lengthening, the contracted tendon is longitudinally split and is allowed to slide into a lengthened position before being surgically repaired. In intramuscular lengthening, the tendinous portion of the muscle–tendon junction is divided and the musculotendinous unit stretches through muscle. In recession, the tendinous portion of the bone is transferred to a more proximal portion of the bone insertion or to the capsule of the joint.

treatment often will be simple and effective if the diagnosis of hip subluxation is made before the subluxation progresses to dislocation with subsequent adaptive changes (e.g., acetabular dysplasia) (Cooperman, Bartucci, Dietrick, & Millar, 1987). However, if this window of opportunity for early intervention is lost, a much more involved and less effective procedure may be required. Hips may dislocate as early as 18 months of age, which stresses the need from the earliest examination for careful scrutiny of the hips of children with cerebral palsy (Tachdjian, 1990). Dislocation of the hip occurs more frequently in nonambulatory children with spastic types of cerebral palsy (Moreau, Drummond, Rogala, Ashworth, & Porter, 1979). Dislocation is more common in children with quadriplegic and diplegic cerebral palsy; however, this condition is rare in children with hemiplegic involvement. The overall prevalence of subluxation or dislocation of the hip in children with cerebral palsy has been reported to fall between 22% and 45% (Root, Laplaza, Brourman, & Angel, 1995). A composite review of the literature comprising four large series of children with cerebral palsy (199 cases) showed that 68% of the children had quadriplegia, 24% had diplegia, and 8% had hemiplegia (Atar, Grant, Bash, &

Lehman, 1995; Erken & Bischof, 1994; Howard, McKibbin, Williams, & Mackie, 1985; Root et al., 1995). In the child with quadriplegia, hip deformities may progress rapidly to painful dislocations (Moreau et al., 1979).

Following the identification of a "hip at risk" or a hip subluxation, some form of intervention is recommended, using either abduction splinting (i.e., keeping the knees apart with either a hip abduction pillow or an orthosis) or surgery. There is some controversy as to whether abduction splinting will prevent hip dislocation. Surgical intervention often is required and most commonly consists of adductor tenotomies-myotomies (i.e., sectioning of a portion of the adductor muscles and tendons [see Figure 7.3]) (Banks & Green, 1960; Silver, Rang, Chaan, & DelaGarza, 1985). In the past, this surgery was performed in combination with dividing the anterior branch of the obturator nerve, which controls the adductor muscles (i.e., anterior obturator branch neurectomy); however, this procedure has been associated with overcorrection of the deformity and can lead to an abduction contracture of the hip, which may interfere with seating (Tachdjian, 1990). Hip flexion contracture, caused by spasticity or contracture of the iliopsoas, may be a contributing factor to the progressive subluxation. At the time of adductor tenotomy, this issue may be addressed by either iliopsoas release or lengthening or by a more proximal iliopsoas recession (see Figure 7.4).

Once the hip subluxation has progressed, osteotomies to redirect the upper femur or acetabulum may need to be combined with soft-tissue lengthening procedures, especially if an increased femoral neck-shaft angle (i.e., coxa valga) or acetabular dysplasia (i.e., a shallow flat cup or acetabulum) exists. In a 19-year follow-up study, Bagg, Farber, and Miller (1993) reviewed 45 children with spastic subluxation of the hip. The study found that soft-tissue procedures with varus (i.e., toward the center of the body) osteotomy prevented dislocation in 45 children. The nine hips that did dislocate later occurred in children with quadriplegia who had not received treatment or who had only muscle releases. Femoral osteotomy usually consists of a varus derotational osteotomy (VDRO) (see Figure 7.5) (Hoffer, 1986; Tylkowski, Rosenthall, & Simon, 1980). In VDRO, the proximal femur is surgically divided and "tipped down" into the acetabulum. The osteotomy is secured with a hip screw and side plate or blade plate.

When acetabular dysplasia exists, a pelvic or an acetabular osteotomy may be needed as part of a combined procedure for hip stabilization. Depending on the location of acetabular deficiency, a variety of acetabular osteotomies can be used. Acetabular dysplasia also can be evaluated well with computed tomography that has three-dimensional reconstructions. Most often the dysplasia is posterior and superior and requires an acetabular osteotomy that augments the area of deficiency, such as a Dega osteotomy (Dega, 1974; Mubarak, Valencia, & Wenger, 1992) (see Figure 7.6).

In general, many late chronic dislocations should be left alone, especially if they are asymptomatic. If pain interferes with sitting or hygiene, several

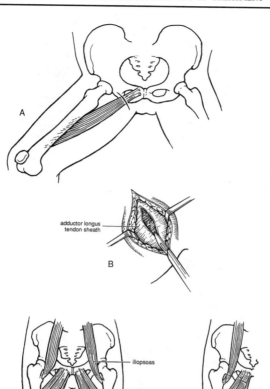

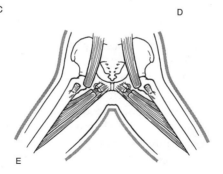

Figure 7.3. Adductor tenotomies-myotomies. A) A transverse incision is used to mark the upper medial thigh. B) The adductor longus is identified and its fascial sheath is opened. C) In the nonambulatory child, the adductor longus, the adductor brevis, the gracilis, and the iliopsoas typically are the most contracted. D) The broken lines indicate the site of division or the site of lengthening of muscle and tendon groups. E) Improved extension and abduction (and balance on the hip joints) following surgery.

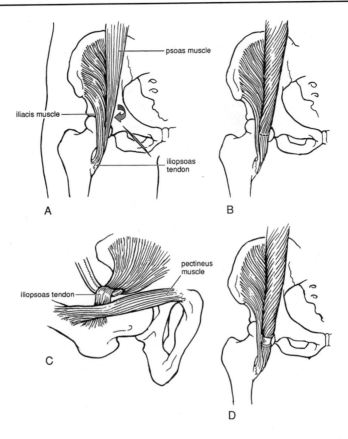

A

B

C

D

Figure 7.4. Iliopsoas lengthening. A) The iliacis and psoas muscles join to form the common iliopsoas tendon. The incision is made well above the level of the lesser trochanter. B) The tendon is identified. C) The tendon is exposed and delivered with a right angle hemostat. D) The contracted tendinous portion is divided, and the muscle tendon unit is allowed to lengthen through the muscle portion. The tendon also can be completely divided when necessary (i.e., nonwalker).

"salvage procedures" may be considered, none of which are entirely satisfactory (see Figure 7.7). A girdlestone osteotomy (i.e., removal of the femoral head and the neck) with muscle or fascia interposition may provide relief (Castle & Schneider, 1978). Other possible solutions for chronic dislocation include valgus osteotomy, total hip replacement, and hip fusion.

Pelvic Obliquity

Pelvic obliquity may be a result of causes above (i.e., suprapelvic) or below (i.e., infrapelvic) the pelvis. Suprapelvic obliquity is often caused by scoliosis and is corrected by spinal fusion to the pelvis (Lonstein & Akbarnia, 1983).

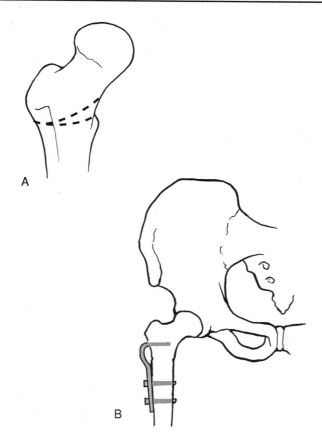

Figure 7.5. Varus derotational osteotomy (VDRO). A) The desired angle of osteotomy is established and the osteotomies are made by removing a medially wedged piece of bone; and B) the osteotomy is closed and secured with the fixation device.

Infrapelvic obliquity is caused by not only an abduction contracture of one hip but also an adduction contracture of the opposite hip as well. This is corrected by soft-tissue release and hip osteotomies. If the problem of pelvic obliquity is not corrected, the hip on "the high side" of the pelvis may become unstable and may dislocate, which can lead to further difficulties with progressive seating (Moreau et al., 1979).

Knee Abnormalities

Problems related to the knee in children with cerebral palsy include flexion deformity usually caused by spasticity or by contracture of the hamstrings, extension deformity caused by spasticity or by contracture of the quadriceps, and

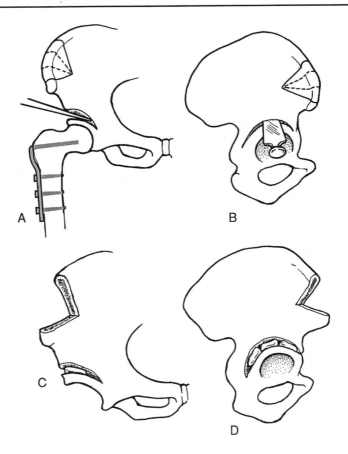

Figure 7.6. Acetabular osteotomy to improve coverage of the femoral head. A) An osteotome is used to make a curved osteotomy over the dome of the acetabulum and down to the triradiate cartilage (with care to avoid the hip joint). B) If the deficiency of coverage is mostly posterior, as is usually the case in nonambulatory children with cerebral palsy, the curved osteotomy is made mostly superiorly and posteriorly. The osteotome is used to apply downward leverage in order to open up the osteotomy site and to improve posterior and superior coverage of the femoral head within the acetabulum. C) A volume-reducing acetabular osteotomy (i.e., the capacity or the volume of the acetabulum is reduced). D) Triangular bone grafts are wedged into the osteotomy site in order to maintain the newly established acetabular position.

genu recurvatum (i.e., hyperextension of the knee) caused by spasticity of the quadriceps muscles (often in combination with equinus deformity as a result of contractures of the Achilles tendon).

Flexion Deformity Flexion deformity may be primary, secondary, or functional. The primary, and most common, type is caused by spasticity and by subsequent contracture of the hamstrings. The secondary type is seen in ambulatory children and occurs in part to compensate for equinus deformity of the

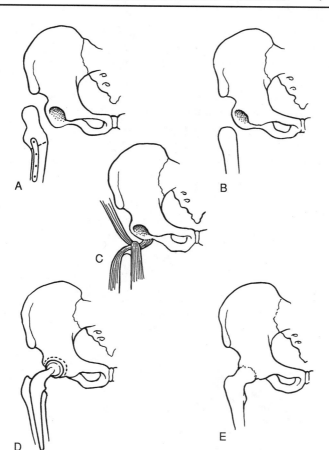

Figure 7.7. Salvage procedures for chronic dislocation: A) valgus femoral osteotomy, B) resection arthroplasty, C) resection arthroplasty with muscle interposition or Castle operation, D) total hip arthroplasty, and E) joint arthrodesis or fusion of the hip joint.

ankle and/or flexion deformity of the hip. Finally, the functional type is caused by an effort to lower the center of gravity in order to achieve balance. In addition, it also is possible for these factors to occur in combination.

Treatment of hamstring contracture is influenced by the functional needs of the child. If the child is nonambulatory and his or her hamstring contracture does not present a functional problem, then no treatment may be necessary. However, if the child does not ambulate and hamstring contractures interfere with his or her ability to transfer or stand in a standing frame or to sit, then more aggressive intervention may be necessary. If the child is ambulatory, then the treatment will depend on the degree of contracture and the presence or absence of functional limitations. Treatment simply may require nonoperative measures such as PT, splinting, casting, motor point blocks, or a combination of these measures. However, if the contracture is significant and limits function, then operative hamstring lengthening may be necessary. Hamstring lengthening can be done proximally or distally. For both ambulatory and nonambulatory children, a distal lengthening of both the medial and the lateral hamstrings is usually recommended (see Figure 7.8). (For nonambulatory children, some surgeons prefer proximal lengthening of the hamstrings, often in combination with hip adductor lengthening [Sharps, Clancy, & Steel, 1984].)

As a result of the gradual tightening of the joint capsule and the cruciate ligaments, knee flexion contracture may present late as a fixed deformity. In

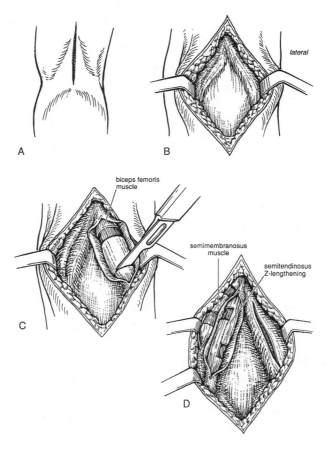

Figure 7.8. Fractional lengthening of medial and lateral hamstrings. A) A midline posterior incision is made. B) The hamstring muscle tendon units and their encasing covering (i.e., peritenon) are exposed. C) The biceps femoris (i.e., lateral) is lengthened by transversely incising the tendon and fascia but leaving the muscle intact. D) The semimembranosus muscle (i.e., medial) is lengthened in a similar fashion. The semitendinosus can be lengthened by Z lengthening the tendinous portion or by doing an intramuscular lengthening.

this situation, hamstring lengthening will not completely relieve the deformity. Although an osteotomy of the femur will change the existing plane of joint motion to a more functional plane with more extension, flexion will be lost, which may interfere with sitting as the child's knees may no longer flex completely.

In ambulatory children, hamstring lengthening in the presence of hip flexion and equinus deformity should be undertaken with caution. One third of hip extensor force is provided by the hamstrings. Lengthening the hamstrings further weakens hip extensor strength, and, as a result, the hip flexion deformity may worsen (Tachdjian, 1990). Genu recurvatum also may follow hamstring lengthening and is caused by equinus deformity as a result of a taut soleus (Rosenthal, Deutsch, Miller, Schumann, & Hall, 1975).

Extension Deformity Extension deformity of the knee is usually caused mostly by spasticity of the rectus femoris, which is the only knee extensor muscle that crosses both the hip and the knee. The spasticity or resulting contracture may limit the ability of the child to bend (i.e., flex) the knee when walking. If this is a significant limitation and has not responded to conservative attempts to improve the situation, then surgery may be necessary. There are several ways to address this problem. The origin of the rectus femoris muscle—where it arises from the pelvis—can be released. If there is no associated rotational malalignment in gait, then surgery can be done distally at the knee, close to where the muscle inserts into the patella (i.e., the knee cap). In ambulatory children with spastic diplegia, hamstring spasticity, and contracture, the excessive activity of the rectus femoris may be used advantageously at the time of lengthening by transferring it to the distal stump of the hamstrings or the sartorius (Perry, 1987; see Figure 7.9). This procedure has been shown to improve knee extension during stance as well as knee flexion during the swing phase of gait (Gage, Perry, Hicks, Koop, & Werntz, 1987). Ounpuu, Muik, Davis, Gage, and DeLuca (1993) reviewed the results of rectus femoris muscle transfer in 98 children and found that in those with less than 80% of typical knee range of motion (ROM) preoperatively, the range was maintained in swing with the transfer; however, the range of motion decreased 10 degrees with only rectus release, and the range decreased 6 degrees with no procedure.

Genu Recurvatum Genu recurvatum in the presence of weak or surgically lengthened hamstrings is usually caused by spasticity of the quadriceps muscle or equinus deformity as a result of contracture of the Achilles tendon. Genu recurvatum is a difficult problem to treat. A fixed molded ankle-foot orthosis (MAFO) or a molded ankle-floor reaction (see Chapter 16) with the ankle dorsiflexed may be beneficial (Rosenthal et al., 1975), and occasionally an orthosis that extends above the knee may be helpful. In order to reestablish knee alignment, adolescents with marked deformity may require an osteotomy of the distal femur.

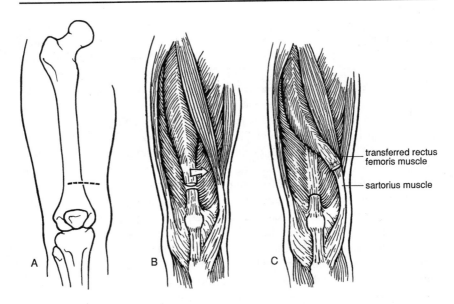

Figure 7.9. Release of the rectus femoris with transfer of its distal end medially to the sartorius. A) A transfer or an oblique incision is made over the distal thigh. B) The tendinous portion of the rectus femoris is divided and moved medially. C) The rectus femoris is sutured to the sartorius.

DEFORMITIES OF THE FOOT AND THE ANKLE

A variety of problems may be encountered at the foot and the ankle in children with cerebral palsy. The spectrum ranges from equinus (i.e., foot-down) and calcaneus (i.e., foot-up) contractures of the ankle and the hindfoot to varus and valgus contractures of the hindfoot and the midfoot. In addition, combinations of problems often occur throughout the spectrum. In spastic diplegia, in general, equinus contractures caused by the overpull of the gastrosoleus group with *valgus* (resulting in an equinovalgus deformity) are more common. In hemiplegia, equinus contractures combined with overpull of the tibialis posterior with *varus* (resulting in an equinovarus deformity) are more common. These problems are in part a result of dynamic muscle imbalance between the evertors and the invertors of the foot and between the tibialis anterior and other ankle dorsiflexors and the plantar flexor muscles associated with the Achilles tendon.

In nonambulators, foot deformity may not be a problem. However, there are situations in which the deformity may require attention (e.g., a deformity that interferes with shoe wear or with foot placement during wheelchair use). In the ambulatory child, consideration must be given to how the foot and the ankle relate to the other joints of the lower extremity and how the deformity influences the other joint deformities and function.

The foot and ankle commonly are forced into equinus contracture as a result of the overpull and the imbalance of the plantar flexors and the heel cord. In addition, depending on the imbalance of the invertors or the evertors, the midfoot may develop a "rocker-bottom" deformity as the foot is pulled either varus or valgus from the midline of the body.

In ambulatory children, it is helpful to selectively test muscles prior to surgery with dynamic electromyography (EMG) in order to determine the motor strength of the overactive muscle and its antagonist (see Chapter 8). In order to prevent the recurrence of an equinus deformity during the postoperative period, it is essential to develop the active voluntary function of the tibialis anterior (i.e., antagonist to the muscles of the Achilles tendon) in gait.

Achilles tendon contracture (i.e., soleus and gastrocnemius muscle and tendon contracture) can be treated with a surgical procedure or with nonoperative measures such as PT, bracing, casting, or motor point blocks. Nonoperative measures such as serial casting are often more successful in younger children with spasticity and with less severe contractures (Banks, 1983). Surgery, usually used only after nonoperative measures have failed, is often reserved for older children who have fixed contracture and functional limitations.

There are many different surgical procedures described for Achilles tendon contracture. In general, operations can be divided into two basic groups: tendon lengthening and intramuscular lengthening (performed at the tendon portion of the musculotendinous junction) (see Figure 7.10). Tendon lengthening can be performed either percutaneously or as an open procedure. At some institutions, surgeons prefer using a percutaneous, two- or three-cut, sliding lengthening procedure for nonambulatory children (see Figure 7.11). A postoperative cast immobilization then is used to promote healing, followed by a solid MAFO to prevent recurrence of deformity. Rang (1990) suggested that heel cord lengthening performed before 4 years of age is associated with a higher recurrence rate; Olney, Williams, and Menelaus (1988) suggested that musculotendinous lengthenings are associated with a higher risk of contracture recurrence. With Achilles tendon lengthening, the range of active motion is diminished but is shifted to a more functional or less problematic arc (see Figure 7.12).

A variety of procedures are available to restore balance to a foot that is being pulled varus or valgus by overactive muscles. The split anterior tibial tendon (SPLATT) transfer, the split posterior tibial tendon (SPOTT) transfer, and the fractional lengthening of the peroneals or the tibialis posterior with distal Achilles lengthening are commonly used procedures that assist with balancing the foot (see Figure 7.13). SPOTT is useful when the tibialis posterior is hypertonic or when the peroneals or the tibialis anterior muscles are weak (Green, Griffin, & Shiari, 1983). This situation most commonly occurs in children with hemiplegia and can be addressed satisfactorily with an Achilles tendon lengthening combined with a SPOTT. However, if there is continuous activity of the anterior tibial muscle on dynamic EMG, then the SPLATT may be used

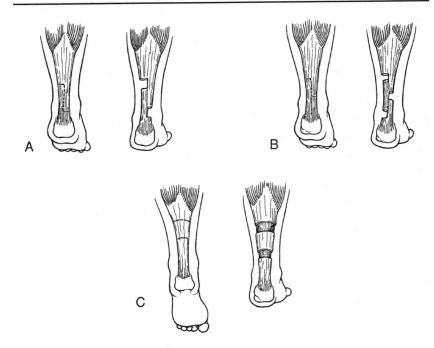

Figure 7.10. The tendon lengthening for the Achilles tendon. A) Two-cut and B) three-cut lengthening out of Z-cut lengthening technique. C) Intramuscular lengthening of soleus and gastrocolminus muscle and tendon contracture.

in combination with heel cord lengthening to correct equinovarus (Hoffer, Barakat, & Koffman, 1985).

Whenever tendon transfer is contemplated, certain general principles must be kept in mind. First, the joint involved should have nearly a full ROM prior to transfer. Second, because the power of the muscle unit attached to the tendon being transferred will be decreased by one level after transfer, only muscles with a nearly typical level of function are useful for transfer.

Subtalar arthrodesis (i.e., surgical fusion of the joint in a corrected position between the talus and the calcaneus) is required when fixed pes valgus deformity is present or is resistant to conservative management or tendon transfers. The surgery is now performed by means of internal stabilization with a screw and an autogenous (i.e., the child's own), cancellous bone grafting (Dennyson & Fulford, 1976) (see Figure 7.14).

SPINAL DEFORMITY

Spinal deformity can take the form of scoliosis (i.e., curvature of the spine in the frontal plane), increased kyphosis (i.e., hunchback), or lordosis (i.e., "sway-

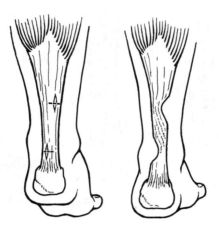

Figure 7.11 A percutaneous, two-cut, sliding lengthening procedure. With this technique, two hemitenotomy incisions are made (the medial half of the tendon is proximally cut, and the anterior half of the tendon is distally cut). The tendon is then stretched through the tenotomy incisions to increase its length.

back"). Kyphosis and lordosis are deformities in the sagittal plane (i.e., in an anteroposterior direction). The incidence of spinal deformity in children with cerebral palsy is approximately 25% (Balmer & MacEwen, 1968), and most of these children are affected by 5–6 years of age. Scoliosis tends to be more severe in children with spastic quadriplegia and to a lesser degree hemiplegia as a result of muscle imbalance related to their spasticity (Rang, 1990; Tachdjian, 1990). Scoliosis may be related to pelvic obliquity that was caused by asymmetrical contracture of hip adductors, hip abductors, or unilateral hip dislocation (Moreau et al., 1979). Scoliosis is often caused by asymmetrical spasticity or by tension athetosis of the trunk musculature. Other causes of spinal deformities include congenital deformities of the vertebrae or idiopathic scoliosis with a similar occurrence rate (e.g., a person without cerebral palsy).

Abnormal kyphosis or lordosis is often related to lower-extremity contractures. For example, if the hamstrings are contracted while a child is sitting, then there can be a loss of lumbar lordosis or a progression to kyphosis of the lumbar spine, which results in a phenomenon called *sacral sitting.* Iliopsoas contracture, however, can lead to increased lumbar lordosis as a result of an anterior inclination of the pelvis.

Treatment of scoliosis can take the form of nonoperative or operative intervention. Nonoperative techniques include bracing and wheelchair support. Although these modalities probably do not affect the natural history (i.e., ultimate prognosis or behavior of the curvature), they may improve comfort and posture in a young child with a flexible but significant curve and may allow for more

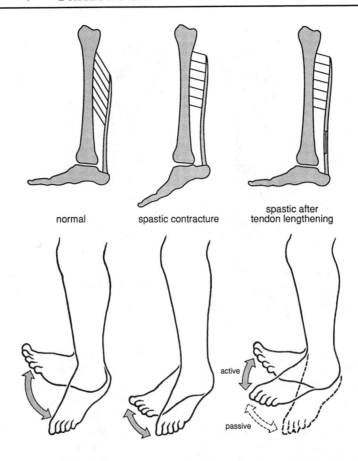

normal   spastic contracture   spastic after
tendon lengthening

active

passive

Figure 7.12. With tendo-Achilles lengthening, the existing arc of active motion is altered to a more functional range; however, the active range is diminished compared with a typical range.

spinal growth before spinal fusion. Most braces are thoracolumbosacral orthoses and ordinarily are not tolerated well by the child with cerebral palsy, in whom cooperation is poor and skin breakdown is frequent. Molded underarm plastic body jackets are the orthoses of choice (Rang, 1990). Wheelchair modifications, especially total contact seating systems, can be used to lessen the likelihood of progressive scoliosis or to delay surgery, allowing for spinal growth prior to fusion. Once a curvature has reached 45–50 degrees in magnitude, it is likely to continue to progress without surgical intervention.

Surgical stabilization can be used to arrest the progression of a curvature and also to obtain correction. Many different techniques of instrumentation have been developed. Segmental instrumentation (Luque, Cotrel-Dubousset, or Texas

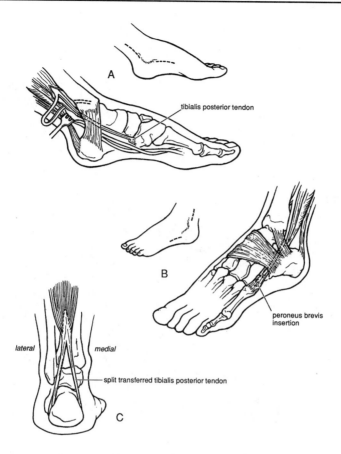

Figure 7.13. Split posterior tibial tendon transfer (SPOTT). A) Half of the posterior tibial tendon is harvested from its insertion site in the base of the medial cuneiform, leaving it attached to the muscle proximally. B) The harvested tendon portion is then rerouted to the lateral aspect of the foot and sutured to the peroneus brevis tendon. C) The end result is a split transferred tibialis posterior tibial tendon that helps provide balance to the foot.

Scottish Rite Hospital [TSRH]) in conjunction with posterior arthrodesis (i.e., fusion) of the spine to the pelvis is the most commonly performed technique for correcting pelvic obliquity. Anterior surgery, which usually consists of removing the spinal discs and packing with bone graft for fusion, combined with posterior instrumentation and fusion can help improve the flexibility of a curvature and is usually reserved for very rigid and severe curvatures (Lonstein & Akbarnia, 1983). At some institutions, doctors prefer the use of the unit rod (i.e., Danek) for correction of these curves (Bulman, Dormans, Ecker, & Drummond, 1996) (see Figure 7.15). This instrumentation device, which al-

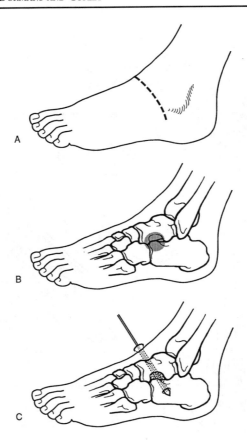

Figure 7.14. Subtalar arthrodesis with internal fixation and autogenous bone graft. A) The subtalar joint is exposed. B) The articular cartilage is identified and a bed of bleeding cancellous bone is established. C) Screw fixation is used to hold the subtalar joint in a stable position, and cancellous bone graft is packed into place in the subtalar joint to promote fusion.

lows for simultaneous correction of scoliosis and pelvic obliquity, is a continuous prebent rod that is fixed to the spine by a series of segmental (i.e., attached to the spine at each level) and sublaminar (i.e., attached to the spine by being passed under the lamina) wires. The end of the rod is inserted to the pelvis in order to stabilize its position with respect to the spine.

UPPER-EXTREMITY ABNORMALITIES

A variety of upper-extremity abnormalities can be seen in children with cerebral palsy. These include control problems, spasticity, contractures, and bony

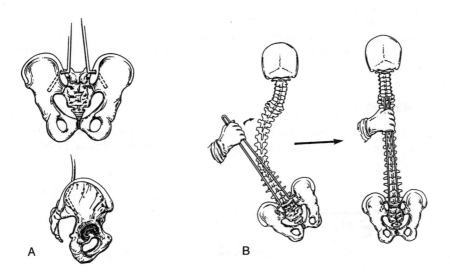

Figure 7.15. Unit rod for correction of spinal deformity and stabilization of the spine to the pelvis. A) The rod first is inserted between the inner and outer tables of the pelvic bone just above the acetabulum and B) progressively levered into position by sequentially attaching and tightening the sublaminar wires to the rod, which provides correction of both the pelvic obliquity and the spinal deformity. (From Bulman, W.A., Dormans, J.P., Ecker, M.L., & Drummond, D.S. [1996]. Posterior spinal fusion for scoliosis in patients with cerebral palsy: A comparison of Luque rod and unit rod instrumentation. *Journal of Pediatric Orthopedics, 16,* 316; reprinted by permission.)

deformities. The following abnormalities are common in spastic paralysis (Tachdjian, 1990):

1. Thumb-in-palm
2. Flexion of the fingers and wrist
3. Pronation of the forearm
4. Flexion of the elbow
5. Adduction and medial rotation of the shoulder

Treatment of upper-extremity abnormalities can involve nonoperative modalities such as occupational therapy, PT, splints, and adaptive equipment (Skoff & Woodbury, 1985). Surgical intervention, which is recommended if functional impairments exist, includes releases, tendon transfers, and osteotomies. Only a small percentage of children benefit functionally from upper-extremity surgery; thus, cooperative, motivated children with good proprioception and two-point discrimination have the best prognoses (Skoff & Woodbury, 1985; Zancolli, Goldner, & Swanson, 1983). A commonly performed upper-extremity tendon transfer is the flexor carpi ulnaris to the extensor carpi radialis, which is used to facilitate the mechanical advantage of the finger flexors for children who lack wrist extension when the wrist is held in a more extended position during grasp (see Figure 7.16).

SUMMARY

There are many variables that have an impact on the orthopedic care of children with cerebral palsy, including age, type and severity of involvement, functional

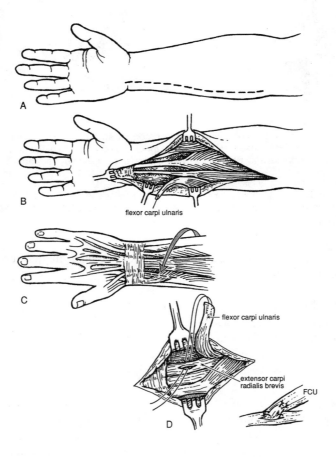

Figure 7.16. Transfer of the flexor carpi ulnaris to the extensor carpi radialis brevis in order to correct contracture and facilitate wrist extension during grasp. A) Skin incision; B) flexor carpi ulnaris is identified and released from its insertion; C) flexor carpi ulnaris is transferred around the ulnar side of the forearm; and D) sutured into the extensor carpi radialis brevis.

abilities, previous treatment, and access to treatment. The overall goal of orthopedic management is the detection of specific orthopedic problems at an early stage so that simple and more effective treatment options may be instituted. Specific deformities must be analyzed in the context of how the child's particular goals relate to function, cosmesis, and prevention of more severe sequelae. Efforts are underway to assess the efficacy of specific interventions. It is clear, however, that a team approach to problems that these children encounter has certain advantages for the child and his or her family. With continued efforts and research, it is hoped that new and better ways will be found to improve the care of these children.

REFERENCES

Atar, D., Grant, A.D., Bash, J., & Lehman, W.B. (1995). Combined hip surgery in cerebral palsy patients. *American Journal of Orthopedics, 24*(1), 52–55.

Bagg, M.R., Farber, J., & Miller, F. (1993). Long-term follow-up of hip subluxation in cerebral palsy patients. *Journal of Pediatric Orthopedics, 13*(1), 32–36.

Balmer, G.A., & MacEwen, G.D. (1968). The incidence and treatment of scoliosis in cerebral palsy. *Journal of Bone and Joint Surgery (British Vol.), 52,* 134–137.

Banks, H.H. (1983). Equinus and cerebral palsy—Its management. *Foot and Ankle, 4,* 149–159.

Banks, H.H., & Green, W.T. (1960). Adductor myotomy and obturator neurectomy for the correction of adduction contracture of the hip in cerebral palsy. *Journal of Bone and Joint Surgery, 42A,* 111–126.

Bleck, E.E. (1987). *Orthopaedic management of cerebral palsy* (2nd ed.). Philadelphia: J.B. Lippincott.

Bulman, W.A., Dormans J.P., Ecker, M.L., & Drummond, D.S. (1996). Posterior spinal fusion for scoliosis in patients with cerebral palsy: A comparison of Luque rod and unit rod instrumentation. *Journal of Pediatric Orthopedics, 16,* 314–323.

Castle, M.E., & Schneider, C. (1978). Proximal femoral resection-interposition arthroplasty. *Journal of Bone and Joint Surgery, 60A,* 1051–1054.

Cooperman, D.R., Bartucci, E., Dietrick, E., & Millar, E.A. (1987). Hip dislocation in spastic cerebral palsy: Long-term consequences. *Journal of Pediatric Orthopedics, 7,* 268–276.

Dega, W. (1974). Osteotomis trans-iliakalna w leczeniu wrodzonej dysplazji biodra. Chir Narz Ruchu Ortop. *Polska, 39,* 601–613.

Dennyson, W.G., & Fulford, G.E. (1976). Subtalar arthrodesis by cancellous grafts and metallic internal fixation. *Journal of Bone and Joint Surgery, 58B,* 507–510.

Erken, E.H., & Bischof, F.M. (1994). Iliopsoas transfer in cerebral palsy: The long-term outcome. *Journal of Pediatric Orthopedics, 14*(3), 295–298.

Gage, J.R., Fabian, D., & Hicks, R. (1984). Pre- and postoperative gait analysis in patients with spastic diplegia: A preliminary report. *Journal of Pediatric Orthopedics, 4,* 715–725.

Gage, J.R., Perry, J., Hicks, R.R., Koop, S., & Werntz, J.R. (1987). Rectus femoris transfer to improve knee function in children with cerebral palsy. *Developmental Medicine and Child Neurology, 29,* 159–166.

Green, N.E., Griffin, P.P., & Shiari, R. (1983). Split posterior tibial-tendon transfer in spastic cerebral palsy. *Journal of Bone and Joint Surgery, 65A,* 748–754.

Hoffer, M.M. (1986). Management of the hip in cerebral palsy. *Journal of Bone and Joint Surgery, 68A,* 629–631.

Hoffer, M.M., Barakat, G., & Koffman, M. (1985). Ten-year follow-up of split anterior tibial tendon transfer in cerebral palsied patients with spastic equinovarus deformity. *Journal of Pediatric Orthopedics, 5,* 432–434.

Howard, C.B., McKibbin, B., Williams, L.A., & Mackie, I. (1985). Factors affecting the incidence of hip dislocation in cerebral palsy. *Journal of Bone and Joint Surgery, 67B,* 530–532.

Lonstein, J.E., & Akbarnia, A. (1983). Operative treatment of spinal deformities in patients with cerebral palsy or mental retardation. *Journal of Bone and Joint Surgery, 65A,* 43–55.

Moreau, M., Drummond, D.S., Rogala, E., Ashworth, A., & Porter, T. (1979). Natural history of the dislocated hip in spastic cerebral palsy. *Developmental Medicine and Child Neurology, 21,* 749–753.

Mubarak, S.J., Valencia, F.G., & Wenger, D.R. (1992). One-stage correction of the spastic dislocated hip: Use of pericapsular acetabuloplasty to improve coverage. *Journal of Bone and Joint Surgery, 74A,* 1347–1357.

Olney, B.W., Williams, P.F., & Menelaus, M.B. (1988). Treatment of spastic equinus by aponeurosis lengthening. *Journal of Pediatric Orthopedics, 8,* 422.

Ounpuu, S., Muik, E., Davis, R.B., III, Gage, J.R., & DeLuca, P.A. (1993). Rectus femoris surgery in children with cerebral palsy: Part II. A comparison between the effect of transfer and release of the distal rectus femoris on knee motion. *Journal of Pediatric Orthopedics, 13*(3), 331–335.

Perry, J. (1987). Distal rectus femoris transfer. *Developmental Medicine and Child Neurology, 29,* 153–158.

Rang, M. (1990). Cerebral palsy. In R.T. Morrissy (Ed.), *Lovell & Winter's pediatric orthopaedics* (3rd ed., pp. 465–506). Philadelphia: J.B. Lippincott.

Root, L., Laplaza, F.J., Brourman, S.N., & Angel, D.H. (1995). The severely unstable hip in cerebral palsy. *Journal of Bone and Joint Surgery, 77A,* 703–712.

Rosenthal, R.K., Deutsch, S.D., Miller, W., Schumann, W., & Hall, J.E. (1975). A fixed-ankle, below-the-knee orthosis for the management of genu recurvatum in spastic cerebral palsy. *Journal of Bone and Joint Surgery, 57A,* 545–547.

Sharps, C.H., Clancy, M., & Steel, H.H. (1984). A long-term retrospective study of proximal hamstring release for hamstring contracture in cerebral palsy. *Journal of Pediatric Orthopedics, 4,* 443–447.

Silver, R.L., Rang, M., Chaan, J., & DelaGarza, J. (1985). Adductor release in nonambulant children with cerebral palsy. *Journal of Pediatric Orthopedics, 5,* 672–677.

Skoff, H., & Woodbury, D.F. (1985). Current concepts review: Management of the upper extremity in cerebral palsy. *Journal of Bone and Joint Surgery, 67A,* 500–503.

Tachdjian, M.O. (1990). *Pediatric orthopedics* (2nd ed.). Philadelphia: W.B. Saunders.

Tylkowski, C.M., Rosenthal, R.K., & Simon, S.R. (1980). Proximal femoral osteotomy in cerebral palsy. *Clinical Orthopaedics and Related Research, 151,* 183–192.

Zancolli, E.A., Goldner, L.J., & Swanson, A.B. (1983). Surgery of the spastic hand in cerebral palsy: Report of the Committee on Spastic Hand Evaluation (International Federation of Societies for Surgery of the Hand). *Journal of Hand Surgery, 8,* 766–772.

CHAPTER 8

Gait Analysis in Cerebral Palsy

Freeman Miller

Walking is the most basic means of human mobility. For parents of children with cerebral palsy, the ability to walk is often a source of great anxiety. If a child does not begin to walk between 12 and 18 months of age, parents may become aware of the fact that there is a significant problem affecting their child's mobility. For some parents, their child's inability to ambulate can cause even more anxiety than if the child had difficulties with eating, failure to gain weight, seizures, or mental retardation, all of which could cause more long-term complications. Parents must be reassured that every effort will be made to maximize their child's ability to walk and that their child will achieve his or her maximum potential. It is important to remember, however, that walking patterns and walking abilities are more dependent on the individual child's level of neurological involvement than they are on the physical therapy (PT), surgery, orthotics, or any medical treatment that he or she may receive. In terms of assisting the child to ambulate, the physical therapist is similar to the coach of a child who is learning to figure skate. Without lessons and practice, the child will not achieve his or her maximum potential; however, not even the best coach can make every child an Olympic athlete.

In order to maximize a child's mobility, it is important to understand the basics of human walking. Walking is neurologically controlled by the cerebral cortex; the cerebellum, brain stem, and spinal cord provide the modifications and input for general control. Perry (1975) described four levels of motor control:

1. Reflex arc, which leads to spasticity and abnormal control
2. Mass limb reflexes, which lead to the abnormal whole limb flexor response
3. Erect posture control and standing stepping movements, both of which are mediated by the brain stem
4. Coordinated volitional movement pattern, which is mediated by the cerebrum

Based on these levels, impairments in the cerebrum will, at various levels, allow the more primitive movements to predominate. The control of the basic walking pattern is thought to be under the control of a gait generator; however, the generator's location and function are not well understood. The presence of a gait generator is supported by the fact that typically developing children begin walking between 9 and 18 months of age when the brain is mature enough to control gait.

All typically developing children have a similar gait pattern when they start walking. No teaching is required for these children to learn to walk, and there is no evidence that suggests that teaching can alter the age or the pattern by which a child starts walking. The ability to modify a typically developing child's gait pattern is not well defined. Although there are a number of different theories on how to change the neurological control of the gait pattern of individuals with neurological control problems, it is unlikely that the basic underlying neurological pattern can be altered.

Considering the basic assumption that the gait pattern cannot be changed, the goal of treating gait problems in children with cerebral palsy is directed at maximizing the function and the efficiency of ambulation given the individual's neurological impairment. For example, the child with a hemiplegic pattern of cerebral palsy (i.e., affecting one side of the body) will always have a hemiplegic gait pattern; the goal of treatment is not to convert the pattern to a diplegic pattern or a symmetric use of the lower limbs but to maximize the child's asymmetric control. In other words, the child's affected limb will always be smaller and weaker than the unaffected limb and because of slower growth will be 1 centimeter shorter in most individuals to enable maximum function. Incorporating this concept of using each child's neurological impairments to maximize his or her ability to ambulate requires careful assessment of the child's pattern of involvement and how his or her associated cognitive and musculoskeletal abilities affect function. In order to maximize the gait for the individual child, a clear understanding of gait and its pathomechanics as well as a careful assessment and an analysis of each individual child is necessary.

DEFINITION OF GAIT ANALYSIS

Gait analysis includes all of the methods of measuring and studying an individual's walking patterns (e.g., movements in sports, movements in the upper extremity, balance). The discussion of gait analysis in this chapter, however, is focused on studying children with cerebral palsy and their ability to walk.

The Gait Analysis Laboratory

The gait analysis laboratory includes a number of devices for measuring different aspects of walking. For children with cerebral palsy, the goal of these measurements is to better understand the abnormalities of gait; this will lead to more effective treatments to manage these abnormalities. Because gait analysis can be extremely difficult to understand, it may be helpful to have an analogy from another field of medicine. Take for instance the treatment program for a leg that was severely damaged in a motorcycle accident. In order to rehabilitate the leg and to reestablish maximum functioning, many different treatments and studies will be necessary; as a group, it is these treatments and studies that make up the discipline of gait analysis.

The walking problems confronted by children with cerebral palsy are not static; they evolve and develop as the child grows and matures. For the child with cerebral palsy, walking may be significantly delayed or may be very atypical. Even after the child begins to walk, his or her walking pattern will change significantly as he or she matures, making repeated evaluation an important aspect of any treatment program. Referring back to the analogy of a severe leg injury, it becomes obvious how important regular examinations are to treatment—healing and rehabilitation can take months if not years to achieve. The treatment options for children under the age of 5 who have walking problems caused by cerebral palsy typically include PT, assistive devices (e.g., walkers, crutches), and simple lower-extremity braces (e.g., ankle-foot orthoses [AFO]). Based on an evaluation made by the child's family and the child's therapists every 6 months, the prescription for these devices is made. (The evaluation should focus on how the child is functioning at home and at school.) These evaluations by the physician, using careful recording of joint ranges of motion (ROM) and observation of the child's gait, are enhanced by the use of standardized clinical videotapes. The videotape, which is usually made approximately every 12 months when the child's gait changes, enables physicians to observe the changes on subsequent clinic visits. This serves the same function as an orthopedist's obtaining X-rays every 2–4 weeks in order to follow the healing of a broken bone. In general, as the child with diplegia reaches a plateau of improvement in walking (usually between 5 and 8 years of age), surgery is often considered. When the child reaches a plateau and is no longer improving his or her gait pattern every 6 months, more sophisticated assessment is needed to determine the surgical changes that are necessary. In terms of the child whose walking has reached a point in which surgery may be necessary, he or she needs to obtain a detailed evaluation to determine the true pathology of his or her gait problem.

Kinematic Evaluation

Kinematic evaluation is the formal portion of gait analysis and includes a number of different evaluations. The kinematic evaluation involves the application of markers (i.e., retroreflexive balls attached to the child with adhesive tape and wraps) to several parts of the child's body and then having the child walk through a room that is equipped with four to six cameras that simultaneously photograph him or her from multiple angles (see Figure 8.1). The video images, usually taken at a rate of 60–120 photographs per second, are fed into a computer, which then combines the different cameras' images into one three-dimensional reconstruction of the child's movement. A detailed measurement of the motion

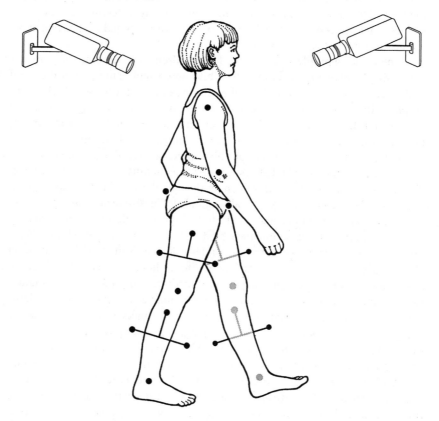

Figure 8.1. During the kinematic evaluation, several cameras simultaneously photograph retroreflexive balls that are attached to the child's body. These video images are fed into a computer and translated into a three-dimensional reconstruction of the child's movement.

of each joint then can be generated as the child walks. These data are generated from two-dimensional images that are obtained from each video camera using triangulation (a method that is similar to the way our brain translates visual perception into three-dimensional images), which enables therapists to create a full three-dimensional reconstruction of each of the child's defined body segments (see Figure 8.2).

There are several commercially available systems that claim to have the ability to produce three-dimensional kinematic data or useful two-dimensional kinematic videotape footage from only one camera. This claim is physically possible only if the assumption that there is a single movement or one deformity in a two-dimensional plane is accepted, and this is almost never the case in the children with cerebral palsy. Therefore, using one video camera to photograph children with cerebral palsy should be limited to making simple videotapes that are useful for subjective assessment (i.e., visually reviewing the child's gait pattern); one video camera is not useful in obtaining valuable quantitative information.

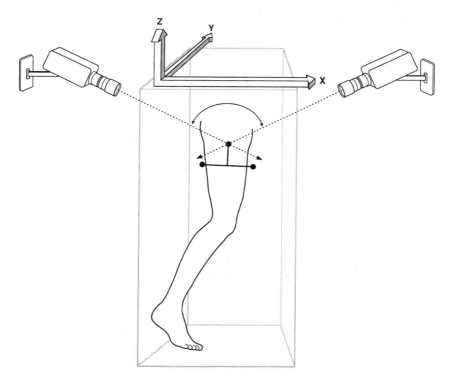

Figure 8.2. Triangulation is a mathematical process in which a computer can combine the images of two cameras (X and Z) to assign a three-dimensional coordinate point (Y). From this point, a full reconstruction and tracking of the extremity being observed can be made through a calibrated space.

Kinetic Evaluation

Kinetic evaluation also is a standard part of gait analysis. In order to assess the child's gait, the kinetic evaluation utilizes a force plate mounted in the floor (see Figure 8.3). The force plate, which the child walks across, is similar to a bathroom scale; however, it is much more sensitive, and, in addition to measuring forces that are vertical to the scale, the force plate also can measure horizontal and torsion forces. These measurements then can be combined with the kinematic data, and the specific amount of force that is used to move each joint can be calculated. The calculations include joint moments, joint power, and joint work. *Joint moment* is defined as the angular force present at a joint and is calculated by multiplying the amount of force from the ground reaction force (GRF; see Figure 8.4) and the distance that the force is applied from the center of motion. For the joint that is in motion, the *joint power* is calculated by multiplying the joint moment and the angular velocity of the joint. The *joint work* is calculated as the amount of joint power that is used over a period of time and, therefore, is the product of joint power multiplied by the time applied. Although these calculated values are combinations of the kinematic evaluation and force

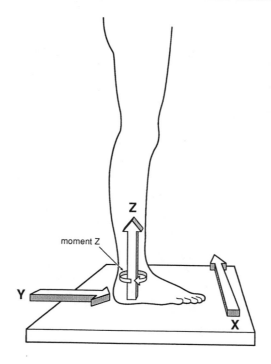

Figure 8.3. The force plate is a scale that is mounted in the floor. It can measure vertical force (Z) similar to a bathroom scale, but it also can measure horizontal forces (X and Y) and torsion force.

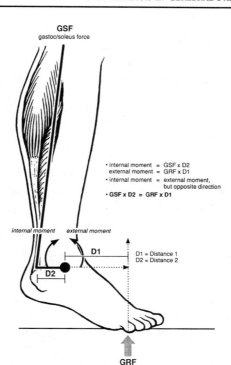

GSF
gastroc/soleus force

• internal moment = GSF x D2
  external moment = GRF x D1
• internal moment = external moment,
  but opposite direction
• GSF x D2 = GRF x D1

internal moment   external moment

D1

D1 = Distance 1
D2 = Distance 2

D2

GRF
ground reaction force

Figure 8.4. The external ground reaction force (GRF) is defined as the force that exists when the foot is in contact with the floor. The internal moment, which is the same as the external moment but in the opposite direction, is defined as gastroc/soleus force (GSF) multiplied by Distance 2 (D2). The external moment is defined as GRF multiplied by Distance 1 (D1). Thus, GSF × D2 = GRF × D1.

plate data (i.e., kinetic evaluation), they provide useful insight into understanding each individual joint.

In addition, it often is useful to perform an electromyogram (EMG), which applies electrodes similar to cardiogram electrodes to the child's muscles. EMGs are very useful in evaluating the muscles' function during actual walking time; this is helpful in determining the muscles that are atypically active or are quiet during specific phases of gait. For deep muscles, such as the tibialis posterior or the iliopsoas, an inserted wire electrode is required.

Pediobarograph

Many children with cerebral palsy also have maladies of their feet (e.g., planovalgus, equinovarus deformities) caused by abnormal muscle pull or poor muscle control. These deformities can be evaluated best with the use of a pediobarograph. The pediobarograph is a device that is placed either inside the child's shoe or on the floor over which the child walks. It measures the pressure of very small sections of the sole of the foot as the child steps on the device. This gives a pressure history of each area of the foot and is very helpful in looking for high pressure points under the sole (see Figure 8.5). The pedio-barograph also is very helpful in monitoring foot posture changes such as the development of planovalgus feet (i.e., the longitudinal arch of the foot is flattened and everted).

Interpreting the Gait Laboratory Tests

In many ways, the interpretation of the gait laboratory tests and deciding how these interpretations fit into determining the appropriate treatment program for the child are more important than the technical aspect of performing the tests. The interpretation is especially important in the gait analysis laboratory because there are large amounts of data that need to be reduced and placed in the context of the individual child's overall improvement, the child's medical history, the child's community, and the family's expectations of cerebral palsy. For this reason, the equipment used in the gait analysis laboratory by itself is relatively useless, unless a team (usually made up of a physician and a physical therapist) with experience in treating cerebral palsy is involved in interpreting the analysis. The detailed gait analysis laboratory data are usually one-time measurements. If repeated videotapes have not been made every 6 months or once a year, then there is no gauge of how the child is changing; this makes choosing a treatment program very difficult. The treatment options that are usually considered include specific recommendations for PT, for bracing, for orthopedic surgery, and for dorsal rhizotomy. Because of the technical nature of the evaluation and the large volume of data generated, the gait laboratory should be considered an interdisciplinary effort that requires the expertise of individuals who have computer and biomechanics training, PT experience, and training

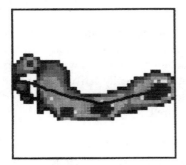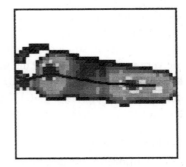

Figure 8.5. The foot pressure measure provides an objective representation of the surface of the foot as it makes contact with the floor. This type of foot-pressure representation is particularly useful when measuring foot deformities such as varus or vulgus positioned feet.

in orthopedics. In most laboratories the data collection is performed by the physical therapist and the biomechanist; the interpretation of the data is performed by a multidisciplinary effort that must include a physician who is experienced in the treatment of children with cerebral palsy.

The Purpose of the Full Gait Analysis Laboratory

The primary purpose of the full gait analysis laboratory is to help determine the most appropriate treatment program for each child with cerebral palsy. However, there is another very important function of the gait analysis laboratory that requires repeat testing. In situations in which the child with cerebral palsy has undergone a major change (e.g., surgery), he or she should be retested in the gait analysis laboratory 1 year after the procedure. The goal of this test should be to document the change that has occurred and to provide a baseline from which to monitor the child as he or she grows. Whether the child will need surgery in the future will be based largely on how the child changes from this baseline measurement.

The actively growing child with cerebral palsy is at high risk for recurrence of gait deformity and, therefore, should receive ongoing monitoring by a physician who is experienced in evaluating and treating gait problems and cerebral palsy. The physician should keep in mind that as the child continues to grow, the use of repeated gait analysis is important to achieving the child's best possible gait. Once the child is completely grown, his or her gait will remain more stable, and close monitoring will no longer be as necessary.

As the surgical options for treating gait problems have evolved from simple single surgeries to single-stage, multiple-level surgeries, the importance of the gait analysis laboratory has increased. Children with cerebral palsy traditionally have had surgery every year while they were growing. At 3 years of age, the child often would have a heel cord lengthening; at 4 years of age, a hamstring lengthening; at 5 years of age, an adductor lengthening; and at 6 years of age, femoral osteotomies. By the age of 7, the child would require the same procedures again. This pattern would continue as the child got older, and, as a result, he or she would seldom go for more than a year without having some minor surgery or having to spend some time in casts. There has been a great shift away from this pattern of excessive surgical treatments to encourage the use of simple bracing and PT to maximize the child's gait pattern. If the child is walking farther and improving his or her control while walking, then surgical treatments are usually not recommended. It is not until a definite plateau in function is reached (typically between 5 and 7 years of age) that surgery is recommended.

UNDERSTANDING GAIT ANALYSIS RESULTS

In order to understand the results gathered from the gait analysis, it is important to have a good understanding of typical gait and gait pathomechanics.

The function of gait is to provide mobility in an energy-efficient way. In typically developing children, gait patterns are extremely energy efficient. In terms of gait, the trunk, the upper extremities, and the head are considered the cargo, which is moved by the locomotion system (i.e., the lower extremities and the pelvis). The goal of energy-efficient movement is for the cargo to have an imaginary center of mass (see Figure 8.6). This center should have minimal movement, except in the direction of motion. In other words, when the child walks forward, the center of mass of cargo should not expend a large amount of energy for up and down or lateral movement (this does not help the child move in the forward direction and, thus, would be wasting energy).

Specific Walking Cycle

The specific walking cycle is broken into right and left steps. A *step* is defined as heel strike to heel strike on the same foot. *Stride* is defined as the cycle of right and left step. *Velocity* is typically quantified in centimeters per second or meters per minute; *cadence* is quantified in steps per minute. *Temporal spatial characteristics* are the parameters of gait that comprise step length and time, stride length and time, and single- and double-limb support time.

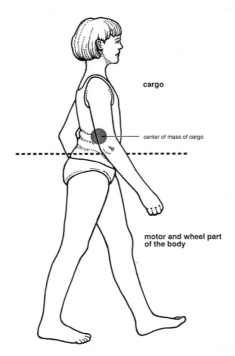

cargo

center of mass of cargo

motor and wheel part of the body

Figure 8.6. With gait analysis, it is useful to think of the arms, the head, and the trunk as the cargo that needs to be moved; it is the pelvis and the legs that are the motor and wheels that actually do the moving.

The most important conceptual separation of the gait cycle, however, is stance and swing phase (see Figure 8.7). The function of these two phases of gait is very different, and problems in each phase must be evaluated and treated separately. In a typical gait pattern, the stance phase takes up 60% of the total time of each step and is defined as the time during which the foot is in contact with the floor. The function of *stance phase* is to support the child's body weight and to provide the energy necessary to propel his or her body forward. This phase has been further broken down by Perry (1992); however, this system has not been adapted nor has it seen widespread use. The subdivisions of stance phase (i.e., first, second, and third rocker; discussed in the next section in this chapter) are used by some therapists (Gage, 1991).

The second part of the gait cycle is termed *swing phase* and is defined as the time during each step when the foot is moving forward relative to the floor (in the typical gait pattern, it is the time when the foot is not in contact with the floor). The function of swing phase is to advance the lower extremity forward and to prepare it for accepting the body's weight.

Problems with Stance Phase

Problems with stance phase need to be considered in relation to the major function of stance phase, which is to support the body weight and to provide a base that directs propulsion force. The first part of stance phase, referred to as the *first rocker,* begins with heel contact and is followed by plantar flexion (i.e., pointing the foot downward) of the ankle in order to bring the foot flat (see Figure 8.8). The first rocker is an important phase during which stability in the limb and the foot is achieved. A common problem for children with cerebral palsy during the first rocker is positioning the foot so that it is flat or so that the heel is striking the ground before the toe (i.e., toe strike). Common causes of toe strike are equinus ankle positioning or lack of terminal knee extension at foot contact. A common mistake made by individuals with little experience with treating children with cerebral palsy and no experience with gait laboratory is assuming that toe strike or toe walking automatically translates into an equinus contraction and, thus, requires heel cord lengthening surgery. However, the real

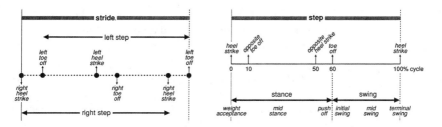

Figure 8.7.   The gait cycle is composed of a right and a left step, which is then divided into a swing and a stance phase.

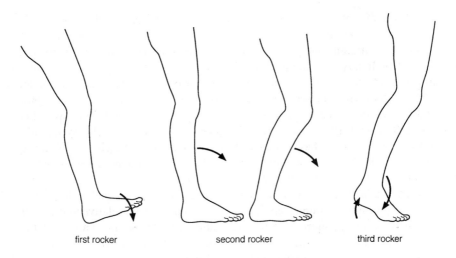

first rocker   second rocker   third rocker

Figure 8.8.   The stance phase of the gait cycle is divided into three stages by the activity of the ankle. During the first rocker, stability is established. During the second rocker, the foot is in contact with the floor and is followed by the tibia's rolling forward. During the third rocker, the foot begins to rise off the floor again.

problem may only be failure of knee extension; wrong diagnosis could lead to severe crouch gait.

The second part of stance phase, referred to as the *second rocker,* begins when the foot is in contact with the floor and is followed by the tibia's rolling forward in order to cause ankle dorsiflexion. The second rocker is sometimes referred to as *weight acceptance* or *midstance.* During this phase, the child who is toe walking may have problems positioning the foot so that it is flat (see Figure 8.9).

Lack of Hip Extension and Force Application   Lack of hip extension and poor force application are additional problems that need to be considered when there is too much hip-knee-ankle flexion (e.g., crouch gait). Force problems are often secondary to poor alignment of the foot with the knee, which may cause lever arm disease (i.e., the poor alignment of the foot that causes flexion of the knee in midstance; see Figure 8.10). This may be caused by planovalgus or equinovarus foot deformities, tibial torsion, or femoral anteversion. Often there is a combination of these deformities, all of which may require separate treatment (e.g., surgical correction of planovalgus foot deformity).

Hyperextension of the Knee   Another problem of midstance is back-kneeing (i.e., hyperextension of the knee; see Figure 8.11), which typically is a result of an imbalance between hamstrings and gastrocsoleus. Back-kneeing also can be a response to severe weakness of all lower-extremity muscles and/or very poor control. A very common error in gait interpretation of midstance phase problems of crouching or of back-kneeing is to mistakenly assume that

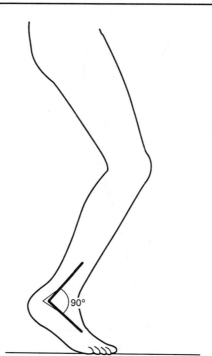

Figure 8.9.   If a child is toe walking, the cause may not always be a contracted Achilles tendon. Often, this type of gait can be a result of insufficient knee extension.

this is a problem related to quadriceps control. However, in children with cerebral palsy, the quadriceps are almost never the cause of this problem; in other words, strengthening or other efforts directed at the quadriceps will not effectively treat crouch gait and attempts to weaken the quadriceps will not have a significant impact on back-kneeing

The third part of stance phase, referred to as *third rocker,* begins when the foot starts to plantar flex (i.e., pointing downward); this is called the "push-off" phase. During this phase, the gastrocsoleus muscles typically exert a large propulsion force to propel the body forward. Premature plantar flexion (i.e., heel rise) is a common problem caused by increased equinus, lack of dorsiflexion ability, or increased knee flexion. Poor push-off leads to less efficient energy use during gait because the power for propelling relies more on the hip musculature.

Problems with Swing Phase

Swing phase also is divided into functions that must occur in order for the child to achieve his or her goal of moving the limb forward. During the first part of the swing phase, the limb has to shorten, which involves hip flexion, knee

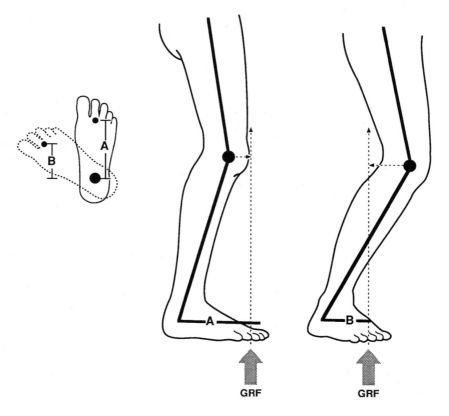

Figure 8.10. In order for the foot and the ankle to work properly to control knee position, the foot must be aligned with the knee joint axis. The type of malalignment shown on the right is called lever arm disease and is a major cause of crouch gait. (GRF, ground reaction force)

flexion, and ankle dorsiflexion. This is accomplished with the force from push-off and the power from active hip flexion, as well as with ankle dorsiflexion. The rectus femoris muscle is an energy transfer muscle that moves energy from knee flexion to hip flexion; however, it commonly has poor timing in children with cerebral palsy and causes toe dragging and stiff-leg gait because it does not allow adequate shortening of the limb. This is specifically determined in gait analysis by evaluating the kinematics of the knee and by evaluating an EMG of the rectus muscle (Southerland, Santi, & Abel, 1990).

The second part of swing phase, or *mid-swing phase,* is the period in which limb advancement occurs. Limb advancement typically occurs with rapid hip flexion, knee extension, and forward rotation of the pelvis. Again, failure of the limb to shorten by inadequate knee flexion in the first period of swing phase will often impede this second aspect of swing. *Circumduction* (i.e., movement in a circular motion) of the limb, which involves increased hip abduction during

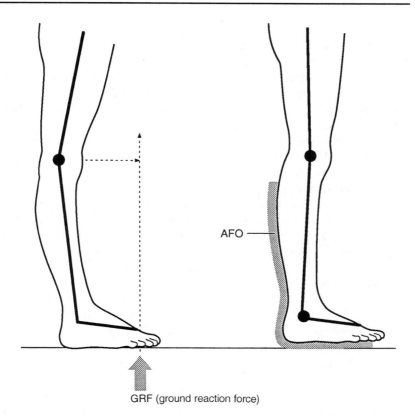

GRF (ground reaction force)

Figure 8.11. Back-kneeing often can be corrected with the use of ankle-foot orthoses (AFOs).

mid-swing phase, is a common component of stiff-knee gait. *Hip hiking* in mid-swing (i.e., an abnormal elevation of the pelvis on the same side as the swing limb) is another maneuver used to improve foot clearance. A common error in interpretation of causes of toe drag or circumduction is the perception that both are caused by equinus foot positioning. (Although equinus foot positioning may be a contributing factor, it is almost never the primary cause.) The primary cause of toe drag or circumduction is a knee problem with firing out of phase by the rectus muscle; this also is the most commonly encountered problem in children with cerebral palsy. Other problems include intrinsic knee stiffness, hip flexor weakness, and fixed quadriceps contractures.

The third part of swing phase involves the pre-positioning of the limb for stable heel strike. In preparation of heel strike, this requires having the knee almost fully extended and the foot in neutral to slight dorsiflexion (i.e., pointing upward). The heel makes contact with the ground before the rest of the foot, similar to an airplane's rear wheels making contact with the ground before the rest of the airplane when landing. Problems in this part of swing phase are most commonly related to insufficient knee extension, which leads to a shortened step length. The causes of insufficient knee extension may be contracture or early initiation of hamstring contraction not allowing full-knee extension. Insufficient knee extension is sometimes caused by short-swing phase resulting from poor supporting ability of the contralateral limb, which is in the stance phase at the same time. Increased knee flexion occasionally may be a result of equinus foot positioning and, therefore, is a secondary adaptive deformity with the primary problem being the foot and ankle position. This can be determined during gait analysis by carefully reviewing the relative position of the foot and knee in terminal swing phase, by evaluating the EMG of the hamstring, and by recording the passive knee and ankle ROM during physical examination. Fixed knee joint contracture also may be a cause of lack of terminal knee extension.

A working knowledge of typical gait and the quantitative measurements of the gait analysis laboratory allow for a more complete understanding of the pathological gait pattern of children with cerebral palsy. This understanding allows for the possibility of more complete one-stage correction by surgery. Some common problems that these children with cerebral palsy exhibit are contracted hamstring muscles; spastic rectus muscle; and a combination of torsional deformities, including increased femoral anteversion, tibial torsion, and planovalgus foot deformity. The careful measurements in the gait laboratory can help identify all of the components of the impairment that contribute to these problems; with hope, this will allow them to be corrected at the same time. Failure to correct one component of the deformity may translate into less overall correction or occasionally no correction at all. The benefits of orthotics and therapy modalities also can be evaluated during gait analysis. For example, there are some children who physicians or therapists believe have a better potential than other children for ambulation when using an orthosis; however, these children (or their families) may feel that they are not doing as well as they would without the use of the device. The laboratory evaluation can be very useful for quantifying the exact changes in the gait pattern that are caused by the orthosis; this allows for a very specific discussion with the child and his or her family. Sometimes the child is able to walk faster without the use of orthosis; however, in this situation, the kinematics of the hip, knee, and ankle may be more abnormal. Although each child is a unique individual and needs to be evaluated as such, there are patterns of involvement that are commonly seen in the gait laboratory. The following section reviews several of these patterns and uses several case examples as illustrations.

Common Gait Patterns   One of the concerns regarding gait in children who have cerebral palsy is that gait is extremely variable and that the detailed analysis in the laboratory is not representative of the child's actual level of function. It has been found that the step-to-step variation and the day-to-day variation in children with cerebral palsy is equal to that of typically developing children. In fact, in some children with cerebral palsy, there is less variation in gait pattern because they have only one true functional means of ambulation (see Figure 8.12).

Hemiplegic Gait Pattern Hemiplegia is the neurological pattern of cerebral palsy that predominantly affects one side of the body. It is the least variable pattern in cerebral palsy and has been subdivided into four subtypes by Winter, Gage, and Hicks, 1987). Subtype 1 has an equinus positioning of the foot but does not have active dorsiflexion of the ankle (see Figure 8.13). Type 2 also has equinus positioning of the foot, which is a result of spastic or contracted gastrocsoleous muscle that overpowers a functioning ankle dorsiflexor. There are important treatment and outcome implications to this separation between children who have Subtype 1 and those who have Subtype 2; for example, if the child has no EMG activity in the tibialis anterior, his or her foot drop will still be present and heel cord lengthening will not alleviate his or her need for a brace. Therefore, with Subtype 1, surgery is recommended only if the contracture is so severe that it prevents placing the foot plantigrade in an AFO. With

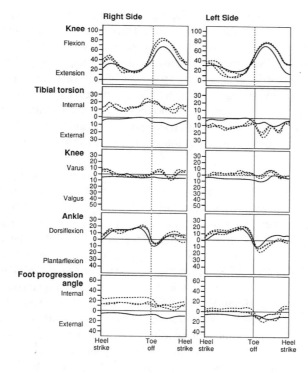

Figure 8.12. The individual gait patterns of children with cerebral palsy are extremely consistent and often show less variation than the gait patterns of typically developing children; this is a result of these children's limited means of ambulation. (Key: ——— = typically developing child; --------- = child with cerebral palsy.)

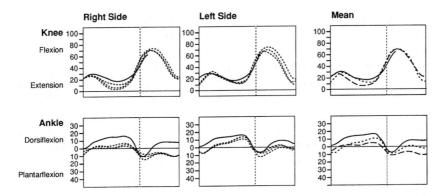

Figure 8.13. The individual has a right hemiplegia in which knee motion is normal in every instance, except during knee extension in stance. As a result of the individual having dorsiflexion in swing, this can be classified as hemiplegia Subtype 2. (Key: ——— = typically developing child; – – – - = right side; --------- = left side.)

Subtype 2, surgical lengthening of the gastrocnemius or Achilles tendon will alleviate the child's need for a brace, and, if the correct lengthening is performed and sufficient neurological control is present, then the child may be able to develop a heel-toe gait pattern. Distinguishing between Subtype 1 and Subtype 2 is achieved by demonstrating the presence of EMG activity in the tibialis anterior muscle during swing phase, especially during early swing phase (which is present in Subtype 2); Subtype 1 has no muscle activity. Children with cerebral palsy more commonly exhibit characteristics of Subtype 2; adolescents with adult pattern closed head injury more commonly exhibit characteristics of Subtype 1.

Hemiplegia Subtype 3 includes all of the characteristics of Subtype 2 with the additional involvement of abnormal knee kinematics and abnormal hamstring or rectus activity. Determining this abnormality is important because an Achilles tendon lengthening when there also is involvement of the hamstring will cause the child to continue walking either on his or her toes because the knee cannot be extended or with a short leg lurch to accommodate for knee flexion. In order to accommodate for the increased functional limb length discrepancy, the child also may develop increased knee flexion on the unaffected side of his or her body. Hemiplegia Subtype 4 includes all of the characteristics of Subtype 3 (thus, all of the characteristics of Subtype 2) with the addition of hip kinematic and hip muscle abnormality (typically increased hip flexor) as well as adductor spasticity or contracture. Again, recognizing these contractures and treating them appropriately is important in order for the child to achieve full hip extension and adequate abduction. It is sometimes very difficult to determine whether the contractures are caused primarily by spasticity or by prolonged adaptive positioning. The secondary contractures develop particularly during late childhood or in teenagers who have not received adequate medical follow-up during the "growing years."

These secondary contractures occur because the gastrocsoleous is compensated for by maintaining knee and hip flexion to equalize leg length, which is caused by ankle equinus. In older and medically neglected children, these secondary contractures are so severe that they occasionally require surgical lengthening. The separation of these four subtypes (i.e., located within the hemiplegic gait pattern) requires a careful physical examination in order to record the amount of static contracture and spasticity, to carefully review the muscle contraction patterns during gait, and to monitor individual joint motion during gait. In addition to these subtypes, hemiplegic pattern involvement also may have transverse plane deformity such as tibial torsion and femoral anteversion, both of which occasionally need to be surgically corrected.

Some children develop foot problems such as equinovarus (i.e., clubfoot), which is the most common problem for children with hemiplegic pattern involvement. The cause of the equinovarus deformity is overexertion of the tibialis posterior or anterior muscles. Because the tibialis posterior is too deep for surface electrodes, determining which muscle is causing the problem requires the use of a wire EMG. This is a very useful test to use with adolescents who are willing to cooperate; however, it is difficult to use with young children who often are frightened of needles and who will stop cooperating if they think a needle will be used. Children with hemiplegia most commonly have a pathological tibialis posterior, whereas adolescents with a closed head injury that exhibits a more adult pattern most commonly have a pathological tibialis anterior. The use of the pediobarograph can be very useful in separating this pathology because the tibialis posterior causes more transfer of the weight bearing to the lateral side of the foot, especially to the fifth metatarsal. Overactivity of the tibialis anterior often causes more of a cavus weight-bearing pattern with increased pressure on the first and fifth metatarsals.

Diplegic Pattern Diplegic pattern involvement is not classified as easily as hemiplegic pattern. The most useful classification is based on age and is described by Rang (1990). This classification is based on the frequently occurring evolution of the diplegic pattern in which the child initially stands with hips, knees, and ankles extended; the child often stands with legs crossed, as well. As the neurological development of the child progresses, better control develops while leg crossing decreases. In addition, the child has an increased tendency to stand with hip and knee flexion as well as with ankle plantar flexion. As the child reaches 5–7 years of age, the neurological maturation starts to plateau and the definite pathological patterns are established. Some of these common patterns include *trunk lurching,* which is an increase in the side-to-side movement of the trunk during gait. Although trunk lurching is a very inefficient gait pattern, it may be the only functional pattern for some children. Lurching has a tendency to become worse after most surgical procedures as well as during periods of rapid growth. The best treatment for lurching is to work on balance and strengthening both the hip and the trunk muscles. Because trunk lurching is usually caused by poor neuromotor control, it seldom can be completely corrected. However, it can be improved with gait training and with strengthening. Many children with diplegic pattern are not completely symmetrical in their pattern, which often can lead to an asymmetric gait pattern. The *asymmetric gait pattern,* in which the child walks almost sideways, also may be called "crab walking." Some crab walking is severe and easy to see, but many children have 20–30 degrees of rotation of the pelvis and because of their clothing covering the trunk and the pelvis, this gait pattern may be very difficult to observe visually. Although the underlying cause for the asymmetry is neurological control, physical problems often can be surgically addressed to improve crab walking. Asymmetric contractures of hip flexors and abductors and asymmetric rotational deformities of the femora are common problems that can be surgically corrected. Hemiplegic pattern, diplegic pattern, and crab walking are some of the most complex gait patterns in children with cerebral palsy; with a working knowledge of the gait laboratory, careful assessment of the different interacting patterns becomes more valuable and more important for planning future surgical corrections.

Scissoring Gait and Internal Hip Rotation   Crossing over of the legs is a common problem in the young child with diplegic pattern cerebral palsy and is typically improved with neurological maturation. There are two causes of the knees crossing over the legs: 1) scissoring, in which the adductors cause hyperadduction during the swing phase; and 2) internal rotation of the hip, usually a result of increased femoral anteversion, which causes adduction with hip flexion and with knee flexion. Although a number of children have either scissoring or hip rotation internal, many may have a combination of both. The evaluation in the gait laboratory is focused on trying to separate how much of the problem is a result of the adductor and how much is a result of the internal rotation. When working with children between 5 and 7 years of age who have had X-rays that illustrate no hip subluxation, gait training walkers and PT should be the focus of treating scissoring and internal rotation. Orthotics offer no long-term benefit for treating scissoring or for treating internal rotation. As the child's neurological maturation reaches a plateau and the scissoring and internal rotation continue to cause functional problems, surgical correction continues to be an option. A very careful gait analysis is required in order to determine how much of the problem is caused by internal rotation of the hip and how much is caused by primary adduction of the hip. Surgically lengthening the adductors when the primary problem is caused by internal rotation is not going to lead to a significant improvement in the child's gait pattern.

Crouch Gait   Crouch gait, which is defined as increased knee flexion in stance phase and is typically associated with increased hip flexion in the young child during equinus positioning of the ankle, is another common diplegic pattern that many children with cerebral palsy exhibit. In the older child with cerebral palsy, there often is hyperdorsiflexion (i.e., increased ankle dorsiflexion in stance) of the ankle. The most common cause of this is the child's neurological pattern, but it may be made worse with Achilles tendon lengthening, especially if the Achilles lengthening were not combined with hamstring lengthening and correction of lever arm disease. In years past, surgery often made crouching worse because of the surgeon's poor understanding of the multiple interacting forces that caused the crouching pattern to get worse. Another common cause of more severe crouching is lever arm disease. Lever arm disease is caused by poor transverse plane alignment, which leads to poor alignment between the foot and the knee; as a result, the GRF is unable to provide stabilization for the knee. Treating crouch pattern requires a careful assessment of the child's torsion alignment (e.g., planovalgus feet, tibial torsion, femoral anteversion).

Wide-Based Gait   Wide-based gait pattern can be observed visually and is characterized during double limb support by the child's feet being separated wider than the width of his or her pelvis. This may be a complication of too much lengthening of the adductors or of poor balance. Treatment for this problem is directed toward balance training and strengthening of the adductors.

Stiff-Leg Gait   *Stiff-leg gait,* defined as decreased peak knee flexion or late peak knee flexion in swing phase, is another common problem for children with diplegic pattern cerebral palsy. As previously discussed with hemiplegic pattern, stiff-leg gait is primarily a result of rectus spasticity or out-of-phase contraction of the rectus (see Figure 8.14). The most common complaint with the stiff-knee gait pattern from the child or from his or her parents is that the child drags his or her toes or wears out the front of his or her shoes every few weeks. Stiff-leg gait often is associated with crouch gait and torsion patterns.

SUMMARY

In diplegic pattern cerebral palsy, numerous problems may be present in the same child; only a very careful assessment, which includes the use of the most sophisticated gait analysis, of these complex problems can clarify and allow a single-stage correction to be obtained. For instance, to maximize the child's function, 10 or more different operative procedures occasionally may be necessary at the same time. Even with the most careful assessment, some children may not achieve the maximum benefit from surgery because of the complex mechanical interactions. Gait analysis provides an excellent tool for the surgeon to learn which procedures work and in which type of child they work best. If there is no quantitative gait analysis, then the surgeon is left with no means for going back and trying to understand why the surgical outcome was not as beneficial as expected. Very few children with diplegic pattern cerebral palsy will be worse off as a result of surgery to improve their gait.

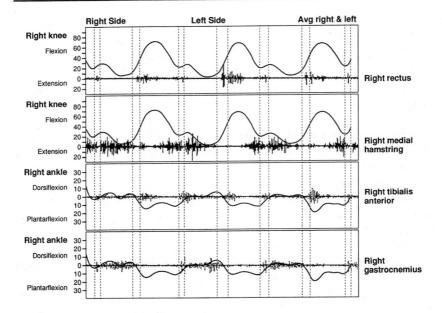

Figure 8.14. A rectus electromyogram (EMG) that shows increased swing phase activity.

Evaluating the benefit of orthotics is another use of the gait analysis laboratory (see Figure 8.15). The data presented in Figure 8.15 compare the difference between a 15-year-old girl who was first tested barefoot while wearing a University of California at Berkeley lab type of in-shoe orthotic and then tested while wearing regular shoes. There were no significant differences found between the two tests, which suggests that the in-shoe orthotic did not change the girl's knee motion or her ankle motion compared with wearing regular shoes. However, there was a significant improvement when shoes were worn as compared with when the girl went barefoot. Therefore, based on this analysis, it is recommended that this girl discontinue orthotic use; however, she should continue to use good, stable, well-constructed shoes. She should avoid shoes that provide no stability because this would be expected to be similar to the barefoot condition in which she does not do well.

In order to maximize the walking function of the child with cerebral palsy, repeated evaluations are required throughout the child's growing years. These evaluations should include physical examinations and documentation of his or her gait pattern with video cameras. After the child reaches a plateau in his or her development, a full three-dimensional gait analysis is helpful to plan surgical correction at one stage. With this treatment option, very few children should have negative effects from surgical corrections; however, it is important to remember that doctors can never be certain that all children will benefit from these interventions.

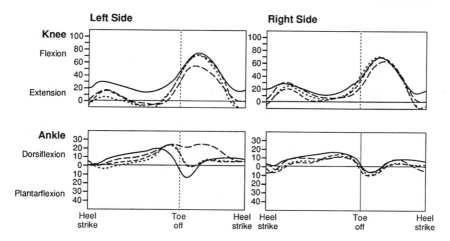

Figure 8.15. Evaluation of orthotics in a 15-year-old girl with cerebral palsy. The child showed no significant difference in gait when wearing regular shoes in comparison with wearing an in-shoe orthotic. This suggests that the in-shoe orthotic did not change the girl's knee motion or ankle motion. (Key: ———— = typically developing child; – – – – = barefoot; --------- = in-shoe orthotic; – · – · – = shoes only.)

REFERENCES

Gage, J. (1991). *Gait analysis in cerebral palsy.* Oxford, England: MacKeith Press.

Perry, J. (1975). Cerebral palsy gait. In R.S. Samilison (Ed.), *Orthopedic aspects of cerebral palsy* (pp. 71–75). Philadelphia: Lippincott Raven.

Perry, J. (1992). *Gait analysis.* Thorofare, NJ: Slack Incorporated.

Rang, M. (1990). In W.W. Lovell & R.B. Winter (Eds.), *Pediatric orthopedics* (3rd ed., pp. 456–506).

Sutherland, D.H., Santi, M., & Abel, M.F. (1990). Treatment of stiff knee gait in cerebral palsy: A comparison by gait analysis of distal rectus femoris transfer versus proximal rectus release. *Journal of Pediatric Orthopedics, 10,* 433–441.

Winter, T.F., Gage, J.R., & Hicks, R. (1987). Gait patterns in spastic hemiplegia in children and young adults. *Journal of Bone and Joint Surgery, 69,* 437–441.

CHAPTER 9

Postsurgical Management of Cerebral Palsy

Sandy McGee,
Johanna E. Deitz Curry, and John P. Dormans

Orthopedic surgery is frequently part of the comprehensive management of cerebral palsy. Regardless of the type of surgery performed (e.g., soft-tissue releases or transfers, bony procedures such as osteotomies), the goals of the surgery and the postsurgical management plan need to be determined, understood, and agreed on by all of the members of the management team, especially the child and his or her family. If the child and his or her family do not understand and commit to the plan, then the desired outcome may not be achieved. Following surgery, the family and the child are as integral to decision making, planning, and goal setting as is the team of professionals.

Surgery is performed most often to prevent deformities (e.g., hip dislocation in nonambulatory children) or to improve functional abilities (e.g., ambulation, transfers, sitting); these improvements may enable the child with severe physical disabilities to use assistive technology devices, or they may make daily caregiving easier. In order to achieve the best results, surgical plans also should include provisions for postoperative rehabilitation (e.g., inpatient or outpatient therapy).

Decisions regarding postsurgical management should begin when the surgery is being planned. The amount and the timing of the surgical intervention, the type of immobilization, and the specifics of the rehabilitation course are determined by the team members, all of whom provide information to ensure that the best decisions are made. A wide variety of options are available, and multiple factors (e.g., the age and functional level of the child, the progression of the child's secondary deformities, the surgeon's experiences and preferences, the family's ability to participate in the postsurgical management) are considered when choosing the best rehabilitation plan for each child.

A large portion of the child's postsurgical rehabilitation is directed by the physical therapist. A thorough preoperative physical therapy (PT) assessment of the child's neuromotor and functional mobility status helps determine the type of postoperative immobilization that should be used. In addition, a PT assessment suggests appropriate assistive devices and assists in planning the rehabilitation phase.

PREOPERATIVE PT EVALUATION AND PARENT EDUCATION

A complete preoperative PT evaluation should be conducted within 2 weeks of the surgery. A PT evaluation includes assessment of posture, gait, range of motion (ROM), muscle strength, muscle tone, reflexes, balance and righting responses, gross motor development, and functional motor skills. Preoperative assessment provides baseline measurements of motor function, assists in setting postoperative expectations and goals, and aids in determining treatment strategies. Ideally, many aspects of the assessment (e.g., gait training) should be videotaped to allow for comparison at various intervals after surgery, thus enabling the therapist to measure the results of the surgical intervention and the rehabilitation.

A posture assessment looks at the alignment of the head, the shoulders, the spine, the pelvis, and the lower extremities while the child is sitting and standing. Asymmetries are noted as either dynamic or static. An assessment for scoliosis and kyphosis also should be done preoperatively during this assessment.

A gait assessment includes an evaluation of static and dynamic postures, stride and step length, cadence, heel strike and push-off, pelvic motion, and arm swing (see Chapter 8). The gait assessment should be conducted with and without the braces and adaptive devices that the child uses on a day-to-day basis. Formal gait laboratory analysis provides information regarding muscle activation and function and assists in planning specific surgical treatments.

A ROM assessment using a goniometer should be conducted following the standardized procedure. (Table 9.1 summarizes ROM testing procedures for the lower extremities.)

It is difficult to test muscle strength in isolated muscles of children with cerebral palsy. Strength testing can be conducted in a gross fashion by selecting

Table 9.1. Testing procedures for ROM in the lower extremities

Motion	Start position	Stabilize	End position	Precautions
Ankle dorsiflexion (relaxed gastroc)	Sitting or supine; knee flexed to 90 degrees; hold heel	At lower leg	Flex ankle toward anterior aspect of leg to end ROM	Keep ankle in neutral in varus or valgus position (flex at heel, not at midfoot)
Ankle dorsiflexion (gastroc at maximum stretch)	Supine; knee extended; hold heel	At lower leg	Flex ankle toward anterior aspect of leg to end ROM	Keep ankle in neutral in varus or valgus position (flex at heel, not at midfoot); do not allow knee to flex
Ankle plantar flexion	Supine; knee flexed or extended; hold heel	At lower leg	Flex ankle away from lower leg to end ROM	Measure at heel, not at midfoot
Knee flexion	Prone; knee extended; hold at lower leg	At buttocks on side tested	Flex knee to end ROM	Do not allow hip flexion or pelvic rotation on same side
Knee extension	Prone; knee flexed; toes off edge of mat; hold at lower leg	At buttocks on side tested	Extend knee to end ROM	Do not allow hip flexion or pelvic rotation on same side; hip at neutral rotation
Popliteal angle	Supine; hip flexed to 90 degrees; hold leg above and below knee	At pelvis and opposite leg	Extend knee to end ROM when opposite leg begins to lift or pelvis begins to rotate	Maintain opposite hip fully extended and pelvis in neutral; maintain hip on side tested at 90 degrees flexion
Hip abduction	Supine; hips and knees extended; hold leg slightly below knee	At pelvis and opposite leg	Move hip away from opposite leg to end ROM when pelvis begins to shift	Maintain hips fully extended; do *not* allow opposite leg to adduct; maintain neutral hip rotation

(continued)

195

Table 9.1. *(continued)*

Motion	Start position	Stabilize	End position	Precautions
Hip adduction	Supine; hips and knees extended; hold leg slightly below knee	At pelvis and opposite leg	Move hip toward opposite leg to end ROM when pelvis begins to shift	Maintain hips fully extended; do *not* allow opposite leg to abduct; maintain neutral hip rotation
Hip flexion	Supine; opposite hip extended and in neutral rotation; hold leg below knee	Opposite leg above the knee	Flex the hip until opposite leg begins to flex or pelvis rotates posterior to end ROM	Do not allow opposite leg to flex or pelvis to shift
Hip extension	Supine; leg off edge of mat; opposite leg slightly flexed at hip and pelvis in neutral; hold at upper leg	Opposite side at pelvis	Extend the hip to end ROM	Do not allow pelvis to shift laterally or anteriorly; maintain the opposite leg flexed at hip and knee to stabilize pelvis
Hip rotation	Supine or sitting; hip and knee flexed to 90 degrees; hold at lower leg	Opposite leg	Rotate the knee in either direction to end ROM	Do not allow weight shift to opposite side; keep pelvis in neutral

196

groups of muscles that function together in a specific movement, which should help the physical therapist to determine whether the muscle group is able to move the joint against gravity or is able to hold it in an antigravity position. If isolated joint movement is not achievable, then the therapist should determine whether the action can be performed in a synergy pattern. For example, when testing ankle dorsiflexion, the therapist should attempt to have the child dorsiflex his or her foot in a sitting position. If the child is unable to perform this exercise, then the therapist should resist hip flexion while the child is sitting and note whether the flexion is accompanied by dorsiflexion (i.e., total flexion of hip, knee, and ankle).

The therapist should test endurance and speed by having the child move by whatever means he or she typically uses for locomotion. Whether the child crawls, rolls, or walks, the distance and the time it takes for him or her to cover a specific distance should be recorded (the same motor skill and the same area should be used over an extended period of time to determine whether there are any changes in the child's endurance or speed). If the child is able to walk on a treadmill, then this can be a very good tool for providing objective data in terms of walking speed and distance.

The physical therapist should evaluate joint integrity and structure. As a result of the muscle imbalances common in children with cerebral palsy, many joints are susceptible to malformation over time. The hip is especially prone to develop subluxation or dislocation as a result of these imbalances (see Chapter 6). The knee joint is generally stable in children with spasticity, but flexion contractures frequently develop in both ambulators and nonambulators. In the ankle, the combination of abnormal forces of muscle pull and abnormal weight-bearing forces contributes to contracture or to deformity.

Assessment of skin integrity is important for children with cerebral palsy. Risk for skin breakdown must be monitored closely in children who wear orthotics, in children in casts, in children with poor nutrition who are nonambulatory, and in children in situations in which care may not be optimal. It is important to remember that children who are at risk for skin breakdown may not be able to shift weight or eliminate pressure from the skin that covers areas of bony prominences and may need assessment to identify areas that are susceptible to breakdown (see Chapter 4).

An assessment of gross motor skills should include changes of position, transfers, movement quality, and the status of functional mobility. Objective gross motor tests can be used to evaluate this information (see Chapter 12).

A neuromotor assessment using a standardized scale (e.g., Ashworth scale) should be used to evaluate muscle tone. Reflexes, balance, and righting responses also should be assessed at this time (see Chapters 2 and 12).

The physical therapist also should evaluate the postsurgical need for adaptive equipment. If adaptive equipment is used before surgery, then it may need to be modified following the procedure. If the child will be in a long-leg cast or a Spica cast, then he or she will need a wheelchair that has elevating legrests, a reclining back, and sufficient width to accommodate the excess hip abduction. If the child travels in a car seat, then it may be necessary for the caregiver to rent a hip Spica car seat from a medical supplier. After surgery, the child may need a hospital bed at home to ensure that optimal care and positioning are provided. In addition, if the child needs assistance in ambulation, then he or she should be evaluated for and trained in the use of crutches, canes, or a walker.

In order to determine the strategies that will optimize the child's functioning following the acute phase after surgery, the team develops a rehabilitation plan before the procedure. The child may be 1) discharged to the family home with a home program and later admitted to a rehabilitation facility on an inpatient basis or to a day hospital for rehabilitation, 2) immediately discharged from acute care to an inpatient rehabilitation facility, or 3) discharged to his or her family home with a home program, which is followed by outpatient therapy services. The option that is selected depends on the individual child's situation, needs, and resources. (The increasing prevalence of managed care also is a factor that influences this decision-making process.)

Physical therapists in the multidisciplinary clinic setting may find a cerebral palsy evaluation form (see Figure 9.1) useful for recording initial and subsequent assessments of the child's neuromotor status, muscle tone, strength, and ROM in the lower extremities. This form concludes with a list of problems and specific goals and recommendations to treat these problems, which can be addressed during the child's subsequent clinic visits.

Preoperative Teaching for the Parent or the Caregiver

Before surgery, it is important for the surgical and rehabilitation team to review the purpose and the goals of the surgery with the child and his or her caregivers. All the members of the team must work together toward the same goal. The primary caregivers should be informed about what to expect after the surgery, especially if the child is going home in casts or if he or she will have restrictions on usual activities. If necessary, parents need to receive instruction in cast care, positioning strategies, ROM exercises, safe transfer techniques, weight-bearing status, and adaptive rehabilitation equipment use.

IMMEDIATE POSTOPERATIVE PT INTERVENTION

Immediately following surgery (prior to discharge from acute care), therapy goals center around management of pain and spasms, positioning for comfort, gentle exercises (if appropriate), procuring or modifying adaptive equipment, and establishing a home exercise program in which the caregiver is the teacher who reinforces the instructions given during the preoperative assessment. (Table 9.2 lists common surgical procedures and PT interventions.)

Name _____ Date of birth _____

Date of evaluation _____

Diagnosis _____

Insurance _____

Insurance identification number _____

History_____

School _____ Level _____

Therapy service _____ Frequency _____

Behavior _____

Posture _____

Reflexes (circle all that apply)

Asymmetric tonic reflexes (ATNR)
Symmetric tonic neck reflex
  (STNR)
Tonic labyrinthine prone (TLP)
Palmar grasp

Tonic labyrinthine supine (TLS)
Startle
Positive support
Plantar grasp

Summary of reflexes:

Righting and equilibrium responses (circle all that apply)

1. Head righting
   Flexion
   Extension
   Lateral (right/left) _____

2. Trunk righting
   Anterior
   Posterior
   Lateral (right/left)
   Landau _____

3. Protective response
   Sitting (anterior, posterior)
   Right
   Left

   Lateral
   Forward parachute

4. Standing balance
   Forward
   Backward

   Left
   Lateral

_____
(continued)

Figure 9.1. PT evaluation form. Very useful for the physical therapist in the multidisciplinary setting for recording initial and subsequent assessments of neuromotor status, muscle tone, strength, and range of motion in children with cerebral palsy.

Figure 9.1. *(continued)*

5. Equilibrium response
   Prone   Quadruped
   Supine   Kneeling
   Sitting

Summary of righting and equilibrium responses:

Motor development skills

1. Supine
   Head centering   Reciprocal kick
   Hands to midline (right/left)   Pelvis rounded

2. Prone
   On elbows   Reaching
   On extended   Pivot
   Crawls

3. Rolling
   Supine to side   Supine to prone
   Prone to supine

4. Sitting
   Assumes   Short sits
   Maintains   Long sits
   W sits   Plays
   Ring sits   Head control in pull to sit
   Pulls with arms in pull to sit

5. Quadruped
   Assumes   Creeps forward
   Maintains   Assumes sitting

6. Kneeling
   Assumes   Pulls to kneel at support
   Maintains

7. Standing
   Pulls to stand at support   Stands at support
   Leg disassociation   Maintains
   Cruises   Stands alone

8. Walking
   One hand held
   Creeps up stairs (on uneven surfaces)

(continued)

Figure 9.1. *(continued)*

Summary of motor development skills:

Gross motor developmental level:

Gait analysis

Gait _____

Assistive device _____

Adaptive equipment (circle all that apply)

Walker	Stroller
Wheelchair	Bath chair
Braces	Lift
Other _____	

Current issues and problems:

Recommendation and plan:

Additional comments:

(continued)

Figure 9.1. *(continued)*

Left			Lower extremities	Right		
Range of motion	Strength	Tone	Motion/muscle groups	Range of motion	Strength	Tone
			Hip flexion			
			Hip extension (Thomas test)			
			Hip abduction (Knee/hip extended)			
			Hip adduction			
			Hip internal position			
			Hip external rotation			
			Knee flexion			
			Knee extension (prone)			
			Popliteal angle			
			Ankle dorsiflexion (knee flexion)			
			Ankle dorsiflexion (knee extend)			
			Ankle plantarflexion			

Key to grading muscle tone: 0 = hypotonic; 1 = normal; 2 = mild hypotonic; 3 = moderate hypotonic; 4 = severe hypotonic; 5 = rigid; 6 = fluctuating tone.

_____

Therapist

Following surgery, pain and spasms are managed during acute care with medications, and an experienced pain team is particularly helpful for assisting with pain management in the early postoperative period. Therapy interventions for pain management include positioning to decrease spasms, teaching relaxation techniques, gentle alternating movements, rocking, gently massaging muscles, and applying ice.

Positioning strategies are established to address issues of pain relief and muscle spasm, to provide gentle stretch to tight muscles, and to optimize function. Children who are unable to initiate position changes should be repositioned every

Table 9.2. Common surgical procedures and PT interventions

Problem	Procedure	Preoperative PT	Postoperative immobilization	Postoperative PT	Rehabilitation phase
Tight heel cords; varus or valgus ankle; muscle imbalance at foot	Tendon Achilles lengthening (TAL); posterior tibialis lengthening; peroneal lengthening; split posterior tibialis transfer (SPTT)	Assessment with video-taping; crutch training; cast care instructions; home program	Short-leg cast for 4 weeks; full-weight bearing with assistive device; measure for braces after surgery (4 weeks); wear bivalve cast until braces fabricated	Discharge to home after 24 hours; review gait training; review home stretching	Outpatient basis: stretch hamstrings, hip flexors, and adductors; gait training; strengthening; home exercise program
Adductor contractures; scissoring of legs; hamstring contractures; hip flexor contractures; excessive hip internal rotation; hip subluxation less than 60%	Adductor longus release; gracilis tenotomy; medial and lateral hamstring tenotomy or proximal release; psoas release	Assessment with video-taping; cast care instructions; positioning instructions; arrange for adaptive equipment needs (e.g., wheelchair)	*Options* <ul><li>Spica cast with spreader bar</li><li>Bilateral long-leg casts with or without spreader bar</li><li>Bilateral knee immobilizers with abduction wedge (SLC if TALs also done)</li></ul>	*For 1 and 2* <ul><li>Review cast care, ROM, and positioning with family</li><li>Modify wheelchair and other adaptive equipment</li></ul> *For 3* <ul><li>PT initiated from first day</li></ul>	Manage pain and spasms; gentle passive ROM; encourage active ROM; muscle strengthening; positioning; transfers; equipment modification; ambulation training; home exercise program
Extension deformity at knee; spastic quadriceps femoris	Rectus transfer	Assessment with video-taping; review ROM exercises; gait training with assistive device	Long-leg knee immobilizer; full-weight bearing	Review ROM exercises; modify adaptive equipment; gait training with knee immobilizers	Manage pain and spasms; *Variables* <ul><li>No ROM 4 weeks</li><li>Early mobilization 1 week (gentle active assisted); ROM at knee; ROM at hip and ankle; strengthening at hip and ankle; gait training</li></ul>

(continued)

203

Table 9.2. *(continued)*

Problem	Procedure	Preoperative PT	Postoperative immobilization	Postoperative PT	Rehabilitation phase
Unstable foot in medial-lateral plane with heel cord tightness; fixed pes valgus	Subtalar arthrodesis; triple arthrodesis	Assessment with video-taping; review ROM at other joints; arrange for wheelchair; review cast care	Long-leg cast for 6 weeks cut to short-leg cast for additional 6–10 weeks; nonweight bearing until cast off; measure for brace and bivalve cast	Cast instructions; check out wheelchair	Initiate at 6 weeks post-operatively; ROM at lower extremities; improve strength; ambulation training that may need knee splint for support
Excess tibial torsion	Distal tibia-fibula derotation osteotomy	Assessment with video-taping; review ROM and transfers; arrange for or modify existing wheel-chair; review cast care	Long-leg cast cut to short-leg cast at 6 weeks or short-leg cast until healing; bivalve cast when healed; measure for braces; weight bearing as tolerated when cast off; splint at knee into extension for initial ambulation and sleeping	Assess for pain and spasms; review cast care; check out wheelchair; gait training with assistive device	When long cast cut to short, stretching to hip and knee flexors; strengthening to hip and knee muscles; *When cast removed* gentle stretch to ankle muscles; ambulation training; no weight bearing without brace

204

Hip dislocation; coxa valga; acetabular dysplasia	Femoral osteotomy (e.g., varus derotation osteotomy [VDRO]); pelvic/acetabular osteotomy	Assessment with video-taping; teach cast care, positioning, transfers, and ROM; arrange for new or modify existing wheelchair	*Options* • Spica cast with spreader bar • Bilateral long-leg casts with or without spreader bar • Bilateral knee immobilizers with abduction wedge (SLC if TALs also done)	*For 1 and 2* Review cast care, ROM, and positioning with family; modify wheelchair and other adaptive equipment; review management of pain and spasms *For 3* PT initiated from second day	Manage pain and spasms; gentle passive ROM; encourage active ROM; muscle strengthening; positioning; transfers; equipment modification; ambulation training; home exercise program
Scoliosis	Spinal instrumentation with or without posterior fusion; anterior fusion if severe	Assessment with video-taping; teach positioning, transfers, and ROM; arrange for wheelchair and, if needed, modify existing wheelchair	Bracing only if bone integrity is not optimal	*Review transfers* No rotation or bending at spine; review positioning; manage pain and spasms; check out equipment	Permanent modifications to wheelchair to accommodate change in posture; stretch to iliopsoas, adductors; positioning for comfort and to stretch tight muscles

ROM, range of motion.

2 hours to prevent excess pressure over bony prominences. In order to stretch hip flexors, children who have knee immobilizers or long-leg casts need to spend periods of time in the prone position (see Figure 9.2). Ideal prone time is between 30 and 60 minutes, three to four times a day. Positioning in the sidelying position often assists in decreasing spasms and promotes reaching (see Figure 9.3). Supine is the least functional position.

Gentle ROM exercises assist in maintaining joint mobility. Rhythmic arcs of motion can promote relaxation and decrease muscle spasms. It is important for the therapist to remember to check with the surgeon before moving joints at surgical sites.

It always should be verified that the child—in addition to his or her caregivers—knows his or her weight-bearing status. If the child is not able to bear weight on the lower extremities after surgery, then he or she (and his or her family) will need instructions on basic wheelchair skills (e.g., folding, propelling, safety, transport). If the child is able to bear his or her full weight and is able to ambulate, then the therapist should assess the child's safety during walking and provide an assistive device if one has not been given to the child during the preoperative visit. If the child has crutches, then the therapist should review crutch training, placing particular emphasis on using them on stairs and on uneven surfaces.

To ensure for proper fit and to address safety concerns, the physical therapist should review all of the equipment that has been ordered and delivered to the hospital for the child. The therapist also should instruct the child's caregiver(s) in the use of this equipment. Manual wheelchairs with elevating legrests and

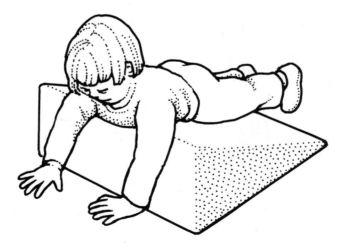

Figure 9.2. Child in prone position. A wedge can be used with a child to promote hip and knee extension. (From Pellegrino, L. [1997]. Cerebral palsy. In M.L. Batshaw [Ed.], *Children with disabilities* [4th ed., p. 512]. Baltimore: Paul H. Brookes Publishing Co.; reprinted by permission.)

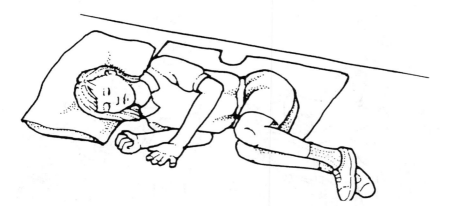

Figure 9.3. Child in sidelying position, which promotes relaxation and assists in reducing muscle spasms. (From Scull, S.A. [1996]. Lifting and transfer techniques. In L.A. Kurtz, P.W. Dowrick, S.E. Levy, & M.L. Batshaw [Eds.], *Children's Seashore House handbook of developmental disabilities: Resources for interdisciplinary care* [p. 281]. Rockville, MD: Aspen Publishers, Inc.; reprinted by permission.)

reclining backs should be adjusted with the child in the chair. The wheelchair must have a safety belt, anti-tippers, and working brakes. Caregivers should learn how to recline the back, elevate and adjust the legrests, position the child properly, and fold the wheelchair for transport.

Appendix A at the end of this chapter provides guidelines for home care following surgery; the physical therapist should review these guidelines prior to the child's surgery to ensure that caregivers can properly lift and transfer the child (see Figures 9.4 and 9.5), position the child, and implement ROM activities and exercises that are appropriate for the child. The therapist also should watch the caregiver(s) perform the various activities that have been recommended; watching the caregivers as they practice the exercise with the child will enable the therapist to provide feedback and to review any contraindications to certain joint motions, positions, or weight bearing. If the child will wear casts following the surgery, then the therapist also should review cast care with the child and the child's family.

A follow-up therapy appointment should be scheduled before the surgery to review the child's progress, to modify the home program, and to provide direct outpatient PT services. The physical therapist should give the caregiver(s) his or her name and telephone number in writing in case the caregiver(s) has any specific questions or concerns.

REHABILITATION COURSE

The timing of the rehabilitative phase (i.e., following the acute postoperative period) is dependent on the surgical procedure(s) and the type of immobilization

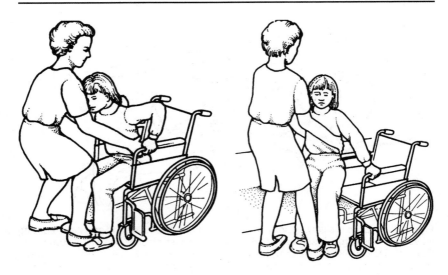

Figure 9.4. Stand-pivot transfer. The caregiver assists the child to stand, turn, and sit down on the bed. (From Scull, S.A. [1996]. Lifting and transfer techniques. In L.A. Kurtz, P.W. Dowrick, S.E. Levy, & M.L. Batshaw [Eds.], *Children's Seashore House handbook of developmental disabilities: Resources for interdisciplinary care* [p. 273]. Rockville, MD: Aspen Publishers, Inc.; reprinted by permission.)

chosen. For the child who is placed in a Spica cast or a long-leg cast(s), the essential part of rehabilitation begins after cast removal. For the child in removable (i.e., bivalve) casts or knee immobilizers, rehabilitation may begin as soon as 2 days after surgery or when the child is able to tolerate the program (see Appendix B at the end of this chapter). Rehabilitation may occur in an inpatient rehabilitation facility, in a day hospital setting, in the community (on an outpatient basis), or in any combination of these alternatives. For the child with transfer and/or functional mobility goals, a 2- to 3-week period of daily, intensive therapy is preferred (either in an inpatient or in a day hospital setting) over a less intensive outpatient program.

Regardless of the timing and the location of the rehabilitation, the goals of the postsurgical rehabilitation remain the same:

- Maintain the correction of the deformity and prevent its recurrence.
- Resume or improve the child's functional level.

Maintain the Correction of the Deformity and Prevent its Recurrence

Regardless of the type of immobilization used following surgery, an important aspect of the rehabilitation phase is to maintain and sometimes to increase the ROM gains achieved during surgery. This is accomplished by positioning, splinting, and therapeutic activities.

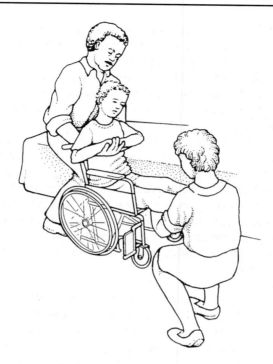

Figure 9.5. Two-person lift. When the child is unable to stand, one person lifts the child's upper body and a second person lifts the child's legs to transfer him or her out of the wheelchair. (From Scull, S.A. [1996]. Lifting and transfer techniques. In L.A. Kurtz, P.W. Dowrick, S.E. Levy, & M.L. Batshaw [Eds.], *Children's Seashore House handbook of developmental disabilities: Resources for interdisciplinary care* [p. 280]. Rockville, MD: Aspen Publishers, Inc.; reprinted by permission.)

Positioning   Prone and standing positions may be used to stretch hip flexors; maintain knee extension and ankle dorsiflexion; and, if combined with an abduction brace, stretch hip adductors. If the child can be positioned with his or her ankles in a neutral dorsiflexion/plantarflexion position and with his or her hips in neutral rotation, then the prone position is usually recommended for sleeping. This usually requires adjusting the child's position on the mattress so that his or her feet can hang over the edge. Prone carts, prone standers, and mobile prone standers enable the child to take advantage of the benefits of the prone position as well as promote the child's interaction with other people and his or her environment.

Long sitting is encouraged in order to maintain or to increase hamstring length. If the child initially is unable to achieve 90 degrees of hip flexion with his or her knees extended, then sitting on a downward sloping wedge in the long-sitting position will enable him or her to maintain a neutral pelvis and an erect spine.

When combined with knee immobilizers to maintain full knee extension, the Nada chair (see Figure 9.6) also can be used to stretch the hamstrings in the long-sitting position. The strap behind the pelvis prevents the pelvis from tilting posteriorly and ensures that the hamstrings are put on maximal stretch.

Splinting   Following surgery, splints are an important adjunct to therapy because they help to maintain the child's increased ROM and to protect the surgical site. In order to maintain the child's ROM and to prevent overstretch of the heel cord, ankle-foot orthoses (AFOs) are prescribed after any surgery involving the foot, the ankle, or the lower leg. The type of lengthening, the functional needs of the child, the presence or absence of previous surgical procedures, and the preferred device affect this decision-making process. For ambulatory children with cerebral palsy, some institutions use solid AFOs 24 hours a day (except for during therapy and hygiene) for a minimum of 6 months after heel cord lengthening or tendon transfers. If appropriate, after 6 months of rehabilitation, the child may be prescribed molded ankle-foot orthoses (MAFOs) with an articulating ankle.

Following surgery at the hip or the knee, a hip abduction orthosis and/or knee immobilizers may be used to maintain the child's ROM and to manage muscle spasms (see Figure 9.7). The use of the hip abduction orthosis and knee immobilizers varies depending on both the type of surgery as well as the surgeon's or the therapist's preference. Following surgery, the hip abduction orthosis is usually worn 24 hours a day for the first 3–4 weeks. After the first month, the hip abduction orthosis generally is worn all night for at least 12 months,

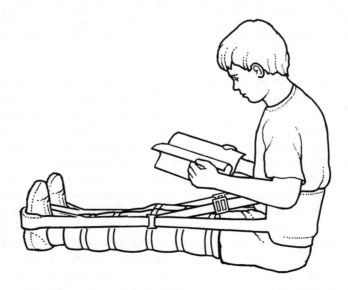

Figure 9.6.   Nada chair. The child's hamstrings are stretched and the pelvis is maintained in neutral alignment using the Nada chair and knee immobilizers.

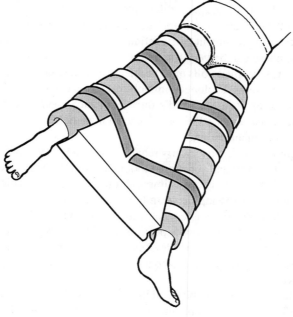
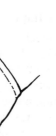

Figure 9.7. Child in prone position with abduction wedge and knee immobilizers.

especially if the child is in a growth spurt. The knee immobilizers generally are worn at night but may be used during the day if the child is experiencing flexor spasms or may be used during gait training until the child's quadriceps are sufficiently strong to actively extend the knee.

Therapeutic Activities Therapeutic activities for children who are not placed in casts following surgery begin 2 days after the procedure; for children who are placed in casts, ROM activities begin on the day of cast removal. The initial focus of these ROM activities is to increase the child's tolerance to passive movement and to encourage active movement, particularly in the muscles that have been lengthened. A heated pool is one of the best environments in which to work on ROM: The warm water relaxes the muscles and the buoyancy of the water supports the limbs, making movement easier. The pool can be used immediately after cast removal; however, for the child entering rehabilitation immediately following his or her surgery, incisions should be healed before he or she exercises in the pool (usually 10–14 days after surgery).

It is important to take precautions to avoid overstretching muscles that have been lengthened. For this reason, active ROM exercises in the rehabilitation phase are more encouraged than is passive manual stretching.

Resume or Improve the Child's Functional Level

Postsurgical rehabilitation of the child with cerebral palsy is a major investment of time and hard work on the part of the child and his or her family. As the child regains strength and learns to incorporate new patterns of movement into functional activities, improvement can continue for as long as 1 year. The early rehabilitation phase can be very frustrating for the child and his or her family because previously learned skills must be relearned using longer, weaker muscles and new motor patterns. Prolonged immobilization in casts also can cause secondary disuse atrophy in the child's muscles, which can weaken them even more than the actual surgery. Preoperative teaching will help the family prepare for this aspect of rehabilitation.

Therapeutic activities in the early rehabilitation phase focus on active ROM, strengthening, balance, and functional mobility. Lengthening a muscle weakens the muscle's strength, and it is important to start with activities that work the muscles without stressing them. Initially, movement in gravity-assisted or gravity-minimized positions is encouraged; as the muscles become stronger, movement progresses to antigravity positions. Stability in a position is achieved before mobility occurs. Assistive devices that were previously not necessary may be necessary as the child learns to incorporate new movement patterns into functional skills.

The child who has severe physical impairment without functional mobility goals has different goals for rehabilitation than does the potential ambulator. A therapeutic plan typically focuses on comfort with position changes as well as on resuming the ability to sit comfortably in a wheelchair during feeding and interacting within the environment. Because the surgical procedure usually results in a change in the child's posture and physical status, all of the child's adaptive equipment must be assessed for appropriateness. For example, the child who has had a unilateral femoral varus derotation osteotomy to correct a dislocated hip will have shortening of the operated leg and may need to have a split-depth seat in his or her wheelchair to properly position the pelvis and the lower body. Children who have had a spinal fusion with instrumentation to correct scoliosis may be more difficult for caregivers to transfer because of a rigid back, and the caregivers may need to obtain a patient lift (e.g., Hoyer lift) for use in the home.

Once the child is able to integrate into his or her regular daily routine, the intensity of therapy services can be reduced from daily therapy sessions to two to three sessions per week on an outpatient basis. If the child receives PT as part of a school program, then the focus is usually on meeting educationally based needs rather than on meeting medical rehabilitative needs. Outpatient PT services in a rehabilitation setting are recommended in addition to school therapy until the child has maximized functional gains.

SUMMARY

A successful outcome following orthopedic surgery for the child with cerebral palsy is enhanced when the procedure and postsurgical management are planned and carried out by a team, including professionals and the child's family. A comprehensive presurgical assessment can assist in goal setting and in planning the postoperative program. Caregiver teaching, which is started in the preoperative phase, is essential to ensure compliance with the postsurgical plan. A period of intensive PT services following the surgery will allow the child to jump-start the rehabilitative process, which can continue for 6–12 months after the surgery.

BIBLIOGRPAHY

Atar, D., Grant, A.D., Bash, J., & Lehman, W.B. (1995). Combined hip surgery in cerebral palsy patients. *American Journal of Orthopedics, 24*(1), 52–55.

Bleck, E. (1987). *Orthopedic management in cerebral palsy.* Philadelphia: J.B. Lippincott.

Campbell, S.K. (Ed.). (1991). *Pediatric neurologic physical therapy.* New York: Churchill Livingstone.

Campbell, S.K. (Ed.). (1994). *Physical therapy for children.* Philadelphia: W.B. Saunders.

Dormans, J.P. (1993). Orthopaedic management of the child with cerebral palsy. *Pediatric Clinics of North America, 40*(3), 645–657.

Etnyre, B., Chambers, C.S., Scarborough, M.H., & Cain, T.E. (1993). Preoperative and postoperative assessment of surgical intervention for equinus gait in children with cerebral palsy. *Journal of Pediatric Orthopedics, 13*(1), 24–31.

Fernandez, J.E., & Pitetti, K.H. (1993). Training of ambulatory individuals with cerebral palsy. *Archives of Physical Medicine and Rehabilitation, 74,* 468–472.

Girolami, G.L., & Hertz, K. (1990). Early mobilization and postsurgical management after hamstring or gracilis muscle release in children with cerebral palsy. *Physical Therapy: Topics in Pediatrics, 8.*

Greiner, B.M., Czerniecki, J.M., & Deitz, J.C. (1993). Gait parameters of children with spastic diplegia: A comparison of effects of posterior and anterior walkers. *Archives of Physical Medicine and Rehabilitation, 74,* 381–384.

Harryman, S.E. (1992). Lower extremity surgery for children with cerebral palsy: Physical therapy management. *Physical Therapy, 72*(1), 16–24.

Hazelwood, M.E., Brown, J.K., Towe, P.J., & Salter, P.M. (1994). The use of therapeutic electrical stimulation in the treatment of hemiplegic cerebral palsy. *Developmental Medicine and Child Neurology, 36*(8), 661–673.

Hoffinger, S.A., Rab, G.T., & Abou-Ghaida, H. (1993). Hamstrings in cerebral palsy crouch gait. *Journal of Pediatric Orthopedics, 13*(6), 722–726.

Kaufman, H.H., Bodensteiner, J., Burkart, B., Gutmann, L., Kopitnik, T., Hochberg, V., Loy, N., Cox-Gasner, J., & Hobbs, G. (1994). Treatment of spastic gait in cerebral palsy. *West Virginia Medical Journal, 90*(5), 190–192.

King, E.M., Gooch, J.L., Howell, G.H., Peters, M.L., Bloswick, D.S., & Brown, D.R. (1993). Evaluation of the hip extensor tricycle in improving gait in children with cerebral palsy. *Developmental Medicine and Child Neurology, 35,* 1048–1054.

Miller, F., & Bacharach, S.J. (1995). *Cerebral palsy: A complete guide for caregivers.* Baltimore: The Johns Hopkins University Press.

Molnar, G.E. (1985). Cerebral palsy. In M.E. Molnar (Ed.), *Pediatric rehabilitation*. Baltimore: Williams & Wilkins.

Pellegrino, L. (1997). Cerebral palsy. In M.L. Batshaw (Ed.), *Children with disabilities* (4th ed., pp. 499–528). Baltimore: Paul H. Brookes Publishing Co.

Rang, M. (1990). Cerebral palsy. In T. Raymond (Ed.), *Pediatric orthopaedics* (pp. 465–506). Philadelphia: J.B. Lippincott.

Rose, S.A., Ounpuu, S., & DeLuca, P.A. (1991). Strategies for the assessment of pediatric gait in the clinical setting. *Physical Therapy, 71,* 961–980.

Scull, S.A. (1996). Lifting and transfer techniques. In L.A. Kurtz, P.W. Dowrick, S.E. Levy, & M.L. Batshaw (Eds.), *Children's Seashore House handbook of developmental disabilities: Resources for interdisciplinary care* (pp. 269–293). Rockville, MD: Aspen Publishers, Inc.

Sutherland, D.H., & Davids, J.R. (1993). Common gait abnormalities of the knee in cerebral palsy: A review. *Clinical Orthopaedics and Related Research, 288,* 39–47.

Thompson, D. (1994). Orthopedic aspects of cerebral palsy: A review. *Current Opinion in Pediatrics, 6,* 94–98.

Wilson, J. (1991). Cerebral palsy. In S.K. Campbell (Ed.), *Pediatric neurologic physical therapy* (2nd ed., pp. 301–360). New York: Churchill Livingstone.

Guidelines for Home Care Following Surgery

Patient _____ Therapist _____

Date _____ Telephone number _____

Equipment/braces

Molded ankle-foot orthoses (MAFOs)

- Check skin daily for redness, which indicates improper fit.
- Wear at all times except during hygiene and therapy.

Knee immobilizers

- When applying, make sure knee is straight and leg is not rotated (i.e., toes point straight up).
- Pull straps tight enough so that knee cannot bend but not so tight that circulation is cut off.
- Keep legs straight when sitting (i.e., elevate legrests of wheelchair).
- Wear at all times except during hygiene and therapy.

Abduction splint/wedge

- Use at all times except during hygiene, therapy, and standing.

Casts

- Check toes daily to make sure skin is warm, child can move toes, child can feel you touch his or her toes, child has no numbness or tingling in toes, and toes are normal size and color.

(continued)

Guidelines for Home Care Following Surgery *(continued)*

- Keep cast dry.
- Keep skin around cast edges clean and dry.
- Elevate legs with pillows when sitting or lying on back or side in bed.
- Change child's position at least every 2 hours.

Prone/supine stander
- Hips and knees should be straight; legs should not be rotated.
- Make sure straps are tight enough to hold child in proper position but not so tight that circulation is cut off.

Specific instructions for equipment/braces:

Positioning (should be changed every 30–45 minutes; not necessary at night)
Prone lying (i.e., on stomach)
- Perform with feet off edge of supporting surface.

Long sitting (i.e., sitting with knees straight)
Standing erect
- Perform in prone or supine stander.

Sleep position
- Lying on stomach is preferred.

Specific instructions for positioning:

Transfers (should use gait belt for all transfers)
- Use wheelchair to move to and from bed or chair.
- Remove legrest closest to transfer surface.
- Place wheelchair as close as possible to a 90-degree angle to transfer surface.
- Lock brakes.
- Swing away other legrest.
- Move child to edge of chair by holding under shoulders and assisting to shift weight to one side and move opposite hip forward.
- Position child's feet flat on the floor.
- Stand in front of child with your hands behind child's back, holding on to gait belt.

(continued)

Guidelines for Home Care Following Surgery *(continued)*

- Bend your knees.
- Tell child to lean forward and push up on armrests to stand.
- Pivot your body and child's body so child is standing parallel to transfer surface.
- Tell child to lean forward and reach back for surface.
- Slowly lower child to surface.

Specific instructions for transfers:

Transporting in car

- Transfer child to seat of car as above and assist child with rotating legs into car (if child is small and rides in toddler car seat, lift child into car seat as described in section on "Lifting/carrying").
- Fasten child's seat belt.
- Fold wheelchair and place in trunk or back seat of car.
- Transfer child out of car, rotate legs out of car, and perform transfer as described in section on "Transfers."

Specific instructions for transporting in car:

Lifting/carrying

- Place one arm under child's thighs and other arm around child's trunk.
- Bend your knees and lift, and keep child close to your body.
- Keep your back straight.
- Complete lift before turning.
- Slowly lower child back down by bending your knees, and keep your back straight.

Specific lifting/carrying instructions:

(continued)

Guidelines for Home Care Following Surgery (*continued*)

Wheelchair mobility (guidelines)
- Always fasten seat belt.
- Be sure child's arms are away from wheels.
- Be sure feet rest on footrests.

Ramps
- Always be sure back of wheelchair is on down side of ramp.

Curbs (up)
- Approach curb in forward direction.
- Tilt wheelchair backward.
- Move wheelchair forward and place front wheels on curb.
- Lift up on handles to bring back wheels onto curb.

Curbs (down)
- Back wheelchair to curb.
- Roll back wheels off curb.
- Keep wheelchair tilted and pull it backward until footrests clear curb.
- Slowly lower front wheels to ground.

Specific instructions for wheelchair mobility:

Walking
- Be sure child wears MAFOs and knee immobilizers for walking.
- Be sure to use appropriate assistive device (e.g., posterior walker, crutches).
- Be sure child wears gait belt.
- Be sure to stand behind and slightly to one side of child while holding on to gait belt.

Specific instructions for walking:

Stairs
- Be sure child is carried either up and down stairs or, if able, bumps up and down stairs (i.e., sitting on stairs—with child's back toward top of stairs—the arms are used to move up and down stairs) with supervision or assistance as needed.

(continued)

Guidelines for Home Care Following Surgery (*continued*)

- Be sure to transfer child to and from stairs (as described in "Transfers" guidelines).

Specific instructions for stairs:

Home exercises

- Be sure to use range of motion (ROM) exercises.
- Other exercises:

Other instructions:

Postsurgery Protocol for Children with Removable Casts or Knee Immobilizers

WEEK 1

GOAL   Increase comfort for ROM exercises by using gentle, passive, and active ROM positioning. If pain and/or spasms are present, medication also may be used.

Equipment   Knee immobilizers and abduction wedge should be applied immediately following the operation and worn at all times, except during hygiene and therapy. If tendon Achilles lengthenings (TALs) were performed, the child should wear either short-leg casts or AFOs at all times (with the previously mentioned exceptions).

PT should be provided twice a day, should begin 2 days after the child's operation, and should consist of the following:

1. Positioning
   a. Prone: The child should be placed on prone cart or bed for 1–2 hours at a time and, if he or she can tolerate, throughout the night. Because the child's ankles are dorsiflexed, adjustments must be made so that his or her feet hang off the supporting surface.

b. Sitting: The child should be seated in a wheelchair that has elevating legrests and a reclining back. The goal of therapy is to promote hip flexion to 90 degrees without posterior pelvic tilt and with the knees fully extended. This may not be achieved for as long as 10 days following surgery.

c. Standing: With the use of casts, AFOs, and knee immobilizers—without the abduction wedge—the child may be able to stand with a prone stander, on a tilt table, or with the parallel bars. The goal of therapy is for the child to stand for at least 30 minutes, twice a day.

2. ROM: Gentle passive ROM is used to maintain the child's range of nonreleased muscles and to gradually increase his or her range of surgically released/lengthened muscles. This therapy must be administered slowly and within the child's tolerance.

3. Strengthening: Active and/or active-assisted ROM therapy to the child's lower extremities should begin when he or she is ready (typically toward the end of the first week following surgery) and should encourage the child to start moving again. Trunk and hip extension strengthening activities (e.g., typically lying prone over a ball) are encouraged because children who have abduction or hamstring length limitations typically have poor back and hip extension.

4. Mobility: Bed mobility, especially rolling and supine-to-sit transfers, should begin as soon as the child can tolerate the therapy.

WEEK 2

GOAL Increase passive ROM in released muscles and improve strength in all trunk and lower-extremity muscle groups.

Equipment The child should continue to wear knee immobilizers at all times, except during hygiene and therapy. If the child's hip abduction range is adequate, the abduction wedge should be removed when he or she is sitting in a wheelchair. However, the immobilizers should continue to be worn when on a prone cart or lying in bed. The wearing schedule for AFOs is determined by the type of surgery performed and the child's heel cord length.

PT should be continued to be provided twice a day, and an emphasis should be placed on the following:

1. Positioning

a. Prone: The child should be positioned on a prone cart or a bed for 1–2 hours at a time. A wedge (placed under the child's chest) and a weight (placed on his or her buttocks) should be used to increase hip extension. The child should be positioned in prone position for sleeping if he or she can tolerate it.

b. Sitting: The child should be placed in a wheelchair with his or her legs elevated. By the middle of the second week (at the latest), the child's back should be fully upright with his or her hips at 90 degrees. The child also should be encouraged to perform long sitting on a solid surface, and it is important that knee immobilizers be worn during this exercise.

c. Standing: Similar to the exercises performed during week 1, the child should continue standing twice a day for 30–45 minutes in a prone stander, a supine stander, or a tilt table.

2. ROM: As the child's pain decreases, passive ROM exercises should become more aggressive, and active and active-assisted exercises should be performed on all of the child's lower-extremity muscles. Full passive ROM of released muscles should be achieved by the end of the second week.

3. Strengthening: In addition to the trunk and the hip extension strengthening activities initiated during the first week, activities to strengthen the child's quadriceps should be added to the program. These exercises should include open-chain as well as closed-chain activities; the physical therapist should take the proper precautions to prevent knee hyperextension.

4. Mobility: Exercises that aim to achieve bed mobility and supine-to-sit transfers should continue if the child has not yet achieved them. Sit-to-stand transfers should be initiated only in therapy. Standing and walking with knee immobilizers and AFOs (or short-leg casts) and assistive devices may begin when the child is ready.

WEEK 3

GOAL Improve strength and increase functional mobility in all lower-extremity muscle groups.

Equipment The child should continue to use knee immobilizers at all times, except during hygiene and therapy. The abduction wedge should be used primarily when the child is in prone position or is in bed. If TALs were performed, the child should continue to wear AFOs or casts at all times.

PT should continue twice a day with the emphasis being placed on the following:

1. Positioning
   a. Prone: The child should be positioned in prone position for 30–60 minutes three times a day and when he or she is sleeping.
   b. Sitting: The child should be seated in a wheelchair and should be wearing knee immobilizers. His or her legs should be elevated, and his or her hips should be flexed to 90 degrees. If the child's hamstring length is adequate, he or she should sit without the knee immobilizers

and should flex his or her knees to 90 degrees for short periods of time (usually during meals). Long sitting on a solid surface with a neutral pelvis, with or without back support, also should continue.

   c.   Standing: The child should be placed in a prone stander for 30–45 minutes every day. If he or she is able, standing with the support of a reverse walker with trunk and hip extension is encouraged for short periods of time several times per day.

2.   ROM: Full passive ROM should have been achieved by this point; as a result, active or active-assisted motion against gravity throughout the full range should be emphasized.

3.   Strengthening: Trunk and hip strengthening exercises should continue. Strengthening of all of the lower-extremity muscles (agonists and antagonists) is encouraged, and particular emphasis should be placed on the quadriceps and the gluteals. Closed-chain activities may be used to improve grading and endurance.

4.   Mobility: For the child who has ambulation goals, walking becomes more important during the third week. Use of an assistive device (e.g., a reverse walker) is recommended to encourage a pattern that incorporates trunk and hip extension. Single-limb stance activities are introduced during this time. For all standing and ambulation activities, AFOs should be worn; however, the knee immobilizers may be removed for short periods of time if quadriceps strength and endurance are adequate. For the child who does not have ambulation goals, the emphasis should be placed on transitions into and out of sitting and independent sitting activities.

CHAPTER 10

Neurosurgical Treatment of Spasticity

Ann-Christine Duhaime and Shirley Albinson-Scull

The management of the physical symptoms associated with congenital or acquired central nervous system (CNS) impairment has a long history in the field of neurosurgery. Interventions to improve outcome in the motor realm range from surgical treatment of hydrocephalus to more direct treatment of spasticity or movement disorders. A variety of surgical procedures that can be performed on the brain and the spinal cord for the direct treatment of spasticity are still in use in specific clinical situations; these procedures are discussed in detail in this chapter.

Since the mid-1980s, the mainstay of neurosurgical treatment for certain patterns of spasticity in some children and adults has been selective dorsal rhizotomy (SDR). This procedure, which involves sectioning selected sensory rootlets at the level of the cauda equina (i.e., bundle of spinal nerve fibers that comprises the roots of all the spinal nerves below the first lumbar vertebrae), requires that children who have cerebral palsy be carefully selected and that a team approach to preoperative evaluation and postoperative care be used. For some children, SDR offers significant long-term improvement in spasticity and can improve functional mobility as well as ease the management of care for these children. This chapter focuses on the use of SDR for the treatment of spasticity and surveys other neurosurgical treatments for motor dysfunction.

HISTORY OF DORSAL RHIZOTOMY

The development of dorsal rhizotomy as a treatment for spasticity is of particular interest in the medical field because it is one of a few operations that arose directly from basic scientific research on animals. In 1898, while studying the pathophysiology of spasticity in cats, Sherrington, a physiologist, found that transection (i.e., cutting across) of the spinal cord or the brain stem resulted in the development of spasticity (i.e., increased tone with velocity dependence and exaggerated reflexes). Sherrington also found that this increased tone could be abolished by transecting the dorsal or the sensory roots below the level of the spinal cord transection. This elimination of increased tone was possible because the spasticity in the cats was in large part caused by overactivity of the typical reflex arc between the peripheral nerves and the spinal cord. This overactivity occurred because the signals that typically arise from the brain, which inhibit the reflex arc, were interrupted. In terms of children with cerebral palsy, perinatal brain damage causes spasticity in the same manner as it was caused in Sherrington's cats: The brain damage in children with cerebral palsy reduces the typical amount of tone inhibition coming from the brain, and, similar to Sherrington's cats, cutting the children's sensory nerves restores a more typical balance to the overactive reflex arc and results in more normal tone.

In 1913, Foerster conducted the same procedure as Sherrington—cutting the sensory nerve roots—on human children with severe spasticity. The operation was successful in reducing spasticity, but, because the sensory nerves were cut, it also led to a loss of sensation, which in many children was associated with symptoms that worsened their overall functional status. For this reason, complete dorsal rhizotomy ("rhizotomy" means cutting or sectioning nerve roots) was essentially abandoned. However, these and other experiments and observations of children with nerve injuries did show that sensation could be preserved if some of the sensory roots were left intact. Thus, the idea of treatment of spasticity with a partial rhizotomy gained favor.

In order to get the most normal tone with the least loss of sensation in children who have cerebral palsy, the problem became defining the nerves that should be cut and the nerves that should be saved. In 1978, Fasano, an Italian neurosurgeon, proposed an answer to this vexing problem. Using electrical recordings taken from individual nerves and muscles in the operating room, Fasano believed that at each level the sensory nerve could be subdivided into nerve rootlets (i.e., individual strands of nerve root), which then could be classified as "normal" or "abnormal" based on the rootlet's response to electrical stimulation. Thus, outcome could be optimized at each level by cutting only the more abnormal rootlets and saving the more normal ones; this was the beginning of the so-called "selective" dorsal rhizotomy (SDR) (Fasano, Broggi, Barolat-Romana, & Squazzi, 1978). Beginning in the 1980s, surgeons in the United States began performing and analyzing the results of SDR (Peacock, Arens, & Berman, 1987).

In the 1990s, surgeons started to question Fasano's belief that intra-operative electrical monitoring helps select the more abnormal rootlets to cut. The exact procedure and the role of the intra-operative stimulation is still being studied (Rivera, Burke, Schiff, & Weiss, 1994). However, because it has proved to effectively decrease tone and to improve function with minimal side effects, the operation itself has been added to the treatment arsenal for spasticity in carefully selected children with cerebral palsy.

One of the major advantages of SDR compared with other treatments for spasticity is that tone in all major muscle groups of the lower extremities can be reduced simultaneously and in essence permanently with a single operative procedure. Postoperative pain is generally short lived and is easy to control, and mobilization can occur early. The procedure often obviates the need for chronic antispasticity medication, thus avoiding the sedation and other side effects associated with this therapy. However, as with other treatments for spasticity, SDR does not improve underlying difficulties with balance, coordination, or strength, which may otherwise limit the child's mobility. Setting clear goals with the family is an important part of the preoperative evaluation.

Some aspects of SDR may be considered as disadvantages when compared with other treatment modalities. First, the procedure causes a permanent reduction in tone, which makes it a poor choice for any child whose spasticity does not appear to be static. Second, some children use spasticity to help with certain functional activities, particularly weight bearing and transferring; reduction in tone may lead to loss of these abilities. Third, the risk of some uncommon but possible surgical complications such as cerebrospinal fluid leak, meningitis, and bladder dysfunction may be unacceptable to some families. These risks are discussed in subsequent sections in this chapter.

SELECTION CRITERIA

The goal of SDR is to reduce spasticity or resting muscle tone. However, the surgery should be planned only if this reduction in tone has a high probability of leading to improvement in function. For the child with spastic diplegia, the procedure should improve the quality and the distance of his or her ambulation. For the child with spastic quadriplegia and more severe gross motor delay, the procedure should make caregiving activities easier and should improve the child's quality of sitting. A secondary benefit of SDR in both types of cerebral palsy is that range of motion (ROM) improves after the reduction of muscle tone.

Reducing muscle tone creates a window of opportunity for the child to learn new movement patterns and new functional skills that were previously impossible. These skills are learned over time and are not present when the tone is suddenly gone. In order to maximize their potential, children with functional mobility goals require intensive rehabilitation for 6 months to 1 year (unless goals are limited to easing activities of daily living [ADLs]).

Selection Criteria for Children with Spastic Diplegia

The ideal candidate for SDR is the young child (3–6 years of age) with spastic diplegia who is an exercise ambulator but seems to have reached a plateau in mobility skills as a result of high muscle tone. For example, for the child with lower-extremity scissoring who has a short stride length and can walk only short distances, using a reverse walker and an ankle-foot orthosis (AFO), SDR may help him or her to achieve functional household ambulation. The most important evaluation finding is that spastic muscle tone interferes with function.

An overview of the selection criteria for the child with spastic diplegia is presented in Table 10.1. In order to ensure that the selection criteria have been met, the child ideally should be examined by a team of professionals, including a neurosurgeon, a physical therapist, and an orthopedic surgeon. The preoperative evaluation should include an assessment of muscle tone, antigravity muscle strength, passive ROM, developmental postures and transitions, righting and equilibrium reactions, gait analysis, and ADLs (Staudt & Peacock, 1989).

In a clinical setting, muscle tone can be graded using the Ashworth scale (see Chapter 12). Tone that is scored at 3 or 4 throughout both lower extremities and especially proximally is a good indication for a rhizotomy. Because involuntary motion may increase if spasticity is reduced, some surgeons suggest that the child should not have a mixed type of cerebral palsy (Peacock et al., 1987).

The child should not have fixed contractures or deformities, which may be difficult to distinguish on clinical examination. ROM should be evaluated with the child relaxed, and a prolonged stretch should be applied in an attempt to determine the child's optimal end range. Slight limitations in ROM may need to be accepted because children with cerebral palsy rarely present with full passive motion.

Table 10.1. Ideal candidate for selective dorsal rhizotomy (SDR) with the goal being ambulation

1. Purely spastic, diplegia distribution
2. Lower-extremity tone (Ashworth score of 3 or 4, especially proximally)
3. Three to six years of age
4. Ambulatory with assistive device for more than 6 months or learning to walk
5. No fixed contractures and/or deformities
6. Antigravity muscle strength–4/5
7. Plateau in mobility skills regardless of physical therapy
8. Independent sitting balance
9. Educable and cooperative with rehabilitation
10. Supportive family
11. Tone interferes with functional skills

If weight bearing is important to function, then strength of the child's anti-gravity muscles, especially the quadriceps, must be sufficient for SDR to be successful. If the child is using extensor tone to stand and has underlying weakness, then weight bearing may become difficult following surgery and the child could lose functional skills. In a clinical setting, quadriceps strength is assessed by asking the child to repeatedly move from a squatting position up to stand while offering him or her support for balance. Hip extensor strength can be assessed in high-kneel posture. Gait evaluation may reveal weakness of specific muscles, such as a Trendelenburg sign (i.e., weakness of the gluteus medius).

Recent radiographs of the child's hips should be reviewed to determine whether subluxation is present and, if so, to what extent. If the child's hips are partially subluxated and could be managed with adductor tenotomy and night-time splinting, then rhizotomy to decrease adductor tone with splinting is theoretically a comparable management plan. Longitudinal studies are needed to determine the optimal management program for hip subluxation in children with cerebral palsy. A history of previous orthopedic surgery is a disadvantage because it is more difficult to predict the effect of SDR on a lengthened muscle.

The child who is at least educable and is willing to cooperate in physical therapy sessions fulfills an important selection criteria. Other limitations that might cause impaired mobility, such as motor planning problems, should be recognized and factored into the child's functional goal setting.

The family must be able to support the child during the inpatient rehabilitation phase as well as have sufficient resources to provide intensive outpatient therapy for up to 1 year after the surgery. Families should have transportation to and from the clinic, have an established record of good attendance, and follow through on managing the child's use of splints and a home exercise program. It is important that the parents have realistic expectations for the outcome of surgery and have discussed specific goals with the team performing the rhizotomy.

Selection Criteria for Children with Spastic Quadriplegia

The benefits of SDR for children with spastic quadriplegia have not been described by medical centers as often as have the benefits for children with spastic diplegia (Peacock et al., 1987). An overview of the selection criteria for the child with spastic quadriplegia is presented in Table 10.2. For this group of children, extensor and adductor muscle tone makes caregiving tasks (e.g., diapering, dressing, holding, carrying, positioning) difficult. Positioning the child in a wheelchair may be difficult; and, thus, customized positioning pads may be required. Some young children may be able to achieve sitting balance if reduced muscle tone allows them to broaden their base of support and flex more easily at the hips and knees. Children who are unable to sit but can show lateral head and trunk righting may have the potential to learn to sit when their legs can

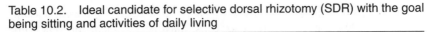

Table 10.2.   Ideal candidate for selective dorsal rhizotomy (SDR) with the goal being sitting and activities of daily living

1. Resting tone interferes with caregiving activities or with positioning
2. Contractures are not fixed
3. Tone is not used for function (e.g., transferring)
4. Parents' goals are realistic

be placed in more optimal alignment. If the child does not have the potential to achieve independent sitting balance, then wheelchair positioning may be achieved more easily and with fewer supports. Because extensor spasticity may be lost following the procedure, it is important to weigh the benefit of improved ROM against the loss of stand-pivot-sit transfers.

SDR Surgical Procedure

SDR is performed under general endotracheal (i.e., with a breathing tube in the trachea) anesthesia. Children are placed in prone position on chest and hip rolls. In the most common version of the procedure, a narrow laminectomy (i.e., removal of the spinous processes and the lamina) or laminotomy (i.e., cutting of these structures, which are then replaced at the end of the operation) is performed extending from L2 to L5 vertebrae (i.e., located in the lumbar region of the vertical column). The dura (i.e., watertight sac containing the spinal cord and the nerve roots) is opened. At each nerve root, from the first or second lumbar root to the first or second sacral root (depending on the child's pattern of spasticity, usually L1–L2 to S1–S2, which are located in the sacral region of the vertical column), the sensory (i.e., dorsal) nerve root is isolated and its rootlets are spread apart using special hooks. Each rootlet is tested with electrical stimulation, and the response is monitored on electromyography (EMG); at the same time, the child's legs and feet are observed for their response to the stimulation. Rootlets with a more normal response pattern to stimulation are saved, and those with an abnormal response pattern are sectioned (see Figure 10.1). (The patterns that are considered normal or abnormal may vary somewhat between medical centers.) The clinical examination, especially gait deviations, also assists in deciding the percentage of nerve roots that should be cut for various muscle groups. Some muscle groups may require more conservative intervention in order to preserve muscle strength. For this reason, some surgeons prefer to have the physical therapist present in the operating room to help with decision making.

In another version of the procedure, the spine is opened at the level of the conus medullaris (i.e., the tapering lower extremity of the spinal cord) and the roots are divided at that level. This procedure has the advantage of a smaller laminectomy, but it makes specific identification of the roots somewhat more difficult.

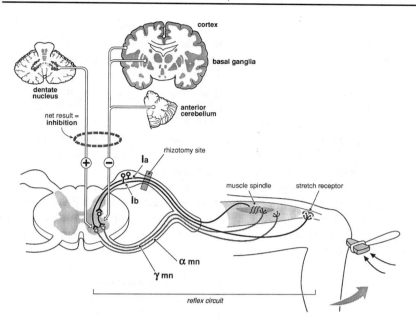

Figure 10.1.   Spasticity is caused by a loss of inhibitory input from neural structures above the spinal level. Selective dorsal rhizotomy helps reduce excess muscle tone by sectioning the dorsal root portion of the over-reactive reflex circuit.

After the abnormal rootlets have been sectioned, the dura is closed. Some surgeons then insert an epidural catheter so that morphine or other analgesic can be administered postoperatively. The incision then is closed and protective dressings are applied. The reduction in tone is evident immediately after surgery.

Postoperative Care

To minimize the risk of spinal fluid leakage through the dural closure, children are kept at bed rest for 3 days after SDR. As previously discussed, although parenteral medications can be used as an alternative, epidural morphine is very effective for postoperative pain management. It is important to keep the incision clean and dry; use of a urinary drainage catheter during the first few days of postsurgical care is useful in this regard. Some children may experience muscle spasms, which generally respond to muscle relaxants and/or positioning with knee immobilizers. Other children may experience transient paresthesias of the feet; however, socks can help minimize this symptom.

Gentle passive ROM exercises are performed from the second day of postoperative management onward. However, because the child has had a laminectomy, passive rotation motion of the lumbar spine is avoided. Straight leg raise and hip flexion above 90 degrees also are avoided because these maneuvers will stretch the dural incision and the lumbar nerve roots.

Splinting is used to maintain ROM. The schedule for wearing AFOs is gradually increased—depending on the child's skin tolerance—until an all-day schedule is resumed. Because sensory nerves have been severed during the surgical procedure, some sensory loss should be expected. If flexor spasms continue to be a problem, then knee immobilizers may be used during nights and naps. If hip subluxation has been identified preoperatively, then the child is positioned in an abduction wedge or an orthosis at night (see Figure 10.2).

During the first 2 weeks of postoperative care, the therapy goals are to resume the child's previous developmental skills. Sitting is initially attempted for 1- to 2-hour blocks three times a day in a recliner wheelchair. By postoperative week 2, the child should be sitting in an upright wheelchair for an entire day. Head control and sitting balance are resumed in prone and short sitting. Bed mobility skills, such as rolling with assistance and moving from supine to sitting, are practiced. The child is taught to sit on a stool with his or her feet on the floor by using upper-extremity support.

By the eighth day of postoperative care, the child typically progresses to standing activities. Depending on the child, this may be achieved on a standing frame (see Figure 10.3) or may be actively achieved with the guidance of the therapist. Contact guard should be provided because the child's weakness can

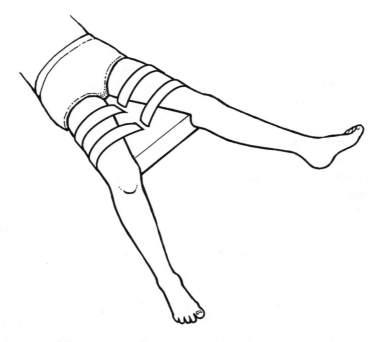

Figure 10.2. Abduction wedge, which holds the child's legs away from the mid-line of the body.

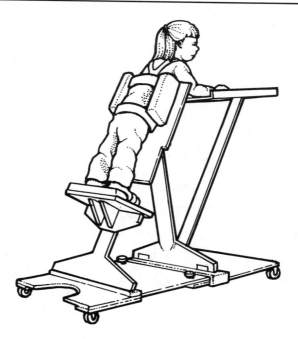

Figure 10.3. Child in prone stander. (From Pellegrino, L. [1997]. Cerebral palsy. In M.L. Batshaw [Ed.], *Children with disabilities* [4th ed., p. 512]. Baltimore: Paul H. Brookes Publishing Co.; reprinted by permission.)

cause sudden collapse during early weight-bearing activities. If possible, then stand-pivot-sit transfers with the therapist assisting are incorporated into the training.

Strengthening activities are initiated in sidelying with active assisted and active lower-extremity flexion and extension motions. As healing and comfort improve, the child may be able to learn to bridge or do other strengthening exercises for hip extensors and abductors as well as knee extensors. Theraband is an inexpensive method of performing resistive exercises that children enjoy. Once the sutures are removed (between postoperative days 10 and 14) and the incision is completely healed, aquatic therapy, if available, may be used as a treatment adjunct. Strengthening activities are often performed more easily in a buoyant environment.

By postoperative week 3, more advanced developmental skills such as crawling or creeping in quadruped may be incorporated into the child's training. Slight hamstring stretch, such as ring sitting, may be tolerated at this time. If this stretch causes discomfort or lumbar flexion, then the child can sit on a wedge with a more open hip angle (see Figure 10.4). Side sitting and transitions from sitting to quadruped may be attempted if the child is comfortable with trunk rotation.

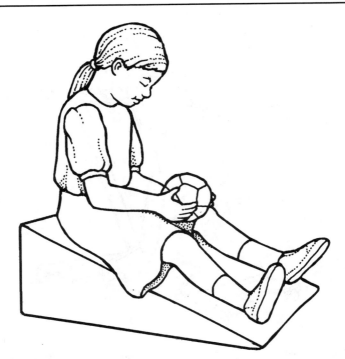

Figure 10.4.   Child sitting on wedge with more open hip angle.

Emphasis on the child's activities to increase muscle strength should continue throughout the training. High-kneeling position strengthens the hip extensors. Cruising sideways at a mat table builds strength of the hip abductors. Children can begin to learn to pedal a tricycle adapted with trunk support and foot loops (see Figure 10.5). Once the child achieves some degree of independence, the adapted tricycle should become preferable to a wheelchair as a mobility device.

Gait training begins with tolerance of standing and then progresses to cruising sideways at a surface. A solid AFO or an articulating joint that is locked out protects the child's foot from assuming a crouched posture and overstretching the heel cords. Ambulation training may progress from the parallel bars to a reverse rollator walker (see Figure 10.6) and perhaps to quad canes. Walking training should advance to longer distances and to elevation activities (e.g., stairs, ramps, curbs). At this time, the wheelchair is reassessed to determine whether all of the positioning devices are still required.

Protocols vary between medical facilities and are also dependent on insurance resources. However, for children who could walk prior to the surgery, some facilities generally recommended 5 days in acute care, followed by 3–6 weeks of intensive daily rehabilitation, with a goal of achieving functional ambulation

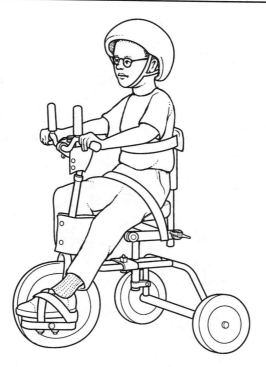

Figure 10.5. Child riding tricycle that is equipped with trunk support and foot loops. It is hoped, as the child progresses, that this mobility device may replace the use of a wheelchair.

prior to discharge. Outpatient therapy continues three to five times a week, supplemented with a daily home exercise program for 6 months to 1 year (Wilson, 1989). Children with spastic quadriplegia require a shorter and less intensive rehabilitation course.

Outcome

Peacock et al. (1987) described the clinical outcome by comparing 60 individual children (ranging in age from 20 months to 19 years) who have had SDRs with their preoperative status. Forty children with more mild impairments (i.e., spastic diplegia) showed reduction in resting muscle tone as well as reduction in power. All but 1 child could bear weight by the eighth postoperative day. Twelve of fourteen children who could walk independently prior to the surgery showed improved gait patterns; five were able to discontinue use of a walking aid. Of 13 children who could walk only with support prior to the surgery, 9 achieved functional ambulation, mostly with assistive devices. Five children who could not walk prior to surgery also progressed in ambulation skills. Functional improvement also occurred in side sitting, reciprocation in creeping, and alignment in

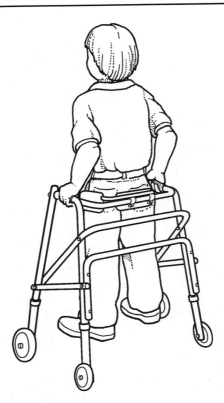

Figure 10.6. Child using a reverse rollator walker.

standing. Nineteen of twenty-eight children showed some improvement in upper-extremity function. Five of 9 children showed improvement in articulation and/or breath control. A possible explanation for these unexpected outcomes is based on ascending collateral branches that may synapse at higher levels. An alternative explanation is that upper-extremity function improved as a result of a more stable sitting base, with less use of the arms for balance.

Peacock et al. (1987) also described outcome in 16 children with more severe involvement of all four limbs. Tone was reduced in the lower extremities postoperatively in all 16 children; in 9 children, tone was graded as normal at rest. ROM was improved. Functional differences also were described, with modest improvement in sitting skills, prone progression, and supported walking. Eleven children showed improvement in upper limb function. The functional goals measured tended to be more appropriate for the higher-level group, and the authors did not report differences in bed mobility, transfer, positioning, or caregiving activities.

Using two-dimensional videography, Vaughan, Berman, Staudt, and Peacock (1988) studied 14 children prior to and approximately 9 months after SDR.

Their study found that improvement was demonstrated in functional gait parameters as well as cosmesis. Stride length increased by more than 20%, walking speed increased by 18%, and hip and knee motion also showed significant improvement. Cadence remained unchanged. In order to assess 11 children who independently ambulated and 8 children who used assistive devices, gait laboratory analysis that was conducted at Newington Children's Hospital (Boscarino, Ounpuu, Davis, Gage, & DeLuca, 1993) used three-dimensional videography and surface electrodes preoperatively and 1 year after SDR. Positive results of the SDR included improved sagittal plane alignment of hip, knee, and ankle, resulting in a plantar-grade foot position at stance. However, the researchers also documented an increased anterior pelvic tilt in the independent ambulators. Coronal plane motion of the pelvis and the hips remained unchanged. At Ranchos Los Amigos, Cahan, Adams, Perry, and Beeler (1990) performed gait analysis on 14 individuals. The study demonstrated improved joint alignment; improved heel strike and foot/floor contact; and improved stride characteristics, including velocity and stride length. However, there was no improvement in the selective control or timing of muscle action on EMG, and Guiliani (1991) corroborated this finding.

Outcome varies among medical centers, as does the operative technique (McDonald, 1991; Peacock & Staudt, 1991). Selection criteria, surgical technique, and postoperative rehabilitation all are variables that are critical to the success of the surgery. Each center should be committed to monitoring the outcome of each child to ensure a successful result. Functional outcome parameters and physical impairments must be measured. Bloom and Nazar (1994) administered the Pediatric Evaluation of Disability Inventory (PEDI) to 16 children (half with diplegia and half with quadriplegia) prior to surgery and 3–12 months following SDR. Modest improvement in self-care, mobility, and social scores were demonstrated in 40%–60% of the individuals. Other studies did not make significant improvements as measured by the PEDI. Parent satisfaction, which is often high, is another significant indicator of outcome.

Multicenter research is under way using the Gross Motor Function Measure (Russell et al., 1989) as an outcome tool. Comparison of whether intraoperative monitoring makes a difference in outcome is of interest to this group. The concern regarding poor reliability of intra-operative monitoring has created this important question. Most teams agree that the EMG alone does not provide the surgeon with adequate, reliable information to determine which nerve rootlets to sever. At some centers, the clinical examination provides a formula for the percentage of nerve roots that should be cut at each level, and this formula is provided by the physical therapist who attends the operative procedure. The selection of the rootlets that should be cut is based on comparing the responses to stimulation on EMG with the responses to overt observation. If a conflict of information occurs, clinical impression outweighs EMG findings.

Complications

The major early complication to monitor with SDR is cerebrospinal fluid leak. This occurs because the closure of the dura is not truly watertight until healing has taken place. Although late leaks can occasionally occur, this problem generally becomes apparent within the first week after surgery. Persistent leaks require intra-operative exploration and dural repair. A leak of spinal fluid is not necessarily a major danger; however, the leak can create a pathway for infection, usually with skin bacteria in the spinal fluid (i.e., meningitis). If infection occurs, treatment with antibiotics will be necessary.

Sensory loss after rhizotomy is usually transient, but some alterations in touch or in proprioception may be more long-standing. However, in general, dyesthesia does not usually appear to have significant functional consequences (Abbott et al., 1993).

Although no motor roots are cut in SDR, underlying weakness that was masked by the spasticity may become apparent after the tone is reduced. In some children with severe impairments in whom the goal of rhizotomy is to improve sitting and positioning, the ability to bear weight for stand-pivot-sit transfers may be lost once the spasticity is reduced. This problem should be anticipated during evaluation and weighed in the decision-making process of whether tone reduction will improve or impair daily functional activities.

Bladder dysfunction has been reported after SDR, but this usually occurs only if sensory roots lower than S1 are sectioned (Abbott et al., 1993). Because the S2 root also participates in gastrocnemius innervation, surgeons must weigh the risks of aggressive sectioning at this level against the likelihood of persistent heel cord tightness. Some surgeons prefer to avoid the S2 root altogether, counseling parents that later lengthening of the Achilles tendon may be necessary. Other surgeons rely on a variety of intra-operative sphincter monitoring techniques to reduce the risk of bladder dysfunction.

Orthopedic complications after SDR may be difficult to assess because the children who require surgery usually have other risk factors independent of the surgical procedure itself for musculoskeletal problems. Late spine complications such as scoliosis are rare. Hip subluxation has been the major abnormality studied, with some researchers reporting an increased incidence after rhizotomy and others reporting an improvement following the procedure (Greene et al., 1991; Heim et al., 1995; Stempien et al., 1990).

Other Neurosurgical Treatments

In addition to SDR, other neurosurgical modalities have been used to improve motor function in children with spasticity. For most of these procedures, children with paraplegia and spasticity caused by spinal cord injury have been more thoroughly studied than have children with cerebral palsy, particularly with respect to long-term outcome.

For children for whom the risk of open surgery is considered too great or for whom selectivity is less important, phenol rhizotomy may be of some use (Nathan, 1959). This procedure involves the injection of phenol into the thecal sac under myelographic (i.e., X-ray visualization of the spinal cord) guidance, which leads to partial denervation of some of the spinal nerves. Like other procedures that involve alcohol, the effect is not permanent; spasticity usually returns between 6 months and 2 years after treatment. Bowel and bladder dysfunction, weakness, and sensory loss also are possible side effects.

The use of implantable pumps to deliver antispasticity medication directly to the CNS has gained popularity since the mid- to late 1980s but has been used more often in adults and adolescents than in young children. Baclofen is the agent most often administered in this manner. The long-term effects of this treatment are still not completely known (Albright, Barron, Fasick, Polinko, & Janosky, 1993).

Cerebellar and spinal cord stimulators also have been advocated as a reversible treatment for some children with spasticity (Maiman, Myklebust, & Barolat-Romana, 1987; Penn, Myklebust, Gottlieb, Afarwal, & Etzel, 1990). Results with these techniques have been mixed, but children appear to benefit considerably in some cases. The treatment of certain movement disorders using stereotactic thalmic lesioning techniques in children with athetoid cerebral palsy has been useful in some children whose abnormal movements cannot be managed by medical means (Gildenberg, 1985).

SUMMARY

For carefully selected children with cerebral palsy, SDR can provide permanent relief from disabling spasticity. The procedure is still evolving as details of child selection, intra-operative monitoring, and outcome are still being studied. Other neurosurgical techniques for motor problems also are available, and these methods must be compared with non-neurosurgical techniques for the management of cerebral palsy. As practitioners who care for children with cerebral palsy work together to understand which children are most likely to benefit from which specific management approach, the next challenge is multidisciplinary planning.

REFERENCES

Abbott, R., Johann-Murphy, M., Shiminski-Maher, T., Quartermain, D., Forem, S.L., Gold, J.T., & Epstein, F.J. (1993). Selective dorsal rhizotomy: Outcome and complications in treating spastic cerebral palsy. *Neurosurgery, 33,* 851–857.

Albright, A.L., Barron, W.B., Fasick, M.P., Polinko, P., & Janosky, J. (1993). Continuous intrathecal baclofen infusion for spasticity of cerebral origin. *Journal of the American Medical Association, 270*(20), 2475–2477.

Bloom, K.K., & Nazar, G.B. (1994). Functional assessment following selective posterior rhizotomy in spastic cerebral palsy. *Child's Nervous System, 10,* 84–86.

Boscarino, L.F., Ounpuu, S., Davis, R.B., III, Gage, J.R., & DeLuca, P.A. (1993). Effects of selective dorsal rhizotomy on gait in children with cerebral palsy. *Journal of Pediatric Orthopedics, 13,* 174–179.

Cahan, L.D., Adams, J.M., Perry, J., & Beeler, L.M. (1990). Instrumented gait analysis after selective dorsal rhizotomy. *Developmental Medicine and Child Neurology, 32,* 1037–1043.

Fasano, V.A., Broggi, G., Barolat-Romana, G., & Squazzi, A. (1978). Surgical treatment of spasticity in children. *Child's Brain, 4,* 289–305.

Foerster, O. (1913). On the indications and results of the excision of posterior spinal nerve roots in men. *Surgery, Gynecology and Obstetrics, 16,* 463–474.

Gildenberg, P.L. (1985). Surgical therapy of movement disorders. In R.H. Wilkins & S.S. Rengachary (Eds.), *Neurosurgery* (pp. 2507–2516). New York: McGraw-Hill.

Greene, W.B., Deitz, F.R., Goldberg, M.J., Gross, R.H., Miller, F., & Sussman, M.D. (1991). Rapid progression of hip subluxation in cerebral palsy after selective posterior rhizotomy. *Journal of Pediatric Orthopedics, 11,* 494–497.

Guiliani, C.A. (1991). Dorsal rhizotomy for children with cerebral palsy: Support for concepts of motor control. *Physical Therapy, 71,* 248–259.

Haley, S.M., Coster, W.J., Ludlow, L.H., Haltiwanger, J.T., & Andrellos, P.J. (1992). *Pediatric Evaluation of Disability Inventory (PEDI): Development, standardization, and administration manual.* Boston: PEDI Research Group and New England Medical Center Hospital.

Heim, R.C., Park, T.S., Vogler, G.P., Kaufman, B.A., Noetzel, M.J., & Ortman, M.R. (1995). Changes in hip migration after selective dorsal rhizotomy for spastic quadriplegia in cerebral palsy. *Journal of Neurosurgery, 82,* 567–571.

Maiman, D.J., Myklebust, J.B., & Barolat-Romana, G. (1987). Spinal cord stimulation for amelioration of spasticity: Experimental results. *Neurosurgery, 21*(3), 331.

McDonald, C.M. (1991). Selective dorsal rhizotomy: A critical review. *Physical Medicine and Rehabilitation Clinics of North America, 2,* 891–915.

Nathan, P.W. (1959, December). Intrathecal phenol to relieve spasticity in paraplegia. *Lancet,* 1099–1015.

Peacock, W.J., Arens, L.J., & Berman, B. (1987). Cerebral palsy spasticity. Selective posterior rhizotomy. *Pediatric Neuroscience, 13,* 61–66.

Peacock, W.J., & Staudt, L.A. (1991). Functional outcomes following selective posterior rhizotomy in children with cerebral palsy. *Journal of Neurosurgery, 74,* 380–385.

Penn, R.D., Myklebust, B.M., Gottlieb, G.L., Afarwal, G.C., & Etzel, M.E. (1990). Chronic cerebellar stimulation of cerebral palsy. Prospective and double blind studies. *Journal of Neurosurgery, 53,* 160.

Rivera, A.D., Burke, T., Schiff, S.J., & Weiss, I.P. (1994). An experimental study of reflex variability in selective dorsal rhizotomy. *Journal of Neurosurgery, 81*(6), 885–895.

Russell, D., Rosenbaum, P., Cadman, D., Gowland, C., Hardy, S., & Jarvis, S. (1989). The Gross Motor Function Measure: A means to evaluate the effects of physical therapy. *Developmental Medicine and Child Neurology, 31,* 341–352.

Sherrington, C.S. (1898). Decerebrate rigidity and reflex coordination of movements. *Journal of Physiology (London), 22,* 319–337.

Staudt, L.A., & Peacock, W.J. (1989). Selective posterior rhizotomy for treatment of spastic cerebral palsy. *Pediatric Physical Therapy, 1,* 3–9.

Stempien, L., Gaebler-Spira, D., Dias, L., Storrs, B., Cioffi, M., & Feathergill, B. (1990). The natural history of the hip in cerebral palsy following selective posterior rhizotomy. *Developmental Medicine and Child Neurology (AACPDM–Abstracts), 32,* 5–6.

Vaughan, C.L., Berman, B., Staudt, L.A., & Peacock, W.J. (1988). Gait analysis of cerebral palsy children before and after rhizotomy. *Pediatric Neuroscience, 14,* 297–300.

Wilson, J.M. (1989). Outpatient-based physical therapy program for children with cerebral palsy undergoing selective dorsal rhizotomy. *Neurosurgery, State of the Art Reviews, 4,* 417–429.

CHAPTER 11

Nutrition and Feeding

Peggy S. Eicher

Adequate nutrition is essential for the optimal growth and development of all children, including children with cerebral palsy. Historically, infants with cerebral palsy were expected to be smaller in size than their age-mates; however, the etiology of their growth failure was not understood. The positive correlation between short stature and degree of motor or mental impairment suggested that the underlying neurological injury in these children directly limited their growth potential (Culley & Middleton, 1969). However, when impaired oral-motor and self-feeding skills were found to exaggerate growth retardation in children with cerebral palsy (Krick & Van Duyn, 1984; Tobis, Saturen, Larios, & Posniak, 1961), attention shifted to nutritional factors. Inadequate nutritional intake is considered a major cause of growth failure in children with cerebral palsy (Shapiro, Green, Krick, Allen, & Capute, 1986; Stallings, Charney, Davies, & Cronk, 1993a).

There are many potential obstacles to adequate nutrition in children with cerebral palsy. Communication difficulties may interfere with requests for food, expressions of hunger, or indications of food preference. Impairments of cognition and fine motor function may limit self-feeding as well as the ability to obtain food independently. Severe oral-motor dysfunction may limit the types and textures of food that children with cerebral palsy can safely ingest (*Growth and Nutrition,* 1990). It has been estimated that one half of all children with cerebral palsy develop a feeding problem that is significant enough to interfere with their nutrition, medical well-being, or social integration (Palmer, Thompson, & Linscheid, 1975). Manifestations of a feeding problem can be subtle (e.g., increased congestion, gagging with meals) or dramatic (e.g., choking, aspirating, failure to thrive). Although the feeding problems associated with cerebral palsy arise in the context of a permanent neurodevelopmental disability, the feeding problems themselves are not irremediable; however, they do not typically resolve spontaneously. A concerted effort by family members and professionals is required in order to recognize feeding problems early and to institute a plan of care that prevents more significant dietary dysfunction. An early plan of management may help to avoid nutritional consequences that could result in pervasive impairments of health and increased risk of early death.

CREATING APPROPRIATE
EXPECTATIONS FOR GROWTH MAINTENANCE

Although children with cerebral palsy are frequently smaller than their age-mates, it is not clear to what extent growth failure is a result of their central nervous system (CNS) disorder. Nonnutritional factors have been shown to play a role in stunting growth, but identification of the involved mechanisms remains unclear (Rempel, Colewell, & Nelson, 1988; Stevenson, Roberts, & Vogtle, 1995; Uvebrandt & Wiklund, 1988). One postulated mechanism is a negative neurotropic effect associated with brain anomaly or injury, which directly influences linear growth, immobility, or lack of weight bearing and indirectly results in poor growth through disuse atrophy or sensory deficit (Tizard, Paine, & Crothers, 1954; Uvebrandt & Wiklund, 1988). In contrast, the adverse effect of inadequate nutrition has been defined more clearly. Inadequate nutrition has been shown to be a major contributor to growth failure in children with cerebral palsy, particularly during early childhood (Stallings et al., 1993a, 1993b). Although longitudinal studies are needed, cross-sectional studies suggest that in the presence of adequate nutrition, the growth rates of children with cerebral palsy approximate those of children without cerebral palsy.

What Is Appropriate Growth for the Child with Cerebral Palsy?

A typical newborn is expected to gain approximately 20–30 grams a day in the first 3 months of life. Body weight typically doubles by 4–6 months of age and triples by 12 months of age. Height increases 50% during the first year of life and doubles by 4 years of age. The brain also grows rapidly during the first 2 years of life. Head circumference increases 1–2 centimeters a month during the first 6 months of life and half of a centimeter per month from 6 to 12 months of age, which reflects the increasing cell numbers. From 12 to 24 months of age, the head grows at .2 centimeters per month as neuronal size and connections increase.

It is imperative to closely monitor the growth parameters of children with cerebral palsy in order to optimize growth for their age as well as to watch their level of physical disability. Frequent monitoring helps to avoid periods of undernutrition and prevent overnutrition, which can also be problematic. The child with cerebral palsy may be more dependent on others for assistance with transfers and mobility, making excessive weight gain undesirable. A helpful goal for children with moderate to severe impairments is to aim for a *weight-for-height ratio* at the 50th percentile in the first 2 years of life and then a ratio at the 10th–25th percentile if they will be dependent on others for transfers and mobility during the ensuing years (Krick, Murphy, Markham, & Shapiro, 1992).

Accurate assessment of growth in children with cerebral palsy can be difficult. Weights must be obtained on an appropriate scale for the child who is unable to stand independently. Measures of length or height are even more difficult to obtain reliably for the child who is unable to stand because of fixed joint contractures, scoliosis, or motor delay. As a result, the lack of reliable length or height assessment prevents use of weight-for-height calculation. Alternative measures of length or height, namely the segmental measures of upper-arm length, lower-leg length, and knee height, have been reliable proxies for height in children with cerebral palsy (Spender, Cronk, Charney, & Stallings, 1989; Stevenson, 1995) (see Figure 11.1). Regardless of the measure that is

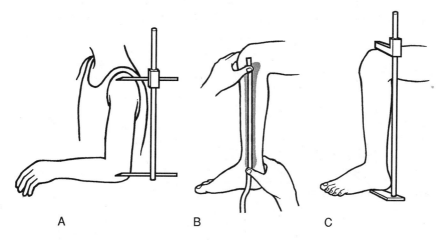

A   B   C

Figure 11.1. Segmental measurements to estimate total body length. A) Upper-arm length is measured with the child sitting or standing upright and the arm relaxed in a resting vertical position with the elbow flexed to 90 degrees; the upper-arm length is measured as the distance from the acromion to the head of the radius using a digital anthropometer (i.e., Harbenden). B) Tibial length is measured from the supermedial edge of the tibia to the inferior edge of the medial malleolus using a flexible steel measuring tape. C) Knee height is measured with the child seated and the knee and ankle both at a 90-degree angle. A Mediform sliding caliper (e.g., Medical Express, Beaverton, Oregon) is used to measure the distance from the bottom of the heel to the superior surface of the thigh over the femoral condyles. (Adapted from Stevenson, 1995.)

chosen, weight needs to be obtained routinely and plotted on the appropriate growth chart in order to facilitate accurate assessment of the child's growth and nutritional status.

As previously discussed, weight-for-height ratios are used to estimate adequate growth and nutrition. An assumption can be made that at any given length, a specific range of weight defines what should be observed in an adequately nourished child, regardless of age. Problems occur when accurate measures of length or height are unavailable. Chronic undernutrition may result in stunted growth (see section on "Failure to Thrive" in this chapter), thus undermining the assumption behind the use of the weight-for-height ratio. In this case, an assessment of the child's fat stores provides a more direct means of determining the adequacy of caloric intake. The clinical judgment that the child "appears well nourished" represents an imprecise and potentially inaccurate estimate of fat stores. Methods using relatively inexpensive equipment are available to reliably and reproducibly measure fat stores (see Figure 11.2).

What Are Abnormal Growth Patterns?

Undernutrition and failure to thrive are major problems for children with cerebral palsy. Failure to thrive involves less-than-adequate weight gain with decreasing weight percentiles. If failure to gain adequate weight persists or worsens, then linear growth and ultimately brain growth also can be affected. The child with failure to thrive may appear thin and wasted. As failure to thrive continues,

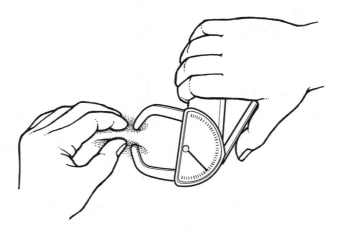

Figure 11.2.   A caliper is used to measure fat stores. A small amount of skin is folded or "pinched" between the ends of the caliper. Measures of skinfold thickness may be obtained at the back of the upper arm (i.e., triceps skinfold) or just below the shoulder blades (i.e., subscapular skinfolds). Charts are available defining typical ranges of skinfold thickness for males and females at different ages. Atypically low measures indicate inadequate caloric intake; high measures suggest superabundant caloric intake.

skin rashes, hair loss, and difficulty fighting off infection may occur. These children become irritable and listless.

Cross-sectional studies conducted by Stallings et al. (1993b) describing the nutritional status of children with cerebral palsy (ranging from 2 to 18 years of age) found that 30% of children with diplegia or hemiplegia were undernourished. In children with quadriplegia, the percentage is even higher. Although undernutrition and growth stunting were already present in the youngest children studied (i.e., 2–3 years of age), both stunting and undernutrition increased over time in children with quadriplegia.

Failure to Thrive Failure to thrive results from inadequate caloric intake, excessive caloric expenditure, or malabsorption of ingested calories and nutrients. However, malabsorption is not more common in children with cerebral palsy. Studies conducted in the 1990s have also shown that spasticity does not increase energy needs. In fact, the energy needs of children with spastic quadriplegia are far lower than the needs of children of similar size who are not affected (Stallings, Zemel, Davies, & Charney, 1996). Thus, the failure to thrive seen in children with cerebral palsy results primarily from inadequate caloric intake, not from malabsorption or excessive caloric expenditure.

Obesity Obesity is the result of overnutrition (i.e., having excess adipose stores). The clinical definition of *obesity* is weight that is 20% more than the standard desirable weight or weight-for-height ratio that is above the 95th percentile. Obesity is a result of excessive caloric intake in relation to expenditure. Children with decreased activity—frequently true of many children with cerebral palsy—are at greater risk of becoming obese because caloric intake exceeds caloric needs. A study of children with diplegia and hemiplegia documented that 8%–14% of these children with paralysis were obese (Stallings et al., 1993b). Obesity also may decrease energy expenditure even further by making mobility, ambulation, transfers, or manual propulsion of a wheelchair more difficult and less often attempted. In addition, the importance of social interaction associated with food is heightened for many children who may have limited opportunity to interact with peers and family in other group activities.

What Is an Appropriate Diet?

In order for children to grow well, they need an appropriate mixture of fats, carbohydrates, protein, water, vitamins, and minerals. The recommended caloric distribution of fats, carbohydrates, and protein is dependent on the child's age. In general, after the child is 2 years of age, 30% of calories should come from fats, 55% from carbohydrates, and 15% from protein (Pipes, 1988).

Proteins Proteins in the human diet are obtained from both animal and vegetable sources. Ingested proteins are broken down by the digestive tract into amino acids, which are then used in the synthesis of new tissue for growth; in repair and maintenance; in the production of hormones, enzymes, and antibodies; and in the production of energy. Dietary protein is useful only if adequate quantities of each of the nine essential amino acids (i.e., threonine, methionine, lysine, valine, isoleucine, leucine, ornithine, arginine, and histidine) are consumed during a meal. The quality of a specific protein is measured by the completeness of its essential amino acid content. In general, animal protein contains larger amounts of the essential amino acids than plant protein. The most important proteins of animal origin are milk and milk products, meats, fish and other seafood, poultry, and eggs. Plant proteins are readily available in cereals, legumes, seeds, and nuts.

Lack of an appropriate mix of the essential amino acids in the child's diet can lead to a reduction in growth rate as well as a failure to develop typical secondary sexual characteristics. To avoid deficiency, it has been recommended that at least one third of total dietary protein should come from animal protein (Burton & Foster, 1988). This is easy to accomplish in an affluent society such as the United States because animal proteins are readily accessible. However, children with cerebral palsy are at higher risk for inadequate dietary protein. If they have immature oral-motor skills, these children frequently do not eat a lot of meat because it is difficult for them to orally process. Milk protein sources may be restricted in children with cerebral palsy because of lactose intolerance, decreased fluid ingestion related to oral-motor problems, or caregivers' belief that dairy products increase congestion or constipation. Thus, unless the appropriate mix of proteins is specifically considered, children with cerebral palsy are at increased risk for protein deficiency.

Carbohydrates   Carbohydrates provide the major source of energy for body and brain metabolism. Although lactose and glycogen are unique to animals, carbohydrates are made primarily through plant photosynthesis. Carbohydrates are grouped according to structure. Monosaccharides (e.g., glucose, fructose, galactose) cannot be broken down further. Disaccharides (e.g., lactose, sucrose) can be broken down into their component monosaccharides. Polysaccharides, which are created from the condensation of a large number of monosaccharides, are found in cereals, grains, potatoes, and corn and are broken down more slowly into simple sugars and fiber. Carbohydrates that are not needed for energy can be stored in the form of glycogen in the liver and in muscle or can be converted into fat and stored as adipose tissue.

Fats   Fats are an important dietary component for several reasons. Adequate dietary fat prevents the breakdown of protein for energy needs. Fat is the sole source of energy that the body can store in quantity and therefore serves as the body's prime fuel reserve. Moreover, fat is the most concentrated energy source that the human diet can provide, yielding 9 calories per gram, compared with 4 calories per gram from carbohydrates and proteins. The high caloric density of fat becomes very important when the child's ability to consume larger volumes of food is limited. For children with cerebral palsy, volume limitation is a common problem, whether related to oral-motor dysfunction or to gastric intolerance. However, fat slows the rate of stomach emptying and decreases intestinal motility. This slowing of gastrointestinal (GI) motility delays the onset of the hunger sensation, increasing the time between meals. Delayed motility also can exacerbate gastroesophageal reflux (GER; see section on "Gastro-esophageal Reflux" in this chapter), which can decrease the child's interest in eating even further.

A balanced fat intake is important to ensure both the necessary supply of essential fatty acids and fat-soluble vitamins as well as minimize the risk of coronary heart disease and atherosclerosis mediated through blood cholesterol. The type of dietary fat is an important factor that influences the level of choles-terol in the blood. In general, saturated fats increase cholesterol, monounsaturated fats have no effect, and polyunsaturated fats decrease cholesterol. The common saturated fats in many people's diets come from meat, dairy products, and coco-nut oil. Monounsaturated fats are exemplified by olive oil and peanut oil. Soy, corn, cottonseed, and safflower oils are polyunsaturated fats because of the lin-oleic acid found within them. A diet designed to lower blood cholesterol is low in saturated fat and high in polyunsaturated fat. To promote a generally bal-anced diet for all healthy individuals over the age of 2 years, no more than 30% of the total calories should be consumed from fat, less than 10% of energy from saturated fat, and less than 300 milligrams should be consumed of dietary cho-lesterol per day (National Cholesterol Education Program, 1990). Because in-fants have a much faster growth rate than adults, the recommended fat intake is increased to 40%–50% of total calories, as provided by breast milk and infant formulas. It is generally recommended that infants make the transition from breast milk or commercial formula to whole cow's milk at around 1 year of age and continue the use of whole milk in the diet until 2 years of age (American Academy of Pediatrics, 1993). At this time, the fat content of the diet can come from more varied sources and can follow the general dietary fat recommenda-tion of about 30% of total calories.

Fiber   Dietary fiber is the part of food that is not broken down in the digestive tract. Plants, fruits, and grains are the primary sources of fiber in most people's diets. An advantage of a high-fiber diet is that it increases stool bulk and discourages constipation. In addition, low-fiber diets have been implicated in everything from cancer to coronary artery disease; however, these assertions remain unproved as of 1997. In fact, excessive fiber is not necessarily good for young children. It takes up room in the child's small stomach and also can interfere with the absorption of certain vitamins. The best recommendation is probably to encourage a common plan in which older infants and children are encouraged to include portions of high-fiber whole grain cereals, breads, fruits, and vegetables in their daily diet (Williams, Bollella, & Wynder, 1995).

Vitamins and Minerals   Vitamins and minerals do not provide calories; however, they do play an important role in the many metabolic processes in-volved in food breakdown and utilization of the energy released as well as the formation and maintenance of body tissues. Essential vitamins and minerals cannot be synthesized by the body and, as a result, must be obtained from the diet. Brief reviews of the essential vitamins and minerals are presented in Tables 11.1 and 11.2, respectively.

Fortunately, vitamin deficiencies are fairly rare in the United States. Vitamins act primarily as cofactors that catalyze enzymatic reactions without being depleted themselves; the human body is able to store the fat-soluble vitamins A, D, E, and K. In addition, many processed foods are supplemented with vitamins. Because of these additives, most children older than 3 months of age receive at least twice the daily requirement of vitamins in their typical food intake.

Although the recommended allowances are the same for children both with and without cerebral palsy, complicating factors may exist that increase the risk of vitamin or mineral deficiencies in children with cerebral palsy. In general, the child with cerebral palsy may be at increased risk for vitamin deficiencies if oral intake is severely limited. In addition, the use of antiepileptic drugs or mineral oil may compound the problem. The antiepileptics phenobarbital and diphenylhydantoin decrease vitamin D availability by increasing the activity of the hepatic microsomal enzymes that metabolize vitamin D. Diphenylhydantoin also can interfere with folate, biotin, and vitamin B_{12} availability, resulting in megaloblastic anemia. Moreover, ingestion of mineral oil can interfere with absorption of the fat-soluble vitamins A, D, E, and K.

Minerals also function as vital constituents of many body tissues, such as the iron in hemoglobin, myoglobin, and cytochromes or the calcium and fluoride in healthy bones and teeth. It is important to remember that the recommended daily mineral allowances do not differ between the child who has cerebral palsy and the child who does not; however, there is increased risk of deficiency for children with cerebral palsy because of drug–nutrient interactions or frequent dietary limitations. Iron deficiency is the most common mineral deficiency. Children with cerebral palsy who have difficulty chewing may consume less meat, poultry, and fish in their diets than children who chew well. Because iron from animal sources is absorbed more readily and to a greater extent than it is from cereals or vegetables, children with difficulty chewing may absorb less dietary iron. Moreover, fiber and antacids that are frequently prescribed for children with cerebral palsy may bind with dietary iron, which further decreases absorption. Unfortunately, the early symptoms of iron deficiency (e.g., weakness and fatigability, dyspnea on exertion, decreased attention span, lag in behavioral and mental development) may be difficult to identify until anemia is present in children with cerebral palsy. At this stage, varying severity of phosphorus depletion can occur related to long-term use of nonabsorbable antacids containing magnesium-aluminum hydroxides. Compensatory increased skeletal demineralization and hypercalcemia occur, which result in clinical osteomalacia accompanied by weakness, loss of appetite, malaise, and stiff joints.

Table 11.1.   Essential vitamins and nutrition

Vitamin	Function	Deficiency	Excess	Source	Risk factors
Biotin	Coenzyme for gluco-neogenesis, fatty acid synthesis, and amino acid metabolism	Hair loss and seborrheic dermatitis		Liver, egg yolk, and cereal yeast	Anticonvulsants impair absorption
Folate	Coenzyme in amino acid metabolism and nucleic acid synthesis	Macrocytic anemia, multi-lobed neutrophils, glossitis, diarrhea, and malabsorption		Breast milk, cow's milk, liver, yeast, leafy vegetables, and legumes	Low-calorie diet that is poor in protein, vitamin, and mineral content with absence of fresh fruits and vegetables, lean meats, eggs, and milk
Niacin	Aids digestion and normal appetite, energy utilization in fat synthesis, tissue respiration, and carbohydrate utilization	Pellagra (i.e., dermatitis, diarrhea, dementia, and death), cheilosis, angular stomatitis, and inflammation of mucous membranes	Dilation of the capillaries and vasomotor instability	Liver, meat, fish, poultry, fortified cereal products, milk, and infant formula	
Pantothenic acid	Part to coenzyme A involved in release of energy from carbohydrate synthesis and degradation of sterols, fatty acids, and steroid hormones	Tiredness; abdominal pain and cramps; nausea, flatulence, and vomiting; parasthesia of the hands and feet		Abundantly available in ordinary foods	Deficiency rare even in marginally adequate diet
Vitamin A (retinol)	Photosensitive pigment in rods, membrane structure and function, integrity of skin and mucous membrane, growth in bony structures and teeth	Nightblindness, follicular keratosis (i.e., chicken skin), xerophthalmia (i.e., dryness of cornea and conjunctiva), and poor growth	Fatigue, malaise, abdominal pain, and headache with increased intracranial pressure	Breast milk, infant formula, fortified cow's milk, liver, carrots, sweet potatoes, green leafy vegetables, peaches, melons, and apricots	Excessive use of mineral oil, which interferes with absorption

(continued)

Table 11.1. *(continued)*

Vitamin	Function	Deficiency	Excess	Source	Risk factors
Vitamin B₁ (thiamine)	Coenzyme in carbohydrate and fatty acid metabolism	Neuritis, edema, anorexia, cardiac failure, loss of vibration sense and deep tendon reflexes, and calf tenderness		Pork, nuts, whole grain and fortified cereal products, breast milk, and infant formula	Chronic vomiting or diarrhea
Vitamin B₂ (riboflavin)	Reactive portion of flavoproteins involved in cellular metabolism	Cheilosis, angular stomatitis, seborrhea, and magenta tongue		Dairy products, liver, lamb, pork, breast milk, and infant formula	Marginal diet devoid of dairy, other animal protein sources and leafy vegetables
Vitamin B₆ (pyridoxine)	Aids metabolism of select amino acids that are essential for adequate function of central nervous system	Seizures, anemia, skin rash, and nerve damage		Chicken, fish, liver, pork, eggs, whole grains, and potatoes	Phenytoin impairs transport
Vitamin B₁₂	Coenzyme for amino acid metabolism, bone marrow, and nerve cell function	Macrocytic anemia, leukopenia, and progressive neurological deterioration ranging from peripheral neuritis to demyelinization of the posterior and lateral columns of the spinal cord		Most animal products, including milk and eggs	Infants of mothers on vegetarian diets fed only on breast milk, KCl interferes with absorption by decreasing ileal pH, and phenytoin impairs transport
Vitamin C (ascorbic acid)	Enhances collagen carnitine and catecholamine synthesis, fibroblast secretion, and cytochrome mixed function oxidase activity	Scurvy (i.e, weakness, swollen tender joints, delayed wound healing, friable gums)	Urinary stones, excessive iron absorption, red blood cell hemolysis, and gastrointestinal disturbances	Breast milk, citrus fruit, strawberries, cantaloupes, raw or minimally cooked vegetables, peppers, broccoli, cauliflower, leafy greens, tomatoes, and potatoes	Exclusive cow's milk-formula diet without vitamin supplementation or access to juices rich in vitamin C

252

Vitamin	Function	Deficiency	Toxicity	Sources	Causes
Vitamin D	Stimulates absorption of calcium and phosphorus from digestive tract and mobilization of both from bone	Osteomalacia, craniotabes, and rachitic changes (i.e., beading of rib ends and widening of distal long bones)	Weakness, lethargy, anorexia, and constipation	Sunlight, cow's milk, infant formula, cod liver oil, fish, and eggs	Inadequate sunlight exposure, deficient dietary intake, decreased absorption related to chronic mineral oil use, and phenytoin
Vitamin E (tocopherol)	Antioxidant and free radical scavenger to stabilize biological membranes	Neuroaxonal disease of brain stem, muscle, and peripheral nerves	Liver, kidney, and red blood cell toxicity at 10–15 times recommended daily allowance	Cereal seed oils, eggs, breast milk, liver, legumes, and butter	Excessive use of mineral oil can interfere with absorption
Vitamin K	Required for the synthesis of four blood coagulation factors	Increased tendency to bleed	Not stored in large quantities	Green leafy vegetables and human intestinal bacterial flora	Excessive use of mineral oil can interfere with absorption

Table 11.2. Minerals and nutrition

Mineral	Function	Deficiency	Source
Calcium	Major component of bones and teeth, essential for blood clotting, nerve and muscle function, hormone and neurotransmitter synthesis and release, and DNA synthesis and enzyme activation	Rickets and osteomalacia, tetany, and cardiac arrythmias	Milk and dairy products, canned sardines and salmon, shellfish, and soybeans
Copper	Component of multiple enzymes involved in skin pigmentation, neurotransmitter synthesis, function of collagen and elastin, and cellular respiration	Severe anemia, bone demineralization, decreased skin pigmentation, neurological abnormalities, decreased white blood cell count, and increased susceptibility to infection	Oysters, cocoa, bitter chocolate, beef liver, mushrooms, nuts, dried beans, and avocadoes
Iron	Component of hemoglobin, myoglobin, cytochrome oxidase, as well as other enzyme systems involved in oxygen transport and cellular respiration	Anemia, weakness, fatigability, decreased attention span and restricted development, and milk intolerance due to decreased gut lactase activity	More available in liver, lean meat, poultry, and fish than in cereal or green leafy vegetable sources
Magnesium	Contributes to normal function of cardiac, skeletal muscle, and nervous tissue; phosphate metabolism; and protein synthesis	Muscle tremor, choreiform movements, weakness, paralysis of specific muscle groups, dysphagia, and vertical nystagmus	Cocoa, nuts, soy and whole wheat flours, barley, wheat, and rice
Phosphorus	Rigidity of bones and teeth, essential to metabolism and function in every cell	Osteomalacia with weakness, anorexia, malaise, and stiff joints	Meat, fish, poultry, eggs, milk and cheese, nuts, and legumes
Zinc	Component of enzymes that catalyze metabolic reactions affecting carbon dioxide exchange, phosphate metabolism, nucleic acid, and protein metabolism	Growth retardation, delayed sexual maturation, loss of taste acuity, anorexia, behavior problems, hair loss, esophageal lesions, and eczematoid dermatitis	Meat, liver, milk, fish, eggs, nuts, and legumes

254

Magnesium deficiency, which may be caused by sustained losses of GI secretions or vigorous diuresis, resembles hypocalcemia. Symptoms include muscle tremor, choreiform movements, weakness, paralysis of specific muscle groups, dysphagia, and vertical nystagmus.

Children with cerebral palsy are especially vulnerable to rickets. Rickets results mainly from vitamin D deficiency and the associated decreased absorption of calcium and phosphorus; it does not result primarily from deficient dietary calcium. Limited mobility; lack of exposure to sunshine; anticonvulsants; and inadequate intake of milk, fish, or eggs contribute to the susceptibility of children with cerebral palsy to vitamin D deficiency. In both rickets and osteomalacia, which are seen in infants, older children, and adults, there is a lack of calcium retention in the skeleton. Children tend to be cranky and have lowered muscle tone, which is difficult to assess in children with cerebral palsy. Although the child's history may include frequent GI upsets and excessive sweating of the head, the diagnostic signs of rickets are skeletal changes. Swelling of the epiphysis of the long bones (i.e., radius, tibia, fibula, and femur) occurs and may be evident first at the wrist, where the radius is affected. Another classic site for swelling to occur is at the costochondral junctions (i.e., "joints" of the ribs) where swelling produces a bead-like appearance referred to as the *rachitic rosary*. As rickets progresses, deformities of the chest lead to the formation of pigeon breast. In young infants, craniotabes often is the first sign of rickets. Craniotabes consists of softened areas of the skull that usually affect the occipital and the parietal bones. The anterior fontanelle (i.e., the "soft spot" at the top of the head and forehead in infants) also is delayed in closing. In severe rickets, there may be bossing (i.e., circumscribed rounded swelling) of the skull at the forehead. Occasionally, the level of serum calcium is reduced enough for tetany to occur. Tetany presents an unmistakable picture of spasm of the hands with the thumb being drawn into the palm. In osteomalacia, pain occurs in the bones of the pelvis, lower back, and legs. Tenderness may be elicited by pressure on the affected bones. Osteomalacia is exaggerated when there is limited weight bearing and mobility.

The diagnosis of rickets is confirmed with radiographs, particularly of the wrists but also of the ends of long bones at other sites. These radiographs usually reveal the characteristic changes in the epiphyses where the outline of the joint is blurred and the epiphyseal line is broadened. The trabeculation of the bone becomes coarse, and there is a decrease in bone density. Blood tests reveal significant elevation of the serum alkaline phosphatase above the typical range, low serum phosphorus, and typical or slight reduction in serum calcium level.

The dose of vitamin D required to prevent rickets or osteomalacia remains unclear. Care should be taken to ensure that the child with cerebral palsy receives the same amounts of vitamin D that are recommended for a child who does not have cerebral palsy. If a child is receiving chronic anticonvulsant therapy, then serum calcium, phosphorus, and alkaline phosphatase should be measured at least annually to assess vitamin D status. Monitoring is conducted to detect any sign of megaloblastic anemia. Other medications should be evaluated for any possible drug–nutrient interactions.

Recognition of Obstacles in Attaining an Appropriate Diet

The child's diet should be judged not only by its caloric and nutrient content on paper but also by its bioavailability to the child. Food intake must be tailored to the child's ability to safely ingest it as well as to adequately metabolize it. For a diet to be appropriate, the child must have the oral–pharyngeal coordination to process and move the food safely from the mouth, past the airway, and into the esophagus. In addition, the GI tract must be able to perform its three major functions: 1) the controlled movement of food from the esophagus to the anus, 2) the digestion of food, and 3) the absorption of nutrients.

FEEDING THE CHILD WITH CEREBRAL PALSY

Feeding is a learned skill that is influenced by multiple factors. For the child to eat successfully, the following prerequisites must exist:

- Oral–pharyngeal competency
- Developmental synchrony
- Stability of medical issues that affect feeding

If there is fluctuation, delay, or abnormality in any of these prerequisites, a disruption may occur in feeding skills, which leads to a feeding problem.

Oral–Pharyngeal Competency

In order to understand what constitutes a feeding problem, one must first understand the typical feeding process. Swallowing can be divided into four phases (see Figure 11.3):

1. The oral preparatory phase in which food in the oral cavity is processed into the appropriate texture and prepared for transport
2. Oral transport of food through the oral cavity
3. Pharyngeal transfer (i.e., movement of the food past the airway to the esophagus)
4. Esophageal transport in which food travels down the esophagus and to the stomach

Neurological Control   Swallowing is a complex act that involves the timed, coordinated action of 27 muscle groups as well as the input from the autonomic and the somatic nervous systems. The swallowing center—the seat of control in the swallowing process—lies in the upper medullary region of the

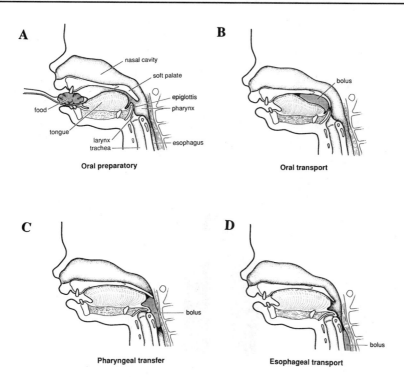

Figure 11.3. The four phases of swallowing. A) Oral preparatory phase in which food in the oral cavity is processed (i.e., the bolus of food is accepted and collected in the mid-tongue region). B) Oral transport phase in which food is pushed backward by the tongue toward the pharynx. C) Pharyngeal transfer stage in which the food is moved past the airway to the esophagus. As swallowing begins, the epiglottis typically folds over the opening of the trachea to direct food down the esophagus and not into the lungs. D) Esophageal transport phase in which food travels down the esophagus and toward the stomach. (From Eicher, P.S. [1997]. Feeding. In M.L. Batshaw [Ed.], *Children with disabilities* [4th ed., p. 622]. Baltimore: Paul H. Brookes Publishing Co.; reprinted by permission.)

brain stem (see Figure 11.4). The medullary region consists of a sensory relay station (i.e., nucleus tractus solitarius), a central rhythm generator, and a motor output station (i.e., nucleus ambiguous). There is a hierarchy of motor control involved in swallowing: local sensory input related to the bolus itself, integrated sensory feedback through the brain stem relay station, automatic control through the central rhythm generator (CRG), and cortical input. The sensory relay station receives taste and tactile information from the mouth and pharynx through cranial nerves V, VII, IX, and X, as well as sensory input from the heart, lungs, stomach, and esophagus. Input also is received from descending projections of cortical centers. Master neurons in the sensory relay station control the coordination of respiration with swallowing and are able to evoke pharyngeal and esophageal swallows. Patterns of output from these master neurons

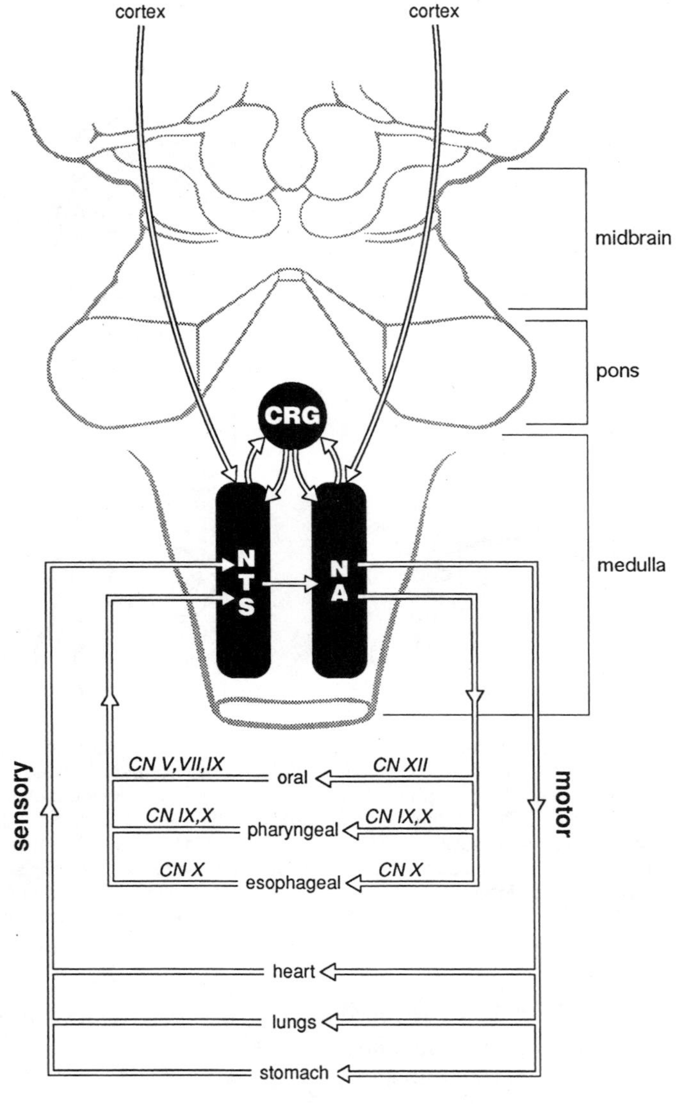

Figure 11.4. Neurological control of the swallowing process. Sensory information is transmitted to the nucleus tractus solitarius (NTS). Patterned output from the NTS activates the central rhythm generator (CRG), which initiates the swallowing cascade. CRG signals are translated by the nucleus ambiguous (NA) into timed motor output signals to the appropriate cranial nerves (CNs). Afferent input from the heart, lungs, or stomach can influence the swallowing process. Likewise, efferent signals from the NA can modify the function of heart, lungs, and stomach. (From Eicher, P.S. [1997]. Feeding. In M.L. Batshaw [Ed.], *Children with disabilities* [4th ed., p. 624]. Baltimore: Paul H. Brookes Publishing Co.; reprinted by permission.)

activate the CRG, which initiates the cascade of movements that results in swallowing. Bursts of activity generated by the CRG are transmitted to the motor area. Signals then are translated and transmitted as timed output to the proper motor neurons at various brain stem levels. Output from the nucleus ambiguous (NA) can be modified directly by sensory feedback from the nucleus tractus solitarius or from descending cortical projections to the NA.

Anatomy Recognizing the structures involved in the digestive process and their relationship to one another is important in understanding the feeding process. The oral cavity is the sole port of ingestion; however, it also plays a supporting role for air entry (i.e., the nose serves as the primary port for air). The ports for food and air meet in the pharynx (i.e., throat). This is divided into three regions: the nasopharynx, the oropharynx, and the hypopharynx (see Figure 11.5). The hypopharynx serves as the gating zone where respiration and ingestion must alternately use the same space. If any anatomical defect involving the oral or nasal cavities occurs, then the pharynx or the esophagus can adversely affect swallowing. Clefts in the lip or palate prohibit sealing off of the oral cavity, which decreases the ability to generate negative pressure and interferes with bolus collection. A structural change that affects coordination between swallowing and inspiration also can be significant (e.g., choanal atresia or adenoidal hypertrophy that renders the child dependent on his or her mouth as an airway).

Ontogeny of Swallowing The process of swallowing is not static in children. It is constantly changing in response to the influence of development and growth. As the nervous system matures, the oral-motor patterns that were initially manifested reflexively are integrated into learned motor patterns through practice. The increased cortical influence allowed by cortical maturation enables more specific and more finely graded movements with more volitional control. This is exactly analogous to the sequential progression that is recognized as underlying gross motor skill acquisition.

The most primitive oral movement is suckling. The suckle pattern involves a rhythmic up-and-down motion of the jaw. The tongue rides with the jaw but also moves out in a similar movement to a wave stripping the nipple. Suckle movements of the tongue and jaw have been seen in fetuses as early as 12 weeks' gestational age. However, suckling is not combined with swallowing until 34 weeks' gestation and only at full term does it become coordinated with breathing to allow for functional feeding. Suckling is initially a reflexive pattern that is elicited involuntarily whenever something enters the child's mouth. With brain maturation, the reflex is inhibited, and the pattern is refined into the voluntary act of sucking.

During sucking, the lips purse, the jaw movements are better controlled, and the tongue is raised and lowered independent of the jaw. This creates a vacuum that pulls food into the mouth. Once an up-down sucking pattern replaces the in-out stripping wave pattern of suckling, the child can progress to

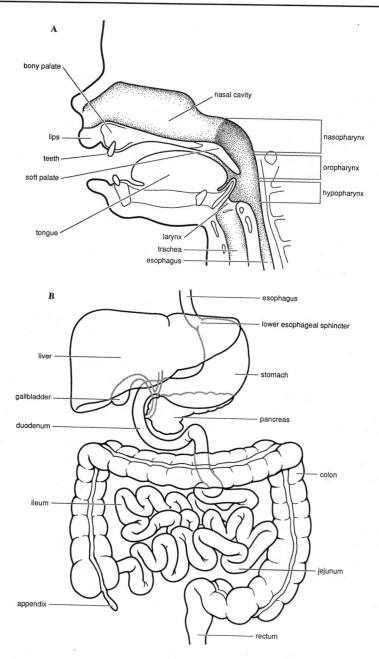

Figure 11.5. The anatomy of feeding. Consideration of the structures involved in the feeding process involves A) the oral, nasal, and pharyngeal cavities as well as B) the entire gastrointestinal system. Food passes down the esophagus, through the stomach, and into the intestines.

spoon feeding. This progression typically occurs at approximately 5 months of age; at this stage the child can begin to eat puréed foods.

The next stage in oral-motor development is munching. During munching, small pieces of food can be broken off, flattened, and then collected for swallowing. Munching consists of a rhythmical bite-and-release pattern with a series of well-graded jaw openings and closings. The emergence of tongue lateralization in this stage enables the child to move food from side to side and back to midline. Chewing food, when it is broken into smaller pieces, does not occur until the child acquires a rotary component to jaw movement. This can emerge as early as 9 months of age, but it is gradually modified with practice to the adult pattern at approximately 3 years of age.

Typically, the attainment of new oral-motor skills is timed to integrate perfectly with the change in oral-motor structures that occurs with growth. The infant, for example, is perfectly equipped for nipple feeding. The buccal fat pads in the cheeks laterally confine the oral cavity. The tongue, soft palate, and epiglottis fill much of the oropharyngeal cavity, making it easier to generate the negative intraoral pressure necessary to draw fluids out of the nipple. The larynx is positioned high and anterior, almost tucked under the tongue, necessitating less intrapharyngeal bolus control to guide it past the airway and into the esophagus. The close approximation of these structures provides positional support (Bosma, 1985) and stabilizes the structures until the infant develops more postural control. As the child grows, the jaw, palate, and teeth enlarge in relation to the soft tissue structures, making the oral cavity larger (see Figure 11.6). Descent and posterior movement of the larynx with growth heightens the importance of postural control for correct alignment and propulsive control, which enables the advanced oral-motor patterns to safely guide the bolus past the airway.

In children with cerebral palsy who have persistent primitive reflex patterns (see Chapter 2), the typical integration of growth and development is disrupted. The child's structures may grow, but the oral pattern may not mature; this may result in decreased efficiency in bottle feeding and increased risk of aspiration for all types of feeding. The texture of the food presented by family members may be based on the child's age rather than on his or her abilities. For example, the child may still have a strong suckle pattern, but he or she may be offered chopped table food that cannot be managed safely. Under these circumstances, meals can become a prolonged, difficult, and at times unsafe chore.

Developmental Influences: Motor
Control, Readiness, and Positive Practice

The act of feeding requires a high level of oral-motor control and coordination superimposed on adequate trunk alignment and support. Atypical muscle tone and persistent primitive reflex activity frequently interfere with body alignment and trunk support. Lack of adequate trunk support greatly hinders rib cage

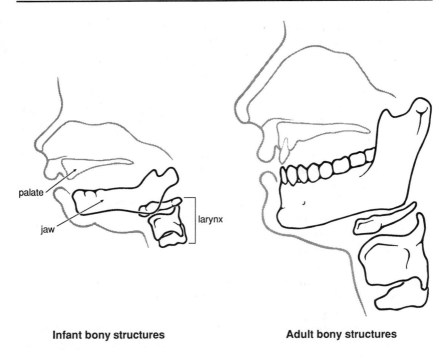

Infant bony structures　　　　　　**Adult bony structures**

Figure 11.6.　Differences between the anatomy and the function of the oral cavity in infants and adults. As the child grows, the bony structures enlarge in relation to the soft tissues, which increase the size of the oral cavity and the pharynx. The larynx descends and moves posteriorly almost 3 vertebral bodies by 8 years of age. These anatomical changes increase the control necessary to guide a bolus safely past the airway and into the esophagus (see Table 11.3). (From Eicher, P.S. [1997]. Feeding. In M.L. Batshaw [Ed.], *Children with disabilities* [4th ed., p. 626]. Baltimore: Paul H. Brookes Publishing Co.; reprinted by permission.)

expansion, which interferes with respiration and increases pressure on the stomach and the abdominal cavity (Nwaobi & Smith, 1986). An unstable posture also limits effective execution of oral-motor patterns. Feeding is best accomplished with the head and trunk neutrally aligned and the extremities in a flexed position (see Figure 11.7). Predominance of extensor patterns anywhere in the body will decrease the child's oral–pharyngeal control.

　　Oral-motor skill acquisition follows a developmental progression similar to that of other motor skills. To be successful, the child must function at a developmental level consistent with the skills required for the texture offered. For example, the child whose skills are at a 6- to 7-month level of development will not have the neurological maturity to adequately chew meats and other hard solids. Because oral skills follow a hierarchical sequence, the child must have experience in every stage of feeding (intermediate stages cannot be skipped).

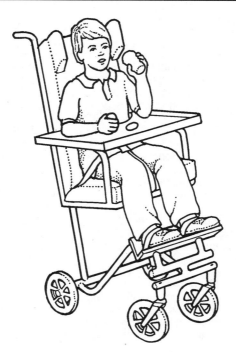

Figure 11.7. Proper positioning for feeding. In order to best promote successful feeding in children with cerebral palsy, the child must be positioned symmetrically and well supported. Typically, a solid seat and back with a 90-degree angle at the hips, knees, and ankles and the feet planted squarely provide a stable base of support. The trunk, shoulder girdle, neck, and head should be aligned squarely over the pelvis. The head and the neck should be in neutral position without extension. If the child has difficulty with maintaining his or her head or trunk in an upright position, the chair may be tilted backward to decrease the work against gravity.

For example, the child cannot make the transition from bottle to table-food solids without experience with purées (see Table 11.3).

Successful progression through the hierarchy of oral-motor skills depends on the ability to practice the new movements until they become learned and incorporated into the child's functional pattern. The amount and the type of practice can clinically enhance or slow the rate of acquisition. Occasionally, the child's experience with eating or drinking may be temporarily disrupted; or eating may become negatively associated with discomfort, which, despite resolution of the initial medical problem, can result in persistent feeding problems. An example of this is the child with an exacerbation of GER secondary to short-term illness. Once the illness has subsided and the reflux is under control, the child may still associate eating with the discomfort experienced in the past. In this type of instance, manipulation of the environment and

Table 11.3. Stages of oral-motor development

Age	Oral-motor pattern	Feeding skill
32–34 weeks' gestation	**Suck/swallow** Swallow initiated after suckle tongue movement but not coordinated with respiration	Nonnutritive suckle on pacifier or fingers
At term	**Suckle** Extension/retraction movement of tongue combined with up–down movements of mandible and coordinated with respiration	Nipple feeding
3–6 months	**Sucking** Up–down motion of tongue independent of graded jaw excursions	Spoon feedings of puréed foods
6–9 months	**Munching** Flattening and spreading of tongue with lateral movement for collection, finely graded and repetitive vertical jaw movements	Advance to small pieces of soft solids and soft finger foods
9–36 months	**Chewing** More controlled tongue lateralization patterns, rotary jaw movements to grind food	Advance to larger pieces of soft solids and more fibrous textures

institution of behavioral interventions may be helpful in managing the feeding problems. If, for medical reasons, oral feeding is precluded for prolonged periods of time, children with cerebral palsy can lose their oral-motor skills (Monahan, Shapiro, & Fox, 1988). If this happens, the child needs to be gradually retrained to eat.

Many feeding transitions typically occur in the first 2 years of life and include the introduction of new textures, new utensils, and new situations. These transitions heighten the importance of both a stable mealtime environment and a consistent interaction between the caregiver and the child. Such consistency imparts a sense of familiarity to the child, which enables him or her to feel comfortable and more tolerant when eating. The child's fine motor and adaptive skills at mealtime influence choice of utensils and level of independence. Cognitive abilities, especially those underlying communication and social skills, shape how the child interacts in the feeding situation. The subsequent sections discuss several factors that can help make meals more interesting for the child with cerebral palsy.

Medical Issues that Affect Feeding

Feeding is especially vulnerable to instability in the primary organ systems that affect eating, namely the respiratory tract, the GI tract, and the CNS. Any medical problem that causes even temporary interruption or disruption of these systems can result in a feeding problem.

Respiratory System   The heart and lungs send information directly to the swallowing center; it is this process that explains why the child with acutely increased respiratory effort (e.g., during pneumonia or wheezing) may start to drool: his or her swallowing frequency is decreased to allow more frequent respiration (Timms, Defiore, Martin, & Miller, 1993). For the child with cerebral palsy who may have a delayed activation of swallowing or more difficulty controlling the food in the oral cavity, any increase in respiratory work may decompensate an already compromised system, resulting in aspiration or food refusal (Rogers, Arvedson, Buck, & Smart, 1994).

Gastrointestinal System   Typically after swallowing, a peristaltic wave guides food down the esophagus and to the stomach, where acids are secreted in order to break down the food (see Figure 11.5). Contractions of the stomach wall mix the food and push it gradually into the duodenum (i.e., the upper part of the small intestine). The lower esophageal sphincter (LES) at the entrance to the stomach functions as a one-way valve to prevent backward flow of stomach contents into the esophagus (i.e., GER). In the duodenum, enzymes and other substances from the pancreas and bile ducts digest food particles into their major components: proteins, fats, and carbohydrates. These components are then further broken down into sugars (e.g., lactose), fatty acids, amino acids, and vitamins. The ileum (i.e., the lower small intestine) absorbs these digested nutrients and all remaining food particles are passed to the large intestine (i.e., colon). Movement through the colon is much slower than it is through the rest of the digestive tract and depends in part on the volume of nonabsorbable nutrients (i.e., fiber) that is contained in the food. If movement is too rapid as with gastroenteritis, diarrhea occurs. Slowed movement allows increased water absorption resulting in hard stools and constipation.

Feedback from the GI tract can affect feeding in several ways. It is obvious that nausea and vomiting could limit caloric intake either through increased losses with vomiting or through decreased intake resulting from food refusal. Bloating or cramping related to constipation or delayed gastric emptying also can decrease the child's interest in eating. Reflux and esophagitis (see section on "Gastroesophageal Reflux" in this chapter) may be associated with pain and discomfort, which also can limit intake.

Digestion   Although cerebral palsy is often associated with oral-motor dysfunction and bowel dysmotility, it is not associated with an increased risk for disorders of digestion or absorption. An exception to this rule occurs in the presence of chronic undernutrition, which can decrease intestinal enzymes and result in malabsorption of nutrients. Occasionally, disorders of absorption can occur in children with chronic undernutrition unrelated to cerebral palsy, and these disorders must be considered in the same manner as they would be in any child with inadequate growth. The most common disorder of malabsorption is lactose intolerance. Food allergies may also interfere with the ability of the GI tract to digest specific foods (Kelly et al., 1995).

Gastroesophageal Reflux   GER is the backward flow of stomach contents into the esophagus. As previously discussed, the LES typically functions as a barrier to prevent the return of stomach contents into the esophagus. GER is very common in individuals with cerebral palsy for several reasons. The esophagus lies, for most of its course, within the thoracic cavity (the most distal end is intra-abdominal and comprises the gastroesophageal junction); the stomach is typically enclosed entirely within the abdomen. Large differences in pressure between the cavities or large fluctuations in pressure within the cavities predispose the child to GER. Increased intra-abdominal pressure related to spasticity of the abdominal musculature or constipation may be sufficient to overcome the barrier posed by the LES, resulting in GER. Because the esophagus enters the stomach posteriorly, prolonged periods in supine positioning, which are common in children with decreased mobility, exaggerate gravitational forces, pushing food up through the LES and into the esophagus. In addition, children who drool may swallow less frequently, decreasing both peristaltic clearance and neutralization of the refluxate by saliva, which acts as a buffer to stomach acid. GER also may be a result of the enteric nervous system (i.e., the specialized system of nerves that controls GI function and motility) being impaired in some way in children who have cerebral palsy, thus directly affecting GI function and motility. Delayed gastric emptying may be one manifestation of such an impairment, resulting in pooling of partially digested foodstuffs in the stomach for extended periods, which further increases the likelihood of GER (Hebra & Hoffman, 1993).

A cycle may develop in which recurrent GER causes chronic irritation and inflammation of the esophagus (i.e., esophagitis), which can result in further impairment of the LES and lead to worsening GER and exacerbating inflammation. Although the primary manifestations of GER are vomiting and abdominal pain, many children with cerebral palsy have GER and even severe esophagitis without these obvious manifestations. Any child with cerebral palsy who has significant feeding or growth difficulties should undergo appropriate evaluation to assess the presence of occult GER.

Bowel Motility and Constipation   In many children with cerebral palsy, constipation is a chronic problem. This is caused by inadequate fluid and fiber intake combined with uncoordinated muscle contractions and poor rectal sphincter control; the result is the retention of stool for prolonged periods of time. The longer the stool remains in the colon, the more water is absorbed, and the harder and more immobile the stool becomes. The end result is constipation (Fitzgerald, 1987). In addition to increasing intra-abdominal pressure and thereby the risk of GER, constipation can be associated with cramping and discomfort that can interfere with appetite, positioning, and sleep.

Overly loose stools also can be a problem. These may be caused by lack of dietary fiber, dumping, overaggressive bowel cleaning, or passage of loose stool around an impaction. If either diarrhea or constipation is a problem, then the child's diet and bowel regimen should be evaluated and adjusted.

Other Medical Conditions   Any medical condition that impairs the baseline function of the respiratory or GI tracts can influence the swallowing process. Reactive airway disease (i.e., asthma) with recurrent exacerbations, uncontrolled seizures, unstable intracranial pressure, renal disease, or metabolic disorders such as cystic fibrosis or a urea cycle defect can be significant contributors to the development of a feeding problem. Cerebral palsy by its very nature presents with nervous system dysfunction on many levels. Feeding represents a complex behavior that is regulated by the nervous system. The degree to which sensory, motor, autonomic, and cognitive systems are affected in an individual with cerebral palsy correlates directly with the likelihood that feeding difficulties will be present.

Diagnostic Procedures

Because of the complexity of the feeding process and the multiple influences on it, evaluating a feeding problem should include a medical history and examination, a neurodevelopmental assessment, an oral–pharyngeal evaluation, a feeding history, and a mealtime observation. The information gleaned by these evaluations may be enough to identify the feeding problem as well as the factors contributing to it; however, diagnostic procedures may be necessary to provide further information to support or to clarify clinical hypotheses.

If aspiration or GER is suspected, several tests are available to further define the problem (Kramer & Eicher, 1993). In GER, an upper GI series may be conducted to rule out anatomical problems in the GI tract. In the upper GI series, a milk-like substance is either ingested by the child or infused into the stomach through an enteral tube. The barium in this substance is visible on X-ray film. Thus, the radiologist can follow the fluid as it courses through the stomach and small intestine, helping to identify structural abnormalities in the esophagus, stomach, and small intestine. Reflux from the stomach into the esophagus also may be seen with this procedure.

In a second procedure, a radionuclide study (i.e., milk scan) provides information about frequency of GER as well as rate of gastric emptying (Heyman, Eicher, & Alavi, 1995). Delayed gastric emptying can lead to vomiting and aspiration; an increased rate of gastric emptying can lead to diarrhea. In a radionuclide study, the child swallows a milk formula that has small amounts of a radioactive tracer, which enables the radiologist to follow the course of the milk through the GI tract as well as determine how fast the formula is moving. The milk scan also is valuable if aspiration from GER is suspected. If radioactive tracer is found in the lung after several hours, then this suggests that aspiration has occurred during a reflux episode.

The final two studies, the pH probe and the gastroesophageal duodenoscopy (i.e., endoscopy), are considered the gold standards in the evaluation of GER and esophagitis (Ross, Haase, Reiley, & Meagher, 1988). In the pH probe study, a nasogastric-like tube is inserted through the nose and passed down the esophagus to just above the junction of the stomach and the esophagus. At the tip of the tube is a small sensor that measures the pH or acidity above the gastroesophageal junction. If acid in the stomach refluxes through an incompetent LES, then the sensor records a sudden drop in the pH level, signaling GER. Reflux is most likely to occur in the hour following a meal or during sleep because the child is reclined. For this reason, the pH probe records for 24 hours to indicate the presence of reflux and the circumstances of its occurrence. This may have important therapeutic implications in terms of positioning after feeding. Endoscopy entails passing a fiberoptic tube through the mouth and into the stomach while the child is sedated in order to visualize the tissues and take small biopsy specimens to examine for irritation and inflammation (i.e., esophagitis).

If aspiration of oral feedings is suspected, then a modified barium swallow with videofluoroscopy is the best test for evaluating GER and esophagitis. In this study, the child is positioned in the usual feeding position and offered foods that contain barium. The radiologist focuses on the pharynx and watches with a videofluoroscope how the food is guided by the muscles past the airway. The texture of the food and the liquids can be changed to evaluate whether the child has more difficulty with one texture than another (Fox, 1990).

Specific Feeding Problems for Children with Cerebral Palsy

There are many obstacles to successful feeding for children with cerebral palsy. Numerous problems related to the child and/or the caregiver need to be monitored closely in order to improve the child's medical, nutritional, and developmental well-being.

Persistent Suckle   It is very common for children with cerebral palsy to have an exaggerated suckle reflex (i.e., spitting out food, increased oral losses, or prolonged feeding time), which is caused by the delayed inhibition of primitive reflex patterns associated with this disorder. This exaggerated reflex precludes advancement to a sucking pattern and interferes with successful spoon feeding because the food rides out on the tongue. As parents thicken the food to keep it in the mouth, the child tends to revert to his or her strongest pattern (i.e., the suckle), which is not efficient for solids and, therefore, prolongs mealtime. Persistence of the suckle pattern eventually becomes medically problematic. First, it is so ineffective for solid-food transport that it becomes difficult for the child to ingest adequate calories. Moreover, as the child grows, the head and the neck elongate and the opening to the esophagus descends and moves posteriorly, requiring a more controlled transport pattern than suckling to guide the food bolus safely past the airway.

Lack of Chewing   As previously discussed, the texture of foods offered to children is commonly determined according to their chronological age rather than by their level of development or their oral-motor function. When oral-motor skills are immature and the child is unable to process chunks or lumps of food, he or she may push the lump into the cheek in order not to choke or gag on it. Compound this situation with the child who has a central pattern of tongue movements, as with sucking or suckling, and the child will not be able to recollect the food back into midline. Food pieces drift into the cheeks because the child is unable to remove them. As a result, each bite is smashed up to the roof of the mouth, gradually becoming a larger and larger bolus until the child has trouble moving the tongue at all. The child will either stop eating, gag, cough, or choke to clear the bolus or will drink to wash the bolus down. This is obviously not an efficient solid-food strategy.

Gagging, Coughing, and Choking   Gagging, coughing, and choking are natural protective responses aimed at keeping the oral airway clear. Each response suggests a different triggering mechanism that may be clinically useful; however, this is not foolproof. Gagging suggests an oral-motor problem in which the food bolus size is not adequately processed, and the child feels that he or she may not be able to swallow it. Coughing suggests that food has entered the airway at some level, triggering a cough in order to clear it out. In children with cerebral palsy, coughing is more typically associated with drinking and thin liquids than it is with solids. Choking suggests that peristalsis of the food past the airway has been stalled and occurs as a forceful expulsion of the trapped food bolus. If gagging, coughing, or choking occur at the end of a meal or after a meal rather than during the meal, GER needs to be considered. If coughing or gagging during meals persists for more than several weeks, this is a serious warning signal and requires thorough, immediate evaluation.

Gagging on the texture of food may be further related to immature or pathological oral-motor transport, hypersensitive gag on a neurological basis, increased gag response associated with GER, or learned refusal. It is not clear how GER heightens the gag response, but it may be related to increased muscle tone. GER frequently enhances extensor posturing through the trunk, the head, and the neck, and this limits oral-motor mobility and can result in loss of bolus control and gagging.

Aspiration   Aspiration refers to the entry of foodstuffs or foreign substance into the airway (see Figure 11.8). It may occur before, during, or after a swallow or as a result of GER. Everyone aspirates small amounts occasionally, but protective responses such as a gag or a cough help to clear the airway without serious consequence. Children with cerebral palsy that affects motor coordination of the oropharynx, larynx, or trachea are at increased risk for recurrent aspiration. Moreover, these children frequently have impaired protective

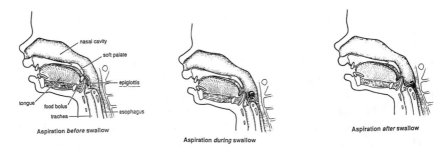

Figure 11.8. Aspiration of food. Aspiration before a swallow can occur if the bolus leaks past the soft palate before a swallow is triggered and flows into the open airway. Aspiration during a swallow can occur if the larynx is not competently closed as the bolus passes. Aspiration after a swallow can occur if food residual in the pharynx is carried into the airway with the next breath. (From Eicher, P.S. [1997]. Feeding. In M.L. Batshaw [Ed.], *Children with disabilities* [4th ed., p. 630]. Baltimore: Paul H. Brookes Publishing Co.; reprinted by permission.)

responses, which limit their ability to clear the airway once aspiration has occurred. Signs of aspiration are influenced by the age of the child. Aspiration in infants may present as *apnea* (i.e., arrest of respiration) or *bradycardia* (i.e., decreased heart rate). In older infants and children, symptoms commonly include coughing, increased congestion, or wheezing during meals. The accumulation of foodstuffs in the airway causes irritation and inflammation. Depending on the amount and the frequency of aspiration, the child can develop recurrent pneumonia, bronchitis, or tracheitis (Loughlin & Lefton-Greif, 1994), all of which can be life threatening and, therefore, must always be considered and ruled out. This ruling-out process can be done by listening to breath sounds and vocal quality for clues of respiratory penetration or puddling in the larynx during a meal (Eicher, Manno, Fox, & Kerwin, 1995). Unfortunately, not all children will cough, choke, or gag when they aspirate. Some children can aspirate without evoking any protective response; this is called *silent aspiration.*

Lack of Interest in Food and Refusal to Eat Some children with cerebral palsy act as if they are very hungry but lose interest in eating and refuse further food after only a few bites. This may be a symptom of several problems. If the child aspirates during a meal, he or she may not want to eat after that point. Children with GER and discomfort after a certain volume of intake will stop at a consistent point in each meal despite how hungry they initially appear. Likewise, constipation can contribute to refusal; as the gastrocolic reflex is stimulated, the child may feel crampy and lose interest in the meal. As noted previously, if eating the food is too much work, the child will stop before attaining adequate caloric intake and will play or dawdle in order to "kill time." It is important to consider how long mealtimes take. It is difficult for anyone to remain interested in meals that last longer than 45 minutes.

Drooling   Drooling is a very frequent problem for children with cerebral palsy. Decreased facial tone and delayed head righting allow gravity to influence the position of the mouth, which enables saliva to roll out. Because of oral-motor difficulty, many children with cerebral palsy may swallow less often or need to swallow several times to clear a bolus. This allows more saliva to pool in the oral cavity. In addition, GER can increase saliva production as the body is signaled to make more buffer to neutralize the stomach acids. This increased production accentuates any swallowing difficulty and may result in drooling. Drooling also may occur as an early presentation of a sore throat or increased work of breathing, which would decrease swallowing frequency.

Overestimation of Caloric Intake   Overestimation of how much the child has eaten is very common and prohibits the reliance on diet recall alone for estimation of caloric intake (Stallings et al., 1996). Contributing factors to overestimation include parental optimism, fear of invasive intervention, estimation bias based on meal duration or effort, and inaccurate accounting of food losses. In the child with inadequate weight gain, efforts to obtain prospective calorie counts or to observe a sample meal to get some idea of typical losses must be accomplished before beginning investigations into less common problems such as malabsorption or increased energy expenditure. Likewise, caregivers must be careful not to be lulled into thinking that the child is obtaining adequate calories for growth based on their best, well-intentioned efforts to remember the amounts of food ingested by the child.

MANAGING FEEDING PROBLEMS

Because feeding difficulties in children with cerebral palsy are typically a result of the interaction of multiple factors, managing them can be difficult, time consuming, and frustrating (Crane, 1987; Helfrich-Miller, Rector, & Straka, 1986). Effective treatment usually requires intervention from more than one therapeutic discipline. The treatment team, including the child's caregiver, needs to prioritize the goals of treatment and outline an integrated plan to approaching these goals. With input from the team, the primary care provider oversees the plan and monitors progress toward the goals. This management is done in the context of the child's medical, nutritional, and developmental well-being. Components of a successful treatment strategy include minimizing negative medical influences, optimizing positioning for feeding, facilitating oral-motor function, improving the mealtime environment, being consistent, and developing an effective plan for monitoring progress. The management recommendations that follow illustrate this approach.

Decrease Gastroesophageal Reflux

GER can adversely affect respiratory and GI function and negatively affect position, oral-motor function, and nutrition. A number of therapeutic interventions, including positioning, meal modification, medications, and surgery, may be necessary to adequately control GER and to prevent these complications (Orenstein, Whitington, & Orenstein, 1983). The goal of treatment is to protect the esophagus from reflux of stomach acid, either by decreasing the amount of food in the stomach at any one time or by decreasing the acidity of the stomach acids.

Small, frequent meals and medications that promote stomach emptying help to decrease the volume of food in the stomach. In addition, studies have found that whey-based formulas also improve stomach emptying and decrease vomiting in children with spastic quadriplegia (Fried et al., 1992). Upright positioning and thickened feedings employ gravity to help keep stomach contents from refluxing into the esophagus. Medications such as urecholine (Bethanechol), metoclopramide (Reglan), and cisapride (Propulsid) increase the tone in the esophageal sphincter, making it harder for reflux to occur (McCallum, 1990). Cimetidine (Tagamet), ranitidine (Zantac), or famotidine (Pepcid) often are added to decrease stomach acidity and thereby lower the risk of inflammation of the esophagus from reflux (Sontag, 1990).

Sometimes GER cannot be controlled by positioning or medication. Prolonged reflux can lead to failure to thrive, recurrent aspiration pneumonia, and gastroesophageal bleeding; surgery then may be necessary. A *fundoplication* (Fonkalsrud et al., 1995) is an operation in which the top of the stomach is wrapped around the opening of the esophagus (see Figure 11.9). This decreases

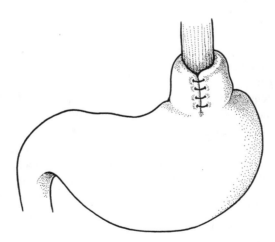

Figure 11.9. Fundoplication for control of GER. Although there are several variations, the basic fundoplication entails freeing the top portion of the stomach, or fundus, and wrapping it around the esophagus to enhance the lower esophageal sphincter and re-create a muscular valve to prevent reflux. (From Eicher, P.S. [1997]. Feeding. In M.L. Batshaw [Ed.], *Children with disabilities* [4th ed., p. 635]. Baltimore: Paul H. Brookes Publishing Co.; reprinted by permission.)

reflux while permitting continued oral feeding. An alternative to surgery is place-ment of a gastrojejunostomy tube (GJ-tube). This tube allows access to the stom-ach as well as the jejunum and allows some portion of the food to bypass the stomach, thereby decreasing the potential for reflux (Albanese, Towbin, Ulman, Lewis, & Smith, 1993).

Avoid and Treat Constipation

Constipation is a long-term problem for many children with cerebral palsy. Hard, infrequent stools that are difficult to pass contribute to increased abdominal fullness. Constipation can be uncomfortable and can lead to poor appetite and increased GER. Bowel evacuation patterns vary among individuals, which makes it very hard to establish an accepted norm. However, a good goal is to aim for no prolonged straining with evacuation. If the child has feeding problems or marginal nutrition, a daily stool helps to increase appetite and thereby oral intake.

Although no cures for constipation are known, the following suggestions may be helpful. As much fluid as possible should be added to the diet. Bulky and high-fiber foods, such as whole grain cereals, bran, and raw fruits and veg-etables, should be included in the child's diet to increase movement through the GI tract (Liebl, Fischer, Van Calcar, & Marlett, 1990). Prune, apricot, or papaya juice can act as a mild laxative. Stool softeners, such as docusate sodium (Colace) or mineral oil–containing drugs (Kondremul), may be used regularly to help coat the stool and facilitate its movement through the intestines. Active or pas-sive physical exercise also is important to aid the movement of the stool.

If bowel evacuation does not improve, laxatives or suppositories may be necessary to facilitate regularity. This group includes magnesium hydroxide (Milk of Magnesia), malt soup extract (Maltsupex), senna (Senokot), bisacodyl (Dulcolax), or glycerin suppositories. Enemas, such as Fleet's pediatric enema, also may help, but constant use of enemas can interfere with typical rectal sphinc-ter control and should be avoided. A combination of these approaches may be needed to establish regular bowel movements.

Ensure Proper Positioning

Appropriate positioning of the child during feeding maximizes his or her ability to eat effectively and safely as well as his or her ability to coordinate the activi-ties of feeding and breathing (Nwaobi & Smith, 1986). The child should be firmly supported through the hips and trunk during feeding to provide a stable base (see Figure 11.7). The head and neck should be aligned in a neutral posi-tion, which decreases extension through the oral musculature while maintain-ing an open airway. This positioning allows better coordination and more control of the steps in oral-motor preparation and transport. This, in turn, allows more positive practice and behavioral reinforcement of appropriate feeding behavior (Kerwin, Osborne, & Eicher, 1994).

Optimize Oral-Motor Function

Facilitating jaw and lip closure when necessary may help make the child's oral pattern more effective as well as accustom him or her to the proper positions for feeding. Spoon placement with gentle pressure on the mid-tongue region can help remind the child to keep the tongue inside the mouth. Chewing may be enhanced by placing food laterally between the upper and lower molars. This input to the molar surface stimulates the child to move the jaw and enhances lateral tongue movement in order to collect the food.

Food textures can be manipulated to facilitate safe, controlled swallowing (Gisel, 1994). Thickening of liquids slows their rate of flow, allowing more time for the child to control the bolus and initiate a swallow. Thickening agents (e.g., Thickit, instant pudding powders) can transform any thin liquid into a nectar-, honey-, or milkshake-like consistency. This provides more options to ensure adequate hydration in children who have difficulty drinking. Almost any food can be chopped fine or puréed to a texture that the child can competently manage.

It is important to remember that the primary goal of eating is to achieve adequate nutrition. Thus, when the child is first learning to accept foods that need to be flattened or ground up by the teeth, these foods should be presented during snacktime when volumes are smaller. At mealtimes, easier textures should be included to ensure consumption of adequate calories during this transition period.

Understand that Eating Is Work

Eating is a motor activity that requires a higher level of coordination between muscle groups than most other motor activities. Atypical sensation, strength, or coordination may result in aspiration, which is unpleasant, frightening, and dangerous. Atypical tone or poor coordination in the upper extremities of the body increases the effort needed to feed oneself with a utensil. If the effort, or work, required to obtain and swallow food is too taxing, the child will avoid eating altogether (Kerwin, Ahearn, Eicher, & Burd, 1995). Therefore, it is important to make eating as easy as possible (Babbitt et al., 1994). The work of eating can be minimized in several ways. First, increase the child's focus on the meal. Let the child know that mealtime is coming so he or she can prepare for the "work" to be done. This may include moving to a special area of the room with less distraction or repositioning and oral stimulation to get the needed muscles ready for eating. Second, include foods in each meal that are easier for the child to control both manually and intraorally. A variety of adaptive utensils is available to facilitate independence and optimize oral-motor function in mealtime, from spoons with built-up or curved handles to specialized cups and bowls with higher sides that will not shift on the table.

The satisfaction the child gets from eating can be increased by social attention during the meal or a favorite food or activity after the meal has been completed (Iwata, Riordan, Wohl, & Finney, 1982). Children with feeding difficulties typically eat better in one-to-one situations or in small groups with less distraction. Undivided attention also makes mealtimes more reinforcing.

Promote Appetite

Some children have little appetite. In addition, they may be unable to communicate that they are hungry. If speech is impaired or limited, signing or using a communication board may prove helpful. If this does not work, a child may be fed at different times of the day to find out at which hour he or she eats best. The child may eat the largest meal for breakfast or lunch rather than for dinner. Foods that the child likes can be paired with less favored ones (Iwata et al., 1982). Regular bowel movements also can improve the child's interest in eating.

Consider Alternative Methods of Feeding

In some cases, oral feeding may not be safe or sufficient to promote adequate nutrition. In these children, nasogastric tube feedings or the placement of a gastrostomy feeding tube is required. Enteral tubes can be very helpful but must be carefully planned to avoid secondary complications (see Figure 11.10).

In nasogastric tube feedings, a tube is passed through the nose down the esophagus and into the stomach. A commercially available formula, such as Ensure or Pediasure, or blended feedings composed of a regular diet combined with milk can be used. However, nasogastric tube feedings should be used only on a temporary basis. The tube may irritate the lining of the nose or the esophagus and can cause aspiration if it is incorrectly placed.

In children who will need tube feedings for a prolonged period, a gastrostomy tube (i.e., G-tube) is recommended. A small hole is made in the abdominal and stomach walls, and a tube is placed through the hole into the stomach. Feeding can then be done through the gastrostomy tube in a manner similar to nasogastric tube feeding. If GER is a problem, a GJ-tube may be a helpful option. The GJ-tube is basically a combination of a G-tube and a J-tube. The J-tube portion travels through the pylorus (i.e., the valve connecting the stomach to the duodenum), the duodenum, and into the jejunum (i.e., the second section of the small intestine) in order to prevent reflux of the nutrients. The placement of a G-tube or GJ-tube does not preclude oral feeding.

A commercially prepared enteral formula can be used with any of these tubes. Although blenderized feedings can be given through an NG-tube or G-tube, they are not appropriate for a J-tube because they will obstruct it. With an NG-tube or a G-tube, feedings can be given in single, large volumes (i.e., bolus) of 3–8 ounces every 3–6 hours or as a continuous drip throughout the day or overnight. J-tube feedings must be given continuously rather than as a bolus. The advantage of large-volume feedings is that they do not interfere with typical daily activities. The feeding itself takes about 30 minutes. However, the large volume may be difficult for the child to tolerate and may lead to vomiting

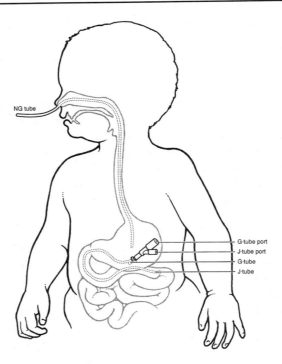

Figure 1 1.10.   Enteral feeding tubes. The nasogastric tube (NG-tube) is placed through the nostril and into the stomach. An NG-tube is helpful if problems with a child's oral function are the primary obstacle to adequate nutrition. A gastrostomy tube (GT-tube) is placed directly through the abdominal wall into the stomach. A GT-tube is helpful if enteral tube feedings are needed for a prolonged period and the child is having difficulty with irritation related to the NG-tube. A gastrojejunostomy tube (GJ-tube) allows access to the stomach as well as directly into the intestine. A GJ-tube can be helpful if the stomach is unable to tolerate the quantity of nutrients needed for adequate growth. (From Eicher, P.S. [1997]. Feeding. In M.L. Batshaw [Ed.], *Children with disabilities* [4th ed., p. 636]. Baltimore: Paul H. Brookes Publishing Co.; reprinted by permission.)

or abdominal discomfort. If this happens, continuous drip feedings can be instituted. A Kangaroo or a similar type pump is used to deliver the formula at a constant rate. Sometimes tube feedings are used to supplement oral feedings. In this case, the tube feedings generally are used at night to ensure that the child's stomach is not filled with the tube feeding during the day.

Once a G-tube or a GJ-tube has been placed, it must be maintained properly. The area surrounding the tube should be washed daily, and the tube should be changed every few months. If the skin around the tube bleeds, it may need to be cauterized using silver nitrate sticks. If the area is inflamed, it means that the area is infected or that stomach acid is leaking. If an infection has been ruled out, the use of Duoderm or another occlusive dressing, such as Vaseline, should help.

SUMMARY

Feeding the child with a developmental disability often requires the implementation of a number of creative approaches and the involvement of a variety of health care professionals. When effective and well integrated, these methods allow the child not only to experience optimal oral feeding experiences with their positive social and developmental ramifications but also to receive the necessary combination of nutrients and fluids to help them grow and remain healthy.

REFERENCES

Albanese, C.L., Towbin, R.B., Ulman, T., Lewis, J., & Smith, S.D. (1993). Percutaneous gastrojejunostomy versus Nissen fundoplication for enteral feeding of the neurologically impaired child with gastroesophageal reflux. *Journal of Pediatrics, 123,* 371–375.

American Academy of Pediatrics. (1993). *Pediatric nutrition handbook* (3rd ed.). Evanston, IL: American Academy of Pediatrics, Committee on Nutrition.

Babbitt, R.S., Hoch, T.A., Coe, D.A., Cataldo, M.F., Kelly, K.J., Stackhouse, C., & Perman, J.A. (1994). Behavioral assessment and treatment of pediatric feeding disorders. *Journal of Developmental and Behavioral Pediatrics, 15,* 278–291.

Bosma, J.F. (1985). Postnatal ontogeny of performances of the pharynx, larynx, and mouth. *American Review of Respiratory Disease, 131*(Suppl.), S10–S15.

Burton, B.T., & Foster, W.R. (1988). *Human nutrition.* New York: McGraw-Hill.

Crane, S. (1987). Feeding the handicapped child: A review of intervention strategies. *Nutrition and Health, 5,* 109–118.

Culley, W.J., & Middleton, T.A. (1969). Caloric requirements of mentally retarded children with and without motor dysfunction. *Journal of Pediatrics, 118,* 399–404.

Eicher, P.S. (1997). Feeding. In M.L. Batshaw (Ed.), *Children with disabilities* (4th ed., pp. 621–641). Baltimore: Paul H. Brookes Publishing Co.

Eicher, P.S., Manno, C.J., Fox, C.A., & Kerwin, M.L. (1995). Impact of cervical auscultation on accuracy of clinical evaluation in predicting penetration/aspiration. *Dysphagia, 10,* 133.

Fitzgerald, J.F. (1987). Constipation in children. *Pediatrics in Review, 8,* 299–302.

Fonkalsrud, E.W., Ellis, D.G., Shaw, A., Mann, C.M., Jr., Plack, I.L., Miller, J.H., & Snyder, C.L. (1995). A combined hospital experience with fundoplication and gastric emptying procedure for gastroesophageal reflux in children. *Journal of the American College of Surgeons, 180,* 449–455.

Fox, C.A. (1990). Implementing the modified barium swallow evaluation in children who have multiple disabilities. *Infants and Young Children, 3,* 67–77.

Fried, M.D., Khoshoo, V., Secker, D.J., Gilday, D.L., Ash, J.M., & Pencharz, P.B. (1992). Decrease in gastric emptying time and episodes of regurgitation in children with spastic quadriplegia fed a whey-based formula. *Journal of Pediatrics, 120,* 569–572.

Gisel, E.G. (1994). Oral motor skills following sensorimotor intervention in the moderately eating-impaired child with cerebral palsy. *Dysphagia, 9,* 180–192.

Growth and nutrition in children with cerebral palsy [Editorial]. (1990). *Lancet, 335,* 1253–1254.

Hebra, A., & Hoffman, M.A. (1993). Gastroesophageal reflux in children. *Pediatric Clinics of North America, 40,* 1233–1251.

Helfrich-Miller, K.R., Rector, K.L., & Straka, J.A. (1986). Dysphagia: Its treatment in the profoundly retarded patient with cerebral palsy. *Archives of Physical Medicine and Rehabilitation, 67,* 520–525.

Heyman, S., Eicher, P.M., & Alavi, A. (1995). Radionuclide studies of the upper gastrointestinal tract on children with feeding disorders. *Journal of Nuclear Medicine, 36,* 351–354.

Iwata, B.A., Riordan, M.M., Wohl, M.K., & Finney, J.W. (1982). Pediatric feeding disorders: Behavioral analysis and treatment. In P.J. Accardo (Ed.), *Failure to thrive in infancy and early childhood* (pp. 297–329). Baltimore: University Park Press.

Kelly, K.J., Lazenby, A.J., Rowe, P.C., Yarkley, J.H., Perman, J.A., & Sampson, H.A. (1995). Eosinophilic esophagitis attributed to gastroesophageal reflux: Improvement with an amino acid–based formula. *Gastroenterology, 109,* 1503–1512.

Kerwin, M.L., Ahearn, W.H., Eicher, P.S., & Burd, D.M. (1995). The costs of eating: A behavioral economic analysis of food refusal. *Journal of Applied Behavior Analysis, 28,* 245–260.

Kerwin, M.L., Osborne, M., & Eicher, P.S. (1994). Effect of position and support on oral-motor skills of a child with bronchopulmonary dysplasia. *Clinical Pediatrics, 33,* 8–13.

Kramer, S.S., & Eicher, P.M. (1993). The evaluation of pediatric feeding abnormalities. *Dysphagia, 8,* 215–224.

Krick, J., Murphy, P.E., Markham, J.F.B., & Shapiro, B.K. (1992). A proposed formula for calculating energy needs of children with cerebral palsy. *Developmental Medicine and Child Neurology, 34,* 481–487.

Krick, J., & Van Duyn, M.A.S. (1984). The relationship between oral-motor involvement and growth: A pilot study in a pediatric population with cerebral palsy. *Journal of the American Dietetic Association, 84,* 555–559.

Liebl, B.H., Fischer, M.H., Van Calcar, S.C., & Marlett, J.A. (1990). Dietary fiber and long-term large bowel response in enterally nourished, nonambulatory, profoundly retarded youth. *Journal of Parenteral and Enteral Nutrition, 14,* 371–375.

Loughlin, G.M., & Lefton-Greif, M.A. (1994). Dysfunctional swallowing and respiratory disease in children. *Advances in Pediatrics, 41,* 135–162.

McCallum, R.W. (1990). Gastric emptying in gastroesophageal reflux and the therapeutic role of prokinetic agents. *Gastroenterology Clinics of North America, 19,* 551–564.

Monahan, P., Shapiro, B., & Fox, C. (1988). Effect of tube feeding on oral function. *Developmental Medicine and Child Neurology, 30,* 7.

National Cholesterol Education Program. (1990). *Report of the expert panel on population strategies for blood cholesterol reduction* (DHHS Publication No. NIH 90–3046). Washington, DC: U.S. Government Printing Office.

Nwaobi, O.M., & Smith, P.D. (1986). Effect of adaptive seating on pulmonary function of children with cerebral palsy. *Developmental Medicine and Child Neurology, 28,* 351–354.

Orenstein, S.R., Whitington, P.F., & Orenstein, D.M. (1983). The infant seat as treatment for gastroesophageal reflux. *New England Journal of Medicine, 309,* 760–763.

Palmer, S., Thompson, R.J., & Linscheid, T.R. (1975). Applied behavior analysis in the treatment of childhood feeding problems. *Developmental Medicine and Child Neurology, 17,* 333–339.

Pipes, P.L. (Ed.). (1988). *Nutrition in infancy and childhood* (3rd ed.). St. Louis: Times-Mirror Mosby.

Rempel, G.R., Colewell, S.O., & Nelson, R.P. (1988). Growth in children with cerebral palsy fed via gastrostomy. *Pediatrics, 82,* 857–862.

Rogers, B., Arvedson, J., Buck, G., & Smart, P.M. (1994). Characteristics of dysphagia in children with cerebral palsy. *Dysphagia, 9,* 69–73.

Ross, M.N., Haase, G.M., Reiley, T.T., & Meagher, D.P. (1988). The importance of acid reflux patterns in neurologically damaged children detected by four-channel esophageal pH monitoring. *Journal of Pediatric Surgery, 23,* 573–576.

Shapiro, B.K., Green, P., Krick, J., Allen, D., & Capute, A.J. (1986). Growth of severely impaired children: Neurological versus nutritional factors. *Developmental Medicine and Child Neurology, 28,* 729–733.

Sontag, S.J. (1990). The medical management of reflux esophagitis: Role of antacids and acid inhibition. *Gastroenterology Clinics of North America, 19,* 683–712.

Spender, Q.W., Cronk, C.E., Charney, E.B., & Stallings, V.A. (1989). Assessment of linear growth of children with cerebral palsy: Use of alternative measures to height or length. *Developmental Medicine and Child Neurology, 31,* 206–214.

Stallings, V.A., Charney, E.B., Davies, J.C., & Cronk, C.E. (1993a). Nutrition-related growth failure in children with quadriplegic cerebral palsy. *Developmental Medicine and Child Neurology, 35,* 126–138.

Stallings, V.A., Charney, E.B., Davies, J.C., & Cronk, C.E. (1993b). Nutritional status and growth of children with diplegic or hemiplegic cerebral palsy. *Developmental Medicine and Child Neurology, 35,* 997–1006.

Stallings V.A., Zemel, B.S., Davies, J.C., & Charney, E.B. (1996). Energy expenditure of children and adolescents with severe disabilities: A cerebral palsy model. *American Journal of Clinical Nutrition, 64,* 627–634.

Stevenson, R.D. (1995). Use of segmental measures to estimate stature in children with cerebral palsy. *Archives of Pediatric and Adolescent Medicine, 149,* 658–662.

Stevenson, R.D., Roberts, C.D., & Vogtle, L. (1995). The effects of non-nutritional factors on growth in cerebral palsy. *Developmental Medicine and Child Neurology, 37,* 124–130.

Timms, B.J.M., Defiore, J.M., Martin, R.J., & Miller, M.J. (1993). Increased respiratory drive as an inhibitor of oral feeding of preterm infants. *Journal of Pediatrics, 123,* 127–131.

Tizard, J.P.M., Paine, R.S., & Crothers, B. (1954). Disturbances of sensation in children with hemiplegia. *Journal of the American Medical Association, 155,* 628–632.

Tobis, J.S., Saturen, P., Larios, G.H., & Posniak, A.O. (1961). Study of growth patterns in cerebral palsy. *Archives of Physical Medicine and Rehabilitation, 42,* 475–481.

Uvebrandt, P., & Wiklund, L. (1988). Hemiplegic cerebral palsy. *Archives of Physical Medicine and Rehabilitation, 42,* 475–481.

Williams, C.L., Bollella, M., & Wynder, E.L. (1995). A new recommendation for dietary fiber in childhood. *Pediatrics, 96,* 985–988.

Optimizing Function of the Child with Cerebral Palsy: Preventing Disability

CHAPTER 12

Promoting Functional Mobility

Johanna E. Deitz Curry

One of the first questions that parents ask after their child has been diagnosed with cerebral palsy is "Will my child be able to walk?" In fact, this issue is part of a larger question—asked or not—regarding all children with cerebral palsy: If walking (i.e., ambulation) is not feasible, how can functional mobility be achieved? *Functional mobility* is any method or means by which a child is able to get from one place to another. *Ambulation* is the ability to walk with or without the aid of caregivers or assistive devices (e.g., braces, crutches, walker). If a child is unable to walk, he or she may be able to achieve functional mobility with the use of a standard manual wheelchair, a power wheelchair, or other specialized methods of transportation (e.g., scooters, mobile standers). Optimizing mobility is of special consideration during the first 5 years of a child's life. In an infant as well as in a young child, many primary tasks of development are centered around mobility and the opportunities for exploration that are generated by increased mobility. Lack of self-directed mobility can lead to withdrawal, passive behavior, apathy, or dependency, all of which may persist into adulthood (Butler, 1991). Mobility also provides the basis for the development of many daily living skills, such as toileting, dressing, and bathing (see Chapter 13). Impaired mobility has implications for all aspects of function and can have a significant impact on a child's ability to participate in a variety of societal settings (e.g., sports, recreational activities).

THE ROLE OF THE PHYSICAL THERAPIST

The physical therapist is a specialist who deals with movement and the components of movement disorders. More important, the physical therapist is concerned with developing management strategies that will enhance long-term mobility. The task of the physical therapist who works with children with cerebral palsy is to define the relationship between gross motor skill acquisition and the development of functional mobility.

First, the physical therapist acts as a clinical consultant to the child with cerebral palsy, to the child's family, and to other professionals involved in the child's care. As part of an interdisciplinary team, the physical therapist assists in decision making regarding a variety of intervention strategies, including orthopedic surgery, medication management of tone, bracing and splinting, equipment needs for activities of daily living, positioning and mobility, the need for direct physical therapy (PT) treatment intervention, and additional testing (e.g., gait analysis, other therapy evaluations).

Second, the physical therapist functions as a professional consultant to outside service providers who work with children with cerebral palsy and to the families of these children. The physical therapist often provides staff training and education to educational personnel, school therapists, visiting nurses, and other professionals outside of the main clinical setting.

Third, the physical therapist serves as a direct provider of treatment in a variety of settings, including the acute care hospital, the rehabilitation center, the outpatient facility, the school, and the home. The optimal location for provision of PT services with a child who has cerebral palsy is in his or her natural environment. The physical therapist also provides parent education instruction, which includes instruction in range of motion and positioning activities, use of adaptive equipment, acute postsurgical management, cast care and related activities, activities during and after rehabilitation management, and general functional gross motor activities.

Finally, the physical therapist engages in research activities either independently or as part of a team effort to explore the rationale behind certain PT treatments and procedures. The physical therapist critically evaluates the current modes of PT practice with the ultimate goal of developing new and effective methods for providing care to individuals who have cerebral palsy and/or other related neuromotor disorders.

GROSS MOTOR SKILLS AND THE
DEVELOPMENT OF FUNCTIONAL MOBILITY

Attainment of the gross motor skills that lead to functional mobility generally follows a logical pattern; however, this pattern does vary. An infant moves from a posture of flexion (i.e., physiological flexion at birth) to extension. Control of movements first occurs proximally at the trunk and the head and then moves distally to the large joints and the extremities. Movement patterns begin primarily with reflexive movements (e.g., asymmetric tonic neck reflex, positive support response, reflexive stepping [see Chapter 2]) and gradually mature into coordinated and voluntary movements (e.g., rolling, creeping, standing, bouncing).

Gross motor milestones are recognized patterns of movement that are attained by a child at specific chronological ages (see Table 12.1). Although there is some variability in the timing at which these milestones appear as well as in the mastery of the movement patterns, there is general agreement in the field in terms of typical ages for appearance and mastery; for instance, a therapist might assume that by 7 months of age, an infant has mastered sitting.

Definitions of functional mobility incorporate information regarding gross motor skill acquisition as well as consider the amount of assistance a child needs to complete a task and the setting in which he or she can perform the task. *Ambulation,* generally the preferred means of mobility, is defined as bipedal locomotion with or without an assistive device. There are three categories of ambulation:

1. *Exercise ambulation:* Ambulation for less than 50 feet
2. *Household ambulation:* Ambulation on level surfaces for 50–150 feet
3. *Community ambulation:* Ambulation on all surfaces and elevations for more than 150 feet

Mastery of ambulation is described in degrees and refers to the amount of assistance a child needs in order to complete a task. A child is considered independently mobile if he or she is able to initiate and complete a task safely (with or without an assistive device) without any assistance from another person. If the child does not require physical assistance or contact to perform a task but does require demonstration, verbal cuing, or close adult proximity for safety, then he or she needs supervision and is not independently mobile. A child who is able to complete more than 75% of a task independently but who requires some physical contact in order to complete the task safely needs minimal assistance. A child who is able to complete 50%–75% of a task needs moderate assistance, whereas a child who is able to complete less than 50% of a task needs maximum assistance. Finally, a child who is able to complete less than 25% of a task is dependent and, as a result, needs full assistance.

MUSCULOSKELETAL AND
NEUROMOTOR PHYSICAL THERAPY ASSESSMENT

The PT assessment is the first step in the process of establishing long-term goals for general mobility or, more precisely, for promoting a child's potential for ambulation (see Figure 12.1 for an example of a PT assessment form). Because the hallmark of cerebral palsy is sensorimotor dysfunction, the PT assessment

Table 12.1. Table of gross motor development

Age (months)	Supine	Prone	Sitting	Standing
Birth to 3	Primarily flexed posture, asymmetrical posture, head lag in pull to sit, reciprocal kicking of legs, and hands to mouth	Protective head turning, flexion posture decreases, prop on forearms, and head raised	Flexed back and head in supported sit with gradual increase in head righting to midline with trunk supported	Primary standing, automatic walking, and total support needed at axilla
3–6	Hands in midline (4 months), no head lag in pull to sit, feet to hands, feet to mouth, bridging, and rolls to side	Prop: extended arms (4 months), reach with one arm while propped on extended arms, pivots in prone, and rolls to supine	Head and upper back straight held in supported sitting, less support needed to maintain trunk, and pulls with arms and leads with head in pull to sit	Maintains head erect and upper trunk in supported stand and bounces in supported stand (5–7 months)
6–9	Rolls to prone (6 months), symmetric positions, and supine equilibrium responses	Crawls forward, assumes hands-and-knees position, reaches while on hands and knees, and prone equilibrium responses	Sits alone propped on arms (6 months), reaches forward in sit with prop (7 months), and sits alone without prop (8 months), protective extension arms forward	Stands when placed at support and support at pelvis (7–9 months)
9–12	Pulls to sit and dislikes supine	Creeps on hands and knees, pulls to kneel at support, and pulls to standing	Sits alone and pivots and plays without support, reaches in all directions, sits in various positions, goes from sitting to quadruped, protective extension with arms to both sides, and trunk righting in all planes	Pulls to kneel then stand at support, lifts leg off ground at support, cruises, and walks with both hands held
12–15		Bear walks on hands and feet	Sit to stand at support, equilibrium reactions in sit, and protective extension of arms to the back	Walks with one hand held, walks alone, and creeps up steps

Background information

Name _____ Date of birth _____ Date of examination _____

Diagnosis _____

Insurance _____ Insurance policy number _____

History_____

School _____ Level_____

Therapy service _____ Frequency of visits _____

Behavior _____

Posture _____

Reflexes (circle all that apply)
- ATNR
- STNR
- TLP
- TLS

- Startle
- Positive support
- Palmar grasp
- Plantar grasp

Summary of reflexes:

Righting and equilibrium responses

Head righting (circle all that apply)
- Flexion
- Extension
- Lateral response R/L _____

Trunk righting (circle all that apply)
- Anterior
- Posterior
- Lateral R/L
- Landau _____

Protective response (circle all that apply)
- Sitting
- Anterior
- Posterior

- Right lateral
- Left lateral
- Forward parachute

Standing balance (circle all that apply)
- Backward

- Left lateral

Equilibrium response (circle all that apply)
- Prone
- Supine
- Kneeling

- Sitting
- Quadruped

(continued)

Figure 12.1. Physical therapy assessment form for children with cerebral palsy.

Figure 12.1.   (*continued*)

Summary of righting and equilibrium responses:

Motor development skills

Supine (circle all that apply)
- Head centering
- Hands on midline R/L
- Reciprocal kick
- Pelvis rounded

Prone (circle all that apply)
- On elbows
- On extended arms
- Reaching
- Pivot
- Crawls

Rolling (circle all that apply)
- Supine to side
- Prone to supine
- Supine to prone

Sitting (circle all that apply)
- Assumes position
- Maintains position
- Short sits
- W sits
- Ring sits
- Long sits
- Plays
- Pulls with arms in pull to sit
- Head control in pull to sit

Quadruped (circle all that apply)
- Assumes position
- Maintains position
- Creeps forward
- Assumes sitting

Kneeling (circle all that apply)
- Assumes position
- Maintains position
- Pulls to kneel at support

Standing (circle all that apply)
- Pulls to stand at support
- Leg disassociation
- Stands at support
- Maintains position
- Cruises
- Stands alone

Walking (circle all that apply)
- One hand held
- Support
- Creeps up stairs
- Creeps on uneven surfaces

Summary of motor development skills:

(continued)

Figure 12.1. (*continued*)

Gross motor developmental level:

Gait analysis:

Assistive device:

Adaptive equipment (circle all that apply)
- Walker
- Wheelchair
- Braces
- Other _____
- Stroller
- Bath chair
- Lift

Left			Lower extremities	Right		
Range of motion	Strength	Tone	Motion/muscle groups	Range of motion	Strength	Tone
			Hip flexion			
			Hip extension (Thomas test)			
			Hip abduction (Knee/hip extended)			
			Hip adduction			
			Hip internal rotation			
			Hip external rotation			
			Knee flexion			
			Knee extension (prone)			
			Popliteal angle			
			Ankle dorsiflexion (knee flexion)			
			Ankle dorsiflexion (knee extend)			
			Ankle plantarflexion			

Key to grading muscle tone: 0 = hypotonic; 1 = normal; 2 = mild hypotonic; 3 = moderate hypotonic; 4 = severe hypotonic; 5 = rigid; 6 = fluctuating tone.

(continued)

Figure 12.1.   (*continued*)

Summary of muscle tone
Upper extremity:

Lower extremity:

Trunk:

Summary of range of motion
Upper extremity:

Lower extremity:

Other:

Summary of strength
Upper extremity:

(continued)

Figure 12.1. (*continued*)

Lower extremity:

Other:

Current issues and difficulties	Recommendation and plan

Additional comments:

describes motor patterns and responses to sensory input, internal stimuli, and external variables. This assessment includes noting the presence of primitive and pathological reflex patterns (see Chapter 2), postural reactions and balance responses, joint range of motion (ROM), motor development, posture, strength, endurance, motor control, and functional mobility. The information attained from the PT assessment is used in several ways: to assess the current status of a child with respect to a normative sample or a specific protocol, to ascertain areas of impairment, to provide a framework for treating and managing motor problems, to establish a prognosis for function, to assess progress, and to aid in the development of new PT treatment techniques.

The components of a PT assessment include the following areas:

- Muscle tone
- Patterns of posture and movement
- Quality of movement patterns
- Effect of sensory input on posture and movement
- Influence of tone and reflexes on movement

Muscle Tone

Muscle tone is defined as the readiness of a muscle to respond to gravity and movement as well as the amount of resistance a muscle gives in response to a stretch. Typical muscle tone is very adaptive, and the tone generated is appropriate for the given task. For example, the muscle tone generated in the leg muscles during walking is fluid and variable. Both flexor and extensor muscle groups have appropriately higher tone in order to maintain a standing position. However, there is lower tone in these muscle groups when movement actually occurs, which enables the advance leg to move during the swing-through phase of gait. During the PT assessment, muscle tone is measured at rest and during active movement. *Active tone* is the power and adaptability of the muscles during spontaneous movement; *passive tone* refers to the resistance of the muscles during movements that are imposed by an examiner.

A complete evaluation of muscle tone (at rest and during movement) and the effect of posture and tone on mobility includes many parameters. Table 12.2 provides a description and measurement of the types and classifications of muscle tone. This table uses a modification of the Ashworth scale (Bohannon & Smith, 1987) that is used in various medical and rehabilitation centers to measure muscle tone.

The distribution of muscle tone is assessed to determine variations in different muscle groups and asymmetries: left versus right side of the body and upper-extremity stimulation versus lower-extremity stimulation. Another reason that tone is assessed is to detect changes during active movement, in various postures, with stress, and with changes in the environment. The effect of movement patterns in relation to tone also is noted. For example, in a supine

Table 12.2. Description and measurement of muscle tone

Grade	Level	Description
0	Hypotonic	Floppy; less than normal muscle tone
1	Normal	No increase in muscle tone
2	Mild hypertonic	Slight increase in tone; minimal resistance to movement in half of the range of motion (i.e., slight "catch" in limb movement)
3	Moderate hypertonic	Greater increase in tone in 50% or more of the range of motion, but limb is easily moved
4	Severe hypertonic	Considerable increase in tone throughout the entire range of motion as well as difficulty in moving the limb
5	Extreme hypertonic	Rigidity of limb in flexion or extension as well as extreme difficulty in initiating movement and throughout the range of motion
6	Fluctuating tone	Variability in muscle tone during movements, ranging from floppy to hypertonic

position, resting muscle tone in the hamstrings (see Chapter 6) may be graded as mild (i.e., slight increase in tone, with a "catch" in the limb movement or with minimal resistance to movement through less than half of the range). However, when tone is assessed in standing position, the muscle tone in the hamstrings may be graded as severe (i.e., considerable increase in tone, making passive movement difficult) as a result of the influence of the positive support response (see Chapter 2). Finally, the impact of sensory input on tone is assessed. Soothing voices, reduced lighting, or bundling a child in a blanket may cause a decrease in high muscle tone. In contrast, loud voices or sudden noises, bright lights, or being placed on a high examining table may dramatically increase a child's resting muscle tone.

Patterns of Posture and Movement

An assessment of motor skills includes an evaluation of the quality of movement patterns while taking into account influencing variables such as tone and posture. The physical therapist should assess postures in different positions (e.g., supine, prone, quadruped, sitting, kneeling, standing; see Table 12.1). In addition, the physical therapist should be aware of the specific patterns of movement that are considered typical for a given age and should note any deviations from the norm. For example, in supine and prone positions, the presence of the tonic labyrinthine reflex should be noted. The physical therapist should note whether this reflex dominates the resting muscle tone and whether it restricts or compromises movement away from the starting position. The physical therapist should determine whether the child has the strength to engage in antigravity movements and whether movements in these positions are smooth and coordinated or jerky and reflexive.

Quality of Movement Patterns

The presence and the quality of typical and atypical movements of the child should be observed by the physical therapist. For example, it is typical for a 6-month-old child to roll from prone to supine with the head and neck turning as a unit (i.e., "log rolling"). By 9 months of age, it is typical for an infant to roll from prone to supine segmentally, with disassociation among the head, the trunk, and the pelvis. Thus, it is considered atypical for a 9-month-old infant to only be able to log roll. Another example of a typical milestone reached by infants is belly crawling. It is typical for a 7-month-old infant to move around by crawling on his or her belly rather than on his or her hands and knees (i.e., creeping). Thus, it would be atypical for a 7-month-old child to crawl using only his or her arms while both legs are stiff in extension. A typically developing 7-month-old infant who is attaining gross motor milestones as expected should have the skills to crawl, although the quality of the crawling pattern may not be developed.

There are motor evaluations that examine both the quality of movement and the typical age for attaining a gross motor skill (see section on "Formal Evaluation of Movement" in this chapter). Asymmetries of movement are assessed to determine whether there is a difference between the right and left sides of the body as well as between the upper extremities and the lower extremities. A child with spastic hemiplegia is expected to show marked differences between the left and right sides of his or her body, whereas a child with spastic diplegia is expected to show more control of the upper extremities of the body than he or she shows for the lower extremities.

Effect of Sensory Input on Posture and Movement

The physical therapist should note the effect of sensory input on the child's posture and movement. This variable indicates the maturity of the child's central nervous system (CNS) and his or her degree of motor control. If a child can safely ambulate with forearm crutches in a quiet and unobstructed area but "stiffens up" and loses control when confronted with obstacles or other people moving around, it is not safe for him or her to walk with forearm crutches in a school environment. This also indicates that PT intervention should focus on teaching the child to use crutches in more crowded areas that are part of his or her daily living environment.

Influence of Tone and Reflexes on Movement

The physical therapist should assess the effect of movement in relation to associated reactions or changes in the child's muscle tone. For example, although a child may be able to sit unsupported on a chair with his or her feet firmly planted on the ground, when he or she reaches down or flexes his or her trunk forward, the legs extend at the knees and cross over one other (i.e., scissoring). This reaction in the legs is not typically seen when bending forward; the overflow of tone means that it is not likely that this child will be able to propel a manual wheelchair independently. When the child leans forward to reach for the large wheels to maneuver the wheelchair, he or she will slide out of the chair. The child's feet need to be secured firmly on the footrest, and the child needs safety supports when learning to propel the wheelchair.

The influence of developmental reflexes and postural reactions on movement are important when assessing a child's readiness to functionally engage in a task. Some children with cerebral palsy retain the primitive stepping reflex and the postural support response throughout their childhood. These patterns of movement sustain a child upright against gravity, and, as a result, the child may move his or her legs forward in response to being tilted forward. However, this is not functional ambulation. These patterns are not controlled and coordinated actions; they are reactions to a given stimulus (i.e., weight on the feet) that are functional only to a parent or a caregiver when moving the child a short distance and when using less effort than carrying the child. This is important for caregiving, but it is not an indication that a child will ever have the skill to perform this movement independently or functionally.

Formal Evaluation of Movement

Several instruments are available for the evaluation of motor performance. Developmental assessments are standardized and tested with a normative sample. They are primarily designed to compare the motor behaviors of a particular child with the motor behaviors of other children who share traits such as age, sex, and socioeconomic status. The results of the evaluations provide age norms for achievement of motor behaviors (hence the name norm-referenced tests) and provide measurements that aid in the identification of motor dysfunction. The instruments measure motor milestones, postural control and reflex integration, and major factors that influence the child's performance. For example, a 15-month-old child whose gross motor performance is evaluated using the Peabody Developmental Motor Scales (Folio & Fewell, 1983) may achieve a percentile score or an age-equivalent score that matches that of a 5-month-old child. Developmental tests are primarily "diagnostic" and are used for establishing the need for intervention. If the test instruments are sensitive enough to detect incremental changes, then they can measure progress over an extended period of time. Several developmental testing instruments claim to be useful for treatment planning and for monitoring progress.

Functional or qualitative assessments are criterion-referenced tests that contain items for measuring how a child performs a certain task. The assessments provide a much longer and more detailed sequence of developmental skills than do quantitative tests and are most often used in program planning (see Table 12.3).

Table 12.3. Tests of gross motor development

Test	Type of test	Age	Areas tested	Number of gross motor items	Gross motor areas tested	Scores	Other
Alberta Infant Motor Scale (AIMS) (Piper & Darrah, 1994; Piper et al., 1992)	Standardized	Birth to independent walking	Gross motor	58	Posture; weight bearing, antigravity; movements in supine, prone, sitting, and standing positions	Developmental age level for performance	Observation only
Revised Gesell Developmental Schedules (RGDSs) (Knobloch, Stevens, & Malone, 1980)	Standardized	4 weeks to 36 months	Gross motor, fine motor, adaptive motor, language, and personal-social	98	Posture reactions, head balance, sitting, standing, creeping, walking, running, hopping, and balance	Developmental quotient for each of the five areas and overall developmental quotient	Parent history, observation and direct testing, no functional skill information for treatment or goal setting
Peabody Developmental Motor Scales (PDMS) (Folio & Fewell, 1983)	Standardized	0–83 months	Gross motor and fine motor	170	Reflexes, balance, nonlocomotion, locomotion, receipt, and propulsion	Standard score and age-equivalent scaled score	Observation and direct handling, good treatment planning, goal setting, and assessment of progress over time
Movement Assessment of Infants (MAI) (Chandler, Andrews, & Swanson, 1980)	Criterion referenced	0–12 months	Gross motor and fine motor	65	Muscle tone, primitive reflexes, automatic reactions, and volitional movements	"Risk" score: at risk for developmental disability and need for further testing	Observation and handling, description of motor behavior, measures progress, and setting treatment goals
Pediatric Evaluation of Disability Inventory (PEDI) (Maley et al., 1992)	Criterion referenced	6 months to 7.5 years	Self-care, bowel & bladder control, motor performance, communication, and social	197 functional, 20 caregiver assistance	Functional skill level, caregiver assistance, and adaptive equipment used	Mastery of task, independence, and maximal function	Uses parent response and interview

Measure	Type	Age	Domain	Number of items	Items	Scoring	Use
Gross Motor Function Measure (GMFM) (Rosenbaum et al., 1990; Russell et al., 1989)	Criterion referenced, and a typically developing 5-year-old can achieve all items	15 months–16 years, and children with cerebral palsy	Gross motor	88	Lying, rolling, sitting, crawling, kneeling, and standing, walking, running, and jumping	Degree of achievement of motor skill	Observation and testing, and use in treatment planning, goal setting, and measuring progress over time
Gross Motor Performance Measure (GMPM) (Boyce et al., 1991; Russell et al., 1989)	Criterion referenced, and a typically developing 5-year-old can achieve all items	15 months–13 years, and children with cerebral palsy	Gross motor	8 activities in each of the following positions: supine, prone, four-point, sitting, kneeling, standing, walking, and climbing	Postural alignment, selective movement, coordination, stability, and weight shift	Five-point scale measuring level of performance in each of the 5 areas (alignment, coordination, stability, movement, and weight shift)	Observation and testing, and use in treatment planning, goal setting, and measuring progress over time
Functional Independence Measure for Children (WeeFIM) (State University of New York at Buffalo, 1993)	Criterion referenced	6 months–12 years	Self-care, sphincter control, mobility, locomotion, communication, and social cognition	18	Mobility and locomotion	Seven-point scale measuring level of caregiver assistance needed to complete task	Measures functional skill, but limited to only 2 areas of mobility locomotion

Neuromotor and Musculoskeletal Assessment

A neuromuscular assessment measures active and passive ROM, muscle strength, endurance and speed, joint integrity, and posture; it also provides an analysis of gait and mobility. When assessing ROM, it is imperative that testing positions remain the same over an extended period of time, that the procedure for testing is standardized, and that a goniometer is used (see Chapter 6).

One method of testing endurance and speed is to encourage a child to move in whatever pattern he or she uses for locomotion. If the child crawls, the physical therapist should note the distance and the time it takes for the child to cover a specific distance. If the child rolls, the physical therapist should note the same information. If a child is ambulatory, the physical therapist should note the distance and time for walking within a prescribed area. The physical therapist should use the same motor skill and the same area in order to assess a child over time; this will assist in determining whether there are any changes in the child's speed or endurance.

The assessment of joint integrity and structure represents an area of overlap between the physical therapist and the orthopedist. The joints most susceptible to malformation are the hip and the ankle. The knee joint is generally stable in children who have spasticity, but the hip and the ankle joints are subject to abnormal forces of muscle pull and improper weight bearing that can contribute to ligamentous laxity (see Chapters 6 and 8).

Postural assessment is another area in which the physical therapist and the orthopedist overlap. If a child ambulates, it is important for the physical therapist and the orthopedist to assess trunk posture in supine, sitting, and standing positions. The physical therapist should note whether the child has scoliosis, kyphosis, or lordosis and whether these deformities are positional (i.e., change with position or are able to be corrected) or structural (i.e., do not change as position changes). See Chapter 7 for a detailed discussion of orthopedic approaches to treatment.

With a child who has cerebral palsy and who is ambulatory, gait analysis should be an ongoing assessment. It can be undertaken in the clinical setting without sophisticated devices, such as using markers over joints or videotaping the child walking in and out of the parallel bars. Gait should be assessed with and without orthotics as well as with and without the assistive device that the child may typically use. See Chapter 8 for a detailed discussion of gait analysis.

TREATMENT OPTIONS AND STRATEGIES

Treatment and intervention strategies vary according to a child's age and functional status. In addition to neurodevelopmental and musculoskeletal issues, treatment strategies need to consider information regarding the child's cognitive abilities and motivation; the resources of the child's family; the goals of the child and his or her family; and other medical issues, such as seizures and sensory impairments (i.e., visual or auditory) that may affect the child.

Treatment strategies are derived from theoretical models of motor development. One outdated treatment model, which is based on maturation of the CNS, specifies that motor development proceeds from reflexive movements to coordinated and deliberate movements in a cephalocaudal direction, from proximal to distal, and from gross movements to fine selective movements.

Another treatment model uses synergy movement patterns. Movement within a synergy is in mass patterns of flexion and extension, which are seen in early fetal life (i.e., reflex patterns). Synergy then moves toward eliciting volitional control of movements out of reflex patterns and finally stimulates righting and balance responses. All of these responses incorporate the use of sensory stimuli. A treatment strategy from this model that is applicable to PT for the child with cerebral palsy is facilitating muscle contraction of weak muscle groups in the synergy pattern to enhance awareness of a movement that is otherwise not able to be elicited.

The techniques of proprioceptive neuromuscular facilitation (PNF) (Knott & Voss, 1968) are based on the observation that motor learning is a combination of voluntary motor control and patterns of movement that are elicited without voluntary effort. Movements are not elicited in mass synergy patterns of flexion and extension; rather, they are elicited in spiral and diagonal patterns that occur in typical movement. When these PNF patterns are applied to typical gross developmental progression, movements are facilitated to encourage transitions by eliciting the inherent movement patterns. These techniques allow for facilitation of functional movements, unlike developmental reflexes and postural reactions that are only reactions to a given stimulus. In order to enhance learning of gross motor skills, PNF also requires repetition and practice, sensory feedback, and motivation. Specific techniques used from PNF in treatment are overflow of movement and tone to reinforce movement in accessory muscle groups (i.e., irradiation); sensory stimuli (e.g., application of touch, pressure, resistance, stretching, traction, compression) to facilitate movement; and relaxation techniques, such as contract–relax and hold–relax, to decrease tone in spastic muscle groups.

In 1972, Rood (cited in Pearson & Williams, 1972) based a PT treatment strategy on neurophysiological principles of the 1950s, which concentrated on the typical sequence of development and organized it into four stages:

1. Mobility (e.g., rolling)
2. Stability (e.g., prone propping on extended arms)
3. Mobility in weight bearing at a fixed distal segment (e.g., rocking in quadruped position)
4. Mobility in non–weight-bearing distal segments (e.g., walking)

According to this model, progress through each of the four stages of development is necessary for higher-level motor function. Rood emphasized that a motor response was a sensory feedback system or a building block for the next level of motor control. A child needed control of the whole sensory environment in order to facilitate the processing of responses to the environment. This treatment strategy was the first approach that viewed motor development in the context of an interactional model between the child and his or her environment. Treatment techniques that are based on Rood's principles and are used with children include icing and brushing to facilitate contraction, joint compression to facilitate co-contraction of muscles around a joint, and activities in given positions to facilitate both mobility and stability.

The neurodevelopmental treatment (NDT) model, formulated by Bobath and Bobath (1972), has roots in neurological principles that were practiced prior to 1950. The key aspect in this treatment approach was to promote motor control by inhibiting reflexive movement patterns and facilitating balance and righting responses within the framework of developmental sequence. Abnormal muscle tone was controlled and modified; postural responses were facilitated through positioning and handling, which emphasized the rotary components of movement. As the rationale for learning movement has changed and theories of motor learning and motor control are based on current neurophysiological research, NDT has been modified to incorporate new principles and outdated techniques have been discarded.

Trends in treatment are based on theories that incorporate principles of motor learning theories, motor control theories, and psychological models of learning. It was proposed in the 1990s that motor development occurs within a dynamic systems model (Thelen, 1995; Thelen & Ulrich, 1991). This theory postulated that there are subsystems that interact together and develop at their own rate, comprising internal components of organization and external contexts that work together to determine the outcome of behavior. These subsystems are the musculoskeletal system, the sensory system, the central sensorimotor integrator, and the entire CNS, as well as the state of arousal, motivation, and environmental influences. Behavior is seen as task specific, and resultant behavior arises from the interaction of all of the subsystems. Control of movement shifts and is dependent on the dominant subsystem.

Movement patterns are more variable during periods of transition, which are sensitive times in development when intervention may be especially effective. Physical therapists use the dynamic systems model as a framework for facilitating motor development. The key is to determine which parameters are dominant and which are able to be manipulated to improve motor outcome (e.g., the speed of movement). In conjunction, the physical therapist needs to determine the components that inhibit subsystem maturation and then focus treatment techniques to address this particular issue. For example, a limitation in walking may be restricted by joint ROM caused by decreased muscle extensibility or tonal abnormality, and it may be this limitation that inhibits the musculoskeletal system. PT techniques should focus on increasing the ROM with stretching, relaxation of spastic muscle tone, and improving muscle extensibility. This can be accomplished by casting a joint, which will increase dynamic stretch to spastic muscle groups; using electrical stimulation to activate antagonistic muscle groups; using contract–relax techniques to stretch the tight muscle groups; or bracing, which will inhibit further loss of joint ROM.

The physical therapist can modify the environment subsystem in order to promote progress. The stimuli are controlled and are conducive to learning new skills by reducing distractions to promote focus on a task and by providing materials that promote performance of a task. The physical therapist can provide a child with opportunities for repetition to practice various components of a functional task, thus improving the child's efficiency and enhancing learning.

COMMON PRINCIPLES OF TREATMENT

Treatment goals must be individualized to each child's needs as well as take into consideration the needs of the child's family. Treatment goals also must address the child's specific limitations and must be modified as different limitations are targeted for intervention. Caregivers need ongoing education that is presented in practical and understandable terms with regard to the child's specific needs and treatments. Families need to be able to integrate the treatment techniques into everyday interactions with the child.

A child's treatment goals should focus on promoting active movement that provides an opportunity to practice the movement patterns as they relate to functional skill development. The goals also should incorporate new skills into the child's daily activities. Following these two guidelines when setting treatment goals will increase the likelihood of the child practicing the skill at home and at school.

In addition, treatment goals should incorporate ways of motivating the child to be an active participant in learning new motor activities, and treatment should be aimed at preventing or minimizing deformities and maximizing function. Finally, the physical therapist and the orthopedist should reevaluate and modify a child's treatment goals periodically.

TREATMENT GOALS AND TECHNIQUES

Treatment techniques change according to a child's age and his or her need for greater function and independence. The techniques should be modified according to the individual child's functional needs as he or she grows and develops. There are a number of books that can assist professionals in understanding cerebral palsy and planning treatment; some examples include

Pediatric Neurologic Physical Therapy (Campbell, 1991) and *Physical Therapy for Children* (Campbell, 1994).

Treatment During Infancy

During infancy and the preschool years, children have the potential for the most development in motor function. This is the time when a child uses his or her sensorimotor experiences to set a baseline for future development. As a result, the time frame from birth to 2 years of age is referred to as the *sensorimotor period of development*. During this stage of development, a child learns how to interact with others, develops an understanding of self and the environment, and begins to explore the environment.

The goals of treatment during infancy are individualized to each child and based on a holistic assessment of the needs of the child and his or her family. The four main therapy goals during the sensorimotor period of development are

1. To facilitate sensorimotor experiences while decreasing functional limitations
2. To develop postural alignment and stability while promoting mobility
3. To promote the parents' and caregivers' ability to handle and interact with the child
4. To educate the parents and caregivers about cerebral palsy

During this stage, there should be an emphasis on promoting the child's mobility, which facilitates his or her play and exploration of the environment as well as promotes his or her social interaction. Development of motor skills also assists with the development of body awareness and spatial perception. The focus of intervention is on promoting head and trunk control in all planes; developing mobility in rolling, crawling, and walking; encouraging transitions of movement; and facilitating righting and balance responses in all planes.

If the child's degree of disability prevents skill attainment, the treatment equipment should be used to promote functional skill development. For instance, an adaptive seat can be constructed or purchased to accommodate a child who has poor sitting balance or insufficient head and trunk control to sit unsupported. While seated in a supported position, the child can use his or her upper extremities for play without needing to control his or her head and trunk. In addition, sitting in an upright position promotes visual attention and encourages practice of head and trunk control within a limited supported range. Other adaptive equipment used during the sensorimotor period of development are rolls and therapy balls to facilitate movement and to practice balance, prone and supine standers to promote weight bearing on the legs and to provide prolonged stretch to tight muscle groups, and floor scooters to promote locomotion (see the appendix at the end of this chapter for more detailed discussion of adaptive equipment).

Treatment During Preschool Years

During the preschool years (i.e., from 3 to 5 years of age), a child develops functional independence in locomotion and in self-care. In addition, a child begins to have interactions with the world outside of his or her home and family environment. Ambulation is the most important goal set by parents and physical therapists in this stage. Independent locomotion is the primary concentration in PT intervention.

PT goals focus on attaining and refining prewalking skills. These skills include postural and skeletal alignment, weight bearing, disassociation of lower extremities, weight shifting in standing, and improving postural stability and balance. Ambulation devices used in accomplishing these goals include walkers and crutches. Posterior walkers are preferred to assist with ambulation in children who have cerebral palsy because they promote upright posture and facilitate a more typical gait pattern. Other adjuncts to ambulation that are used to assist in gait may include braces and splints (see Chapter 16).

If ambulation is ineffective or unattainable as a result of the severity of motor disability, physical therapists should provide alternative means of functional mobility. Children can learn independence in mobility with the use of an adaptive tricycle; a manual wheelchair; or a power mobility device, such as a wheelchair or a scooter (see the appendix at the end of this chapter for detailed discussion of alternative mobility products). PT activities should be incorporated into play activities that are appropriate for the child's level of cognition. Kicking a ball in a sitting position is a good way to improve quadriceps strength and eye–foot coordination while keeping a child interested in the activity.

Physical therapists should include the child's parents and siblings in PT activities and in home programs. Children are often motivated by family members; thus, teaching therapeutic activities to family members can assist in bringing these activities into the home as well as into outdoor activities. The home program needs to be realistic and tailored to fit into the family constellation. Parents often do not have a lot of extra time to devote to a specific home program, so the physical therapist should devise a program that is workable for the particular family involved. Books that help formulate a home program and assist the parents in understanding cerebral palsy include *Handling the Young Cerebral Palsied Child at Home* (Finnie, 1975), *Cerebral Palsy: A Complete Guide for Caregivers* (Miller & Bacharach, 1995), and *Home Program Instruction Sheets for Infants and Young Children* (Jaeger, 1987).

Treatment During School Age and Adolescence

During school age and adolescence, a child with cerebral palsy is coping with developing independence from the family, integration with peers, and a variety of social and emotional issues. In this stage, a child with cerebral palsy is aware of the extent and impact of his or her disability, which may add to the typical stresses of adolescence. Issues addressed in PT at this stage are the lack of independent mobility, decreased endurance and speed in performing tasks (including ambulation), increasing contractures, lack of social independence, and limited opportunities to participate in sports and social activities.

During adolescence, the goals for PT intervention are more remedial and attempt to refine the basic skills acquired during the early formative years. This is a time of rapid physical growth, and the focus is to prevent any postural deformities or secondary muscular impairments that would hamper progress or cause regression of motor skills. In certain instances, surgical intervention may be necessary and PT goals must then focus on rehabilitation of functional motor skills (see Chapter 7 for a detailed discussion of orthopedic approaches to treatment). Because children need to travel longer distances in school and at social events during adolescence, the PT goals in this stage are aimed at maximizing endurance and efficiency of movement, improving the speed and efficiency of gait, increasing joint ROM as contractures are caused by growth or decreased physical activity, improving muscle extensibility to preserve joint integrity and prevent secondary joint changes that occur with aging, improving physical fitness, and overcoming barriers to independent access (e.g., curbs, getting on and off buses). With individuals who have extensive physical impairment, goals for PT focus on attempts to maximize caregiver ease and minimize child deformity. The child must be fully included in setting his or her goals for PT.

Therapeutic activities used with adolescents may include isokinetic exercises, weight training to improve strength, or treadmill exercise to increase cardiovascular fitness. In addition, these exercises may include gait pattern and endurance, electric stimulation to muscle groups to increase muscle force and decrease spasticity, casting to improve joint ROM and muscle extensibility, and splints or orthotics to compensate for muscle imbalance or weakness.

Independent ambulators require high energy expenditure, and, as a result, the fatigue combined with travel over long distances may require school-age children to use secondary adjuncts to mobility (e.g., a manual wheelchair, a power wheelchair, a scooter) to conserve energy. Using one of these adjuncts in school or during recreational activities will assist in maximizing function and preserving energy and attention for tasks other than walking.

Adjuncts to Physical Therapy Treatment

Throughout all stages of development, adjuncts to therapeutic activities can be used to supplement direct PT. Splints and orthotics are used to provide correct postural alignment of the foot, ankle, and knee for activities such as positioning, standing, and ambulation. Biofeedback is useful in enhancing cognitive awareness of muscle contraction and in grading muscle tone. Functional electrical stimulation assists in temporarily reducing spasticity and in enhancing muscle contraction and power. Serial casting and splints can improve joint ROM by providing a constant stretch to spastic muscles. Casting can be done in conjunction with motor point blocks. Aquatic therapy can provide relaxation and decrease gravitational forces on movement as well as provide joint conservation in practicing motor activities. Therapeutic horseback riding (hippotherapy) has the advantage of enhancing motor development while using the motion of the horse to provide both relaxation and facilitation of balance and righting reactions.

PROGNOSIS AND OUTCOMES

Predicting whether a child with cerebral palsy will walk is difficult because ambulation potential involves a multitude of factors, including cognitive status, motivation, interest, and the presence of other complicating medical issues such as seizures, sensory involvement, family compliance, and environment. The severity of involvement and the type of cerebral palsy also may influence the child's potential for ambulation. Children with hemiplegia have a greater probability of walking than children with other types of cerebral palsy. One study (Molnar, 1985) found that most children with spastic hemiplegia walk by 3 years of age. This study also found that if children with spastic diplegia were going to walk, they usually attained this skill by 3 years of age. Of all the children in this study who were diagnosed with spastic diplegia, 65% were ambulatory without assistive devices, 20% were ambulatory with some assistive device, and 15% relied solely on wheelchairs and were not functional ambulators. Children who were diagnosed with ataxia had a longer latency period than children with spastic hemiplegia or diplegia, but most of these children walked by 8 years of age. Only 25% of children with athetosis were nonambulators; the remaining 75% walked either independently or with an assistive device. Children who had spastic quadriplegia were the least likely to walk, with only 65% of the children achieving some sort of ambulatory potential.

Researchers have attempted to demonstrate a relationship between ambulation potential and the persistence of pathological or primitive reflexes. The primitive reflexes most associated with poor ambulation potential include the Moro reflex, the asymmetric tonic neck reflex, the symmetric tonic neck reflex, the extensor thrust (i.e., the positive supporting reaction), and the neck righting reflex.

In 1975, an orthopedist developed a scale of seven variables that used the presence of five primitive reflexes and the absence of two postural responses as the criteria for ambulation (Bleck, 1975). If a child had a score of 2 or more (i.e., retention of primitive reflexes or absence of balance responses) at 3 years of age, he or she had a minimal chance of being a functional ambulator. The scale defined *functional ambulation* as walking independently on a level surface for a minimum of 15 meters. The only assistive device this scale would allow was forearm crutches. Another study demonstrated a high correlation between the persistence of primitive reflexes at 2 years of age and the inability to walk at 8 years of age (Watt, Robertson, & Grace, 1989). This study also found that the ability to sit independently by 2 years of age was highly correlated with the potential to ambulate. A similar study also conducted in the 1990s (Trahan & Marcoux, 1994) supported the theory that the persistence of primitive reflexes past the first 2 years of life was highly correlated with the inability to functionally ambulate.

A third area that researchers have investigated as a predictor of ambulation in children who have cerebral palsy is the age at which gross motor skills are first attained. A study conducted in the 1990s examined gross motor skills and how they correlate with attainment as a predictor of ambulation (Campos da Paz, Burnett, & Braga, 1994). The skills assessed by this study were head balance in prone, independent sitting, and crawling symmetrically or reciprocally. Every child who had head balance in prone by 9 months of age was ambulatory with or without an assistive device; however, the children who achieved this skill later than 20 months of age never became ambulators. If a child achieved independent sitting by 24 months of age, he or she was able to walk; however, few of the children who achieved this skill later than 36 months of age were able to ambulate. All children who achieved symmetrical crawling by 30 months of age were ambulators, but no child who achieved crawling later than 61 months was an ambulator.

A general principle may be applied when considering the ambulation potential for a child who has cerebral palsy: The earlier that gross motor skills are acquired, the better the correlation for ambulation. For example, sitting independently without support by 2 years of age was highly correlated with the potential to ambulate. The persistence of primitive reflexes and the absence of postural reactions (e.g., balance, righting responses) by 2 years of age and beyond were indicators that a child would not ambulate. Almost all children with spastic hemiplegia will ambulate, and more than 85% of children with spastic diplegia will achieve ambulation; however, most children with spastic quadriplegia will not achieve ambulation.

Willy's Story

Willy is a 13 year old boy with a mixed type of cerebral palsy (he has generalized spasticity, involving the right side of his body more than the left, and involuntary, athetoid movements, especially of his arms). The cause of his cerebral palsy is unknown. He was born at full term following an uncomplicated pregnancy, labor, and delivery. (Willy was evaluated by an interdisciplinary team; the results of these evaluations is summarized in this and subsequent chapters in this section.

(continued)

Willy's Story–continued

Willy arrived for a PT assessment in a manual wheelchair that he had outgrown and that did not fit him well. Willy was unable to functionally propel his manual wheelchair. Apart from rolling, which was not appropriate in a variety of settings, Willy had no functional mobility skills. He was unable to sit without support and was unable to make transitions to antigravity positions.

Willy had flexion contractures at the hips and knees, limited abduction at the hips, and planovalgus feet; he could not be held in a supported standing position as a result of the contractures. Willy's family reported that he had never crawled or walked.

Willy was quite intelligent and his cognitive skills were nearly age appropriate. In spite of his speech difficulties, Willy communicated a desire to use a power wheelchair. In conjunction with the occupational therapist in the seating clinic, a power wheelchair assessment was performed.

Willy was measured for a seating system that would support his postural instability and provide for optimal use of his left arm and left hand in order to use the power wheelchair controls. He was fitted with a solid seat and a back that was mounted to the wheelchair frame with adjustable depth hardware to allow for 3 inches of linear growth. Swing-away lateral trunk supports were mounted on the back of the wheelchair to control lateral trunk flexion, and a chest harness was added for anterior trunk control. On the seat, a flip-down abduction pommel was added to control adduction, which worsened when Willy was stressed or excited. In addition, a flip-down headrest was mounted on the back of the wheelchair to ensure safety during transportation.

The necessity for a power mobility system was determined by Willy's need for multiple parameter adjustability while learning to control the power wheelchair and his need for adaptations to his athetoid movements. In addition to financial constraints, transportability of the wheelchair was an issue of concern for Willy's family. They did not have access to a van. Unfortunately, Willy needed a heavy-duty wheelchair as well as sophisticated control mechanisms that were not found on easily transportable power wheelchairs. A manual wheelchair with a power add-on unit would not satisfy Willy's needs nor would his needs be met with a power wheelchair that was capable of being disassembled.

Willy received an Everest and Jennings Kidz Power Wheelchair with a remote mount joystick control for left hand use that was mounted on a retractable mount for versatility in positioning. He had a tray on his

(continued)

Willy's Story–continued

wheelchair with a cutout for the power controls. Willy used the tray as a work surface and put his right hand under the tray to control the athetoid movements while driving the power wheelchair.

With three sessions of training, Willy became proficient in using his power wheelchair indoors and outside on all terrain and in a variety of settings. He used the power wheelchair both at school and in his neighborhood to play with his peers. Willy has become more assertive and outgoing because he has some control over his environment and has achieved independent mobility.

Unfortunately, Willy's home was not accessible to a power wheelchair. A temporary ramp was made to get the power wheelchair into the house, but the rooms were quite small and crowded. Willy had limited use of power mobility in his home and usually changed to a manual wheelchair when he came indoors.

Although Willy would probably not be a functional ambulator, he also participated in PT treatment to prevent further deformity and contractures and to promote trunk control in sitting. Willy was issued knee immobilizers and an abduction wedge that his family was instructed to use after Willy did ROM exercises. If he could tolerate immobilizers and a wedge at night, Willy was to wear them all night when sleeping. Willy was fitted for solid ankle-foot orthoses to control progression of plantar flexion deformity and to assist in controlling his feet while learning stand-and-pivot transfers and while wearing knee immobilizers. Willy was placed in a prone stander in PT to assist in weight bearing, to stretch out tight hip flexors, and to promote trunk control in an upright position. There was no room at his house for a prone stander, but he was placed in the stander daily for 45 minutes or more in school. He also engaged in therapeutic activities in a pool during PT to encourage relaxation and active movement that was also carried out in school.

SUMMARY

Children with cerebral palsy need to and want to be mobile. It is not an easy task to make this desire a reality, but mobility concerns should be paramount in setting treatment goals for children with cerebral palsy. As technology advances and knowledge of movement development increases, better opportunities exist for training children who have cerebral palsy to acquire prewalking skills and functional motor skills. For the child who has more severe physical impairments, technology exists to provide alternative means of mobility, and refinement of these alternatives will only continue with time. Mobility means exploration, and exploration means learning. Mobility means freedom and independence. Mobility opens up the world to individuals who have dysfunctional mobility skills.

REFERENCES

Blanchet, D., & McGee, S.M. (1996). Orthotics. In L.A. Kurtz, P.W. Dowrick, S.E. Levy, & M.L. Batshaw (Eds.), *Children's Seashore House handbook of developmental disabilities: Resources for interdisciplinary care* (pp. 465–488). Rockville, MD: Aspen Publishers, Inc.

Bleck, E.E. (1975). Locomotor prognosis in cerebral palsy. *Developmental Medicine and Child Neurology, 17,* 18–35.

Bobath, K., & Bobath, B. (1972). Cerebral palsy. In P.A. Pearson & C.E. Williams (Eds.), *Physical therapy services in the developmental disabilities.* Springfield, IL: Charles C Thomas.

Bohannon, R.W., & Smith, M.B. (1987). Interrater reliability of a modified Ashworth scale of muscle spasticity. *Physical Therapy, 67,* 206–207.

Butler, C. (1991). Augmentative mobility: Why do it? *Physical Medicine and Rehabilitation Clinics of North America, 2*(4), 801–815.

Butler, P.B., Thompson, N., & Major, R.E. (1992). Improvement in walking performance of children with cerebral palsy: Preliminary results. *Developmental Medicine and Child Neurology, 34,* 567–576.

Campbell, S.K. (Ed.). (1991). *Pediatric neurologic physical therapy.* New York: Churchill Livingstone.

Campbell, S.K. (Ed.). (1994). *Physical therapy for children.* Philadelphia: W.B. Saunders.

Campos da Paz, A., Burnett, S.M., & Braga, L.W. (1994). Walking prognosis in cerebral palsy: A 22 year retrospective analysis. *Developmental Medicine and Child Neurology, 36,* 130–134.

Chandler, L., Andrews, M., & Swanson, M. (1980). *The Movement Assessment of Infants.* Rolling Bay, WA: Rolling Bay Press.

Finnie, N.R. (1975). *Handling the young cerebral palsied child at home* (2nd ed.). New York: E.P. Dutton.

Folio, M., & Fewell, R. (1983). *Peabody Developmental Motor Scales.* Hingham, MA: DLM.

Jaeger, D.L. (1987). *Home program instruction sheets for infants and young children.* Tucson, AZ: Therapy Skill Builders.

Knobloch, H., Stevens, F., & Malone, A.F. (1980). *Manual of developmental diagnosis* (Rev. ed.). New York: Harper & Row.

Knott, M., & Voss, D.E. (1968). *PNF: Patterns and techniques.* New York: Harper & Row.

Miller, F., & Bacharach, S.J. (1995). *Cerebral palsy: A complete guide for caregivers.* Baltimore: The Johns Hopkins University Press.

Molnar, G.E. (1985). Cerebral palsy. In G.E. Molnar (Ed.), *Pediatric rehabilitation.* Baltimore: Williams & Wilkins.

Russell, D.J., Rosenbaum, P.L., Cadman, D.J., Gowland, C., Hardy, S., & Jarvis, S. (1989). The Gross Motor Functional Measure: A means to evaluate the effect of physical therapy. *Developmental Medicine and Child Neurology, 31,* 341–356.

State University of New York at Buffalo. (1993). *Guide for the Uniform Data Set for Medical Rehabilitation for Children (WeeFIM), version 4.0–inpatient.* Buffalo, NY: Author.

Thelen, E. (1995). Motor development: A synthesis. *American Psychologist, 50*(2), 79–95.

Thelen, E., & Ulrich, B.D. (1991). Hidden skills: A dynamic systems analysis of tread-mill stepping during the first year. *Monograph of the Society for Research in Child Development, 56*(1), 1–98.

Trahan, J., & Marcoux, S. (1994). Factors associated with the inability of children with cerebral palsy to walk at six years: A retrospective study. *Developmental Medicine and Child Neurology, 36,* 766–773.

Watt, J.M., Robertson, C.M.T., & Grace, M.G.A. (1989). Early prognosis for ambulation of neonatal intensive care survivors with cerebral palsy. *Developmental Medicine and Child Neurology, 31*(6), 766–773.

ADAPTIVE EQUIPMENT TO ENHANCE FUNCTIONAL MOBILITY

If the severity of a motor disability is so severe that functional mobility is ineffective or unattainable, then adaptive equipment can assist in building independence in mobility for children with cerebral palsy.

STANDERS

Standers are adjustable wooden devices that provide support in an upright position and weight bearing on lower extremities. They have the potential to enhance musculoskeletal development as well as provide proper alignment and weight bearing on lower extremities, which can help with molding the acetabulum and assist in proper hip formation. The weight-bearing forces to the long bones assist in bone calcification and may assist in preventing osteoporosis. Prone standers provide maximum stretch to the hip flexors and maintain the knee in extension and the ankle in neutral dorsiflexion, which is necessary for future ambulation. Prolonged stretch to the lower-extremity flexor muscles aids in controlling the development of contractures, deformities, and pain, all of which diminish the chance for functional locomotion. There are three main types of standers: prone standers, supine standers, and a variation of the parapodium stander.

Prone Standers

Prone standers provide support across the anterior surface of the body (see Figure 10.3). The angle can be adjusted to vary the degree of weight bearing on the extremities. Prone standers provide trunk support and allow a child to work on improved head and trunk control in an antigravity posture. Several companies make prone standers that come with a variety of adaptations. A tray attached to the stander can provide a child with a work surface (see "Willy's Story" in this chapter). Trunk supports can be added to prevent lateral trunk flexion. An abduction pommel (i.e., medial thigh support) and a hip stabilizer can be added for preventing adduction and hip flexion. The foot support can be angled to vary the plantarflexion and dorsiflexion angle. The foot support generally has straps with which to secure the feet. Other straps are located at the pelvis and the trunk to secure a child and ensure his or her safety. Some prone standers have a wheeled base so that they can be easily moved around the environment by a caregiver.

There are some difficulties that can occur with prone standers. Because a child must be lifted onto the prone stander, larger and heavier children may require the assistance of two people to ensure their safety. Prone standers are cumbersome and difficult to store, and they can be expensive and may not be covered on some medical insurance plans.

Supine Standers

Supine standers (see Figure 12.2) provide support across the back (i.e., posterior surface of the body) in a manner similar to a tilt table. They support the entire body through the back (i.e., dorsal surface). Additional positioning features on the supine stander include straps to control the trunk and the pelvis, trunk supports to prevent lateral trunk flexion, adjustable foot boards to accommodate foot deformities, and straps to secure the feet. A wheeled base is

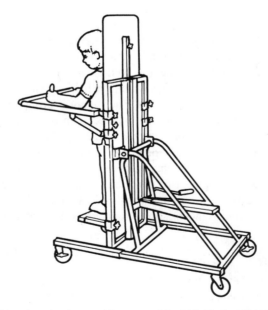

Figure 12.2. A supine stander provides support for individuals without adequate head control while providing lower-extremity weight bearing.

optional, making it easily transportable. A tray or an adjustable height table can also provide a work surface.

There are difficulties that can be encountered with supine standers. The supine stander does not provide positioning to allow a child to practice head and trunk control. The child's arms are not in a gravity-assisted position for function and play. It is cumbersome and difficult to store, and it can be expensive and may not be covered on some medical insurance plans.

Parapodiums and Freestanding Standers

Parapodiums and freestanding standers provide support up to the waist (see Figure 12.3). The frame is mounted on a base with straps to hold the ankles, knees, hips, and pelvis in position. It allows lower-extremity weight bearing for children who have good head and trunk control but do not stand in correct alignment. Parapodiums have been used mainly with children who have spina bifida or spinal cord injury.

Freestanding standers are easier to store than prone or supine standers and are usually less expensive. They can be set up at a regular table or at the sink. However, one difficulty that can occur with freestanding standers is that they do not provide a lot of trunk control.

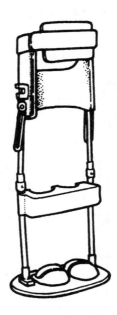

Figure 12.3. A parapodium (freestanding stander). (From Blanchet, D., & McGee, S.M. [1996]. Orthotics. In L.A. Kurtz, P.W. Dowrick, S.E. Levy, & M.L. Batshaw [Eds.], *Children's Seashore House handbook of developmental disabilities: Resources for interdisciplinary care* [p. 474]. Rockville, MD: Aspen Publishers, Inc.; reprinted by permission.)

GAIT-TRAINING DEVICES

Gait-training devices are alternative mobility products that build independence in functional mobility. There are seven main types of gait training devices: anterior or posterior walkers, ring walkers, crutches, quad canes, manual wheelchairs, and power wheelchairs.

Anterior or Posterior Walkers

Walkers are light metal frames with four legs that provide support while walking (with or without wheels) and are able to stand alone. Walkers that are pushed with the frame in front of the body are *anterior walkers* (see Figure 12.4); walkers that are pulled with the frame behind the body are called *posterior walkers* (see Figure 12.5).

Although anterior walkers require less energy to use than posterior walkers, a child is often flexed at the hips during use, and this is discouraged because it can contribute to hip flexor tightness and prevent use of hip extensor muscles. In contrast, posterior walkers promote an extended trunk and a more upright posture.

A walker can have four legs and be equipped with two wheels or four wheels. If a child has hemiplegia or poor upper-extremity control but is able to use a frame walker, a forearm support can be added to the walker to support the child's arm, which will enable him or her to grip the handle on the walker.

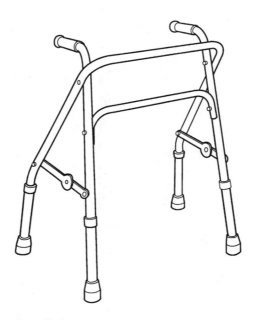

Figure 12.4. Anterior walker.

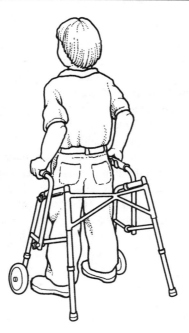

Figure 12.5. Posterior walker.

Ring Walkers

Ring walkers (i.e., walking frames) provide maximum support to a child's trunk and upper extremities. They are used primarily as an ambulation training device when a child is gaining postural control. They also serve as an alternative for a child who has severe motor impairments and who may be capable of using this device as a means of self-directed mobility. Controversy exists as to whether this type of device will reinforce abnormal tone or posture and, thus, jeopardize a child's ability to gain prerequisite skills for more independent ambulation. For example, a walker may reinforce scissoring or a crouched posture in standing. The benefits of improved functional mobility, enhanced motivation, and self-confidence must be weighed against the risk of exacerbating underlying motor impairments on a case-by-case basis.

Walkers provide maximum support and safety for assisted ambulation. They can be modified for use with individuals who have limited upper-extremity control. Walkers with wheels require less energy expenditure to use, particularly if there are swivel wheels in the rear.

Difficulties that can occur with walkers include not being accessible to ambulate up and down steps and being cumbersome to transport. Although a child who is in a wheelchair may be able to use a walker, it is still difficult to carry and gain access to. In addition, walkers are more expensive than crutches.

Crutches

There are two main types of crutches. Axillary crutches provide support under the arm with pads, and weight bearing is provided on a horizontal bar between the two uprights (see Figure 12.6). Forearm crutches (i.e., Loffstrand crutches) have one upright, a cuff that fits around the forearm, and weight bearing is provided on a horizontal projection below the cuff (see Figure 12.7). Crutches require more trunk control and balance than does a walker. The user's arms must be strong enough to bear a substantial portion of his or her body weight. Fair righting and balance responses in standing are necessary to use crutches.

Crutches are more versatile than a walker. They can be used for support when going up and down steps. The cost is not overly expensive, and they can be carried on the back of a wheelchair. However, crutches tend to promote hip flexion, which displaces the center of gravity more anterior and requires less reciprocal lower-extremity movement when children do a swing-through gait pattern.

Quad Canes

Quad canes (see Figure 12.8) provide support for individuals who need more support than the forearm or axillary crutches can provide. The quad cane has a horizontal handle and a large base with four short legs for additional support, rather than one continuous leg as in a regular cane. Quad canes often are used as a training device when transferring from a walker to crutches.

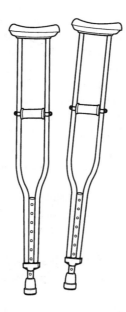

Figure 12.6.   Axillary crutches.

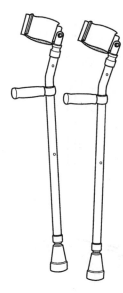

Figure 12.7. Forearm or Loffstrand crutches.

Manual Wheelchairs

Children need to explore their environment. When a child has limited to nonexistent functional ambulation, a wheelchair is an effective alternative to walking. Parents may presume that getting a wheelchair for a child who may have the potential for ambulation will deter the child from ever walking. In other words, parents may presume that the child will become "lazy" and depend on the wheelchair. However, anecdotal reports cite that children who are in a wheelchair have a greater motivation to walk.

As a child with cerebral palsy grows and gains weight, his or her muscles appear to get tighter. In addition, the energy expended in walking with braces and an assistive device may be too costly. A child may suffer in his or her educational and social activities because he or she is too tired to participate and because he or she uses so much effort to walk. Providing a child with alternative means of mobility allows him or her to engage in other activities with more energy and vigor.

Children with severe motor impairments, poor sitting balance, and little to no functional mobility need a wheelchair that is both a mobility device and a proper positioning system. For a child who has insufficient control or strength to propel a manual wheelchair, power mobility provides an alternative means of exploring his or her environment. Specialty transport and mobility wheelchairs offer positioning and safe transport for small children who are unable to use conventional strollers or a wheelchair.

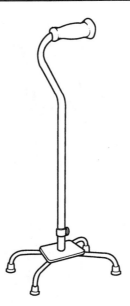

Figure 12.8. Quad cane.

Wheelchairs come in many shapes and sizes that meet the varied needs of children with diverse interests and levels of function. A properly fitted wheelchair meets the needs of a child and his or her family and the specific settings in which the wheelchair is used. Wheelchairs are an important component in the rehabilitation of a child who has motor impairments. The prescription and fitting for a wheelchair should be undertaken in consultation with knowledgeable professionals, such as a physical or occupational therapist, a wheelchair vendor who deals with pediatric rehabilitation equipment, and the child's physician.

An adaptive seating system aims to provide a stable and secure base of support for sitting and adequate postural support that maximizes a child's potential for educational experiences and provides the independence to explore his or her environment and facilitate social interaction. The system can assist in decreasing the influence of abnormal muscle tone, pathological reflexes, and poor motor control. It also can prevent or minimize contractures and deformities while facilitating developmental skills.

Manual wheelchairs are used with children who can propel a wheelchair by maneuvering the wheels. Wheelchairs allow a child to be at the same height as his or her peers, to keep up with other children in social and recreational interaction, and to develop independence.

The manual wheelchair frame provides the base for the seating support system and is a means of mobility and transportation for a caregiver if a child is unable to propel independently. Manual wheelchairs can accommodate a growing child by changing its seating system and/or altering its frame. They can be transported in a bus or van with a tie-down system, and most manual wheelchairs are partially or fully funded by third-party payers.

Manual wheelchairs are propelled by using upper-body strength. Manual wheelchairs have a metal frame, large rear wheels, small front wheels, sling seat and sling back, some type of footrest, and push handles (see Figure 12.9). For proper positioning, it is generally recommended that wheelchairs have a solid seat and a solid back. Additional positioning pieces, such as trunk supports, chest supports, head supports, pelvic supports, abduction pommel, or adductor pads, may be added to a solid frame.

Several varieties of manual wheelchairs are on the market, and these are classified by weight, the child, or the child's functional abilities. Ultralightweight wheelchair frames are under 25 pounds in weight and are made of high-strength material. These are generally used for sports as well as everyday use by individuals who need less postural support and a lighter weight wheelchair for propelling longer distances with less fatigue. A tilt-in-space wheelchair component is used for individuals who need to recline while maintaining a fixed hip angle (see Figure 12.10). Wheelchairs with large wheels in the front are used with children who cannot propel the chair with large rear-positioned wheels. Wheelchairs with a one-arm drive mechanism are used with individuals who have functional use of only one arm and one hand to propel the wheelchair.

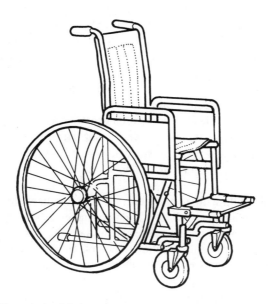

Figure 12.9. Manual wheelchair.

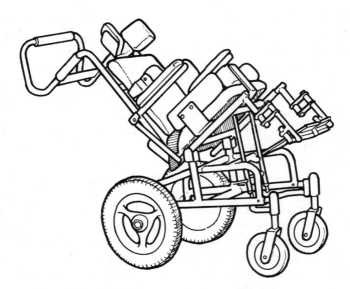

Figure 12.10.   Tilt-in-space wheelchair with postural supports.

Power Wheelchairs

Children who have the capability to propel a manual wheelchair but insufficient strength or endurance to functionally use the wheelchair or engage in typical activities of daily living are candidates for power mobility (i.e., a power wheelchair) (see Figure 12.11). These children may also walk with assistive devices, but this ability is classified as an exercise or household ambulation (i.e., without the potential to functionally ambulate for distances). An example is a child with spastic diplegia who can push a manual wheelchair for short distances but is unable to use the wheelchair without assistance for mobility in school, outdoors, or in recreational/social settings.

Power mobility is indicated for children who do not have the strength, control, or endurance to propel a manual wheelchair but have the cognitive capabilities to understand and use a power wheelchair. Power wheelchairs allow independent exploration of the environment and the ability to keep up with peers.

A 2-year-old child without a disability is able to run, explore the environment, and interact with other children. Toddlers and preschool children who are mobile can learn, explore, and socialize and, as a result, develop independence and a healthy concept of self in relation to others. To promote overall development and not merely compensate for a neuromuscular disorder, power wheelchairs have been successfully used with children as early as 2 years of age. The key to successful use is minimal cognitive impairment combined with the motivation of the child and his or her family.

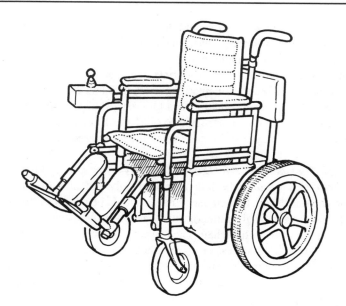

Figure 12.11. Power wheelchair.

Power wheelchair use requires sufficient cognition to safely manage the controls. There is a great variety of controls that are easily accessible to children who are not severely affected as well as to children who are severely physically limited. The newer controls on power wheelchairs are capable of fine adjustments for speed, acceleration and deceleration, turning speed, and tremor dampening. These controls can be mounted wherever a child has the most access and control to maneuver the wheelchair: at the head, chin, face, shoulder, elbow, hand, knee, or foot. The most widely used control is the joystick, which is mounted for use with the hand.

Power wheelchairs have either gel cell or lead acid batteries that supply power to the motor. Power wheelchairs are made with either a direct drive or a belt-driven system. The batteries need to be recharged on a regular basis, and these wheelchairs are quite heavy in order to accommodate the power mechanism and other adaptive devices that may be added to the wheelchair.

The standard design for power wheelchairs is a wheelchair frame mounted on top of a base that contains the motor. Power wheelchairs can be ordered with a variety of components, such as a reclining or tilt back, which can be operated by the same controller that is used to drive the power wheelchair. The legrests can elevate and the headrest can be adjusted to accommodate changes in position.

Although there is a power wheelchair system that can be disassembled and placed in a car, this is not an easy process, and the weight of the wheelchair without the batteries is more than 45 pounds. These "lightweight" power wheelchairs usually come in adult sizes, and the smallest width is 14 inches. These wheelchairs are only available to older and larger children, unless an insert system is added to support a smaller child.

Manual wheelchairs are able to be converted to power wheelchairs with the addition of power pack attachments. These wheelchairs can be disassembled and put into a car, but they are heavy. An additional disadvantage is that manual wheelchair frames are not constructed to hold all of the additional weight of the power units and may sustain more breakdowns and require more frequent repairs.

Special Considerations for Power Mobility Because children grow in length, depth, and weight, wheelchairs that have the potential to convert their frame and seating system to their user's needs should be chosen. Children need to have a power wheelchair with controls that can be adjusted as they master maneuvering the power wheelchair. The drive parameters should be adjustable to accommodate either progress or regression in skill and control.

The power wheelchair's control system should be able to interface with various other devices that a child may require for independence in his or her environment. Several of the sophisticated control systems have the ability to interface the power control mechanism with augmentative communication devices and environmental control units. These systems increase exponentially in cost as the degree of sophistication increases.

Once the appropriate system is identified for a child, the challenge is to find the finances to purchase the system. The equipment can range anywhere from $800 to more than $20,000. Most families do not have the resources to cover the total cost of a wheelchair. Other resources for funding need to be explored, such as private health insurance, government programs for those qualifying for medical assistance, private nonprofit organizations and service clubs, leasing equipment, or loans.

CHAPTER 13

Promoting Function in Daily Living Skills

Lesley A. Geyer, Lisa A. Kurtz, and Lynette E. Byarm

For children with cerebral palsy, the ability to actively participate in meaningful daily routines is central to their ability to adapt to home, school, and community settings. Children with cerebral palsy vary widely in their capacity to perform adaptive (i.e., self-care) activities, including dressing, feeding, and managing personal hygiene. This variation is in part a result of the severity of the motor impairments that the child may develop, but it also relates to the presence of associated cognitive and sensory limitations (Case-Smith, 1994; Fraser, Hensinger, & Phelps, 1990). For example, the child who has typical cognitive skills and mild spastic hemiplegia should be capable of developmentally appropriate independence, with only minor modifications to his or her daily routine. In contrast, the child who has more significant impairments will likely remain dependent on caregivers for many aspects of self-care well into adulthood. A variety of rehabilitation interventions may be used to minimize the impairments and the functional limitations that commonly result from cerebral palsy and often contribute to limitations in self-care. Examples of these interventions include specialized seating or positioning equipment designed to promote stable posture, special handling techniques (e.g., neurodevelopmental therapy [see Chapter 12]) designed to influence muscle tone and to control movement needed for self-directed reach and grasp, splinting designed to improve hand function, and a variety of adapted aids and equipment designed to promote self-care. In addition, for many children with cerebral palsy, environmental and societal limitations represent serious obstacles to independence in daily living skills. These limitations serve to remind professionals that interventions that focus exclusively on the child may be ineffective in optimizing functional independence; suboptimal characteristics of the child's real-life settings also must be addressed in a carefully constructed program for habilitation.

It is critically important to encourage children and their families to identify the daily routines that most affect their lives and to prioritize the goals of intervention according to their unique personal and/or cultural values. If more than one reasonable option exists for addressing a problem, families should have a clear voice in selecting their preferred intervention approach. It is always important to acknowledge the influence of choice in empowering individuals to take charge of their lives and to retain a sense of ownership and control over daily activities. For example, many professionals remember to allow the child to select the preferred flavor of toothpaste for routine dental hygiene, knowing that this may increase the child's motivation. However, they may forget to build choices into the many other aspects of this task, such as the time of day when toothbrushing occurs, the temperature of the water, or the firmness of the bristles on the child's toothbrush. Despite the proliferation of literature supporting the benefits of family-centered therapy practices, there is evidence to suggest that many therapists working with young children who have cerebral palsy continue to concentrate their efforts more on the establishment and achievement of rehabilitative goals than on addressing the family's needs and priorities (Hinojosa, Anderson, & Ranum, 1988). Studies suggest that mothers of young children with cerebral palsy spend significantly more time than do mothers of typically developing preschoolers in dressing, feeding, washing, and toileting routines, a factor that may contribute to the responsibility of care involved in parenting a child with a disability (Johnson & Deitz, 1985). When activities have been selected to be nonstressful and enjoyable to both the child and the caregivers, parents are more likely to integrate therapy principles and techniques into their typical daily routines (Hinojosa & Anderson, 1991; Johnson & Dietz, 1985). Although many of the interventions provided by medical, rehabilitative, or educational specialists support the development of self-care skills, it is often the occupational therapist who focuses effort on this aspect of the child's development. Occupational therapists are trained to evaluate and treat functional limitations that affect fine motor performance, cognitive and perceptual development, and psychosocial adjustment as they relate to the child's ability to function in play, in adaptive skills, and in school performance, which are the primary occupations of childhood (Kurtz & Scull, 1993).

ASSESSMENT OF DAILY LIVING SKILLS

A child's activities of daily living (ADLs) typically include self-care skill activities, play, and engagement in school endeavors, which for older children include participation in prevocational activities. It is commonly accepted that children acquire ADL skills at widely varying individual rates and that ages for specific skill acquisition cannot be definitively predicted. A general sequence of skill acquisition that is common to typically developing children is delineated in Table 13.1.

Family Interview

The daily living skills assessment may address any or all of the child's ADLs that are performed in the home, in the school, or in other community settings. The assessment process often begins with a family interview (with the child present) in order to determine which areas are appropriate to address. For example, the school-age child who is already receiving intensive school-based intervention for issues related to school performance may not require an evaluation of school performance and prevocational skills when he or she visits a hospital clinic to obtain recommendations to improve self-care skills. In addition, this child may need only a cursory screening for problems related to play skills. During the initial family interview, the therapist attempts to acquire an understanding of the family's priorities for the focus of intervention, and the assessment process is usually guided by the information obtained in this interview. The therapist may find it necessary to work with family members in order to help establish goals for ADLs that are compatible with the child's motor skills, cognitive level, and perceptual abilities. The therapist also needs to establish an understanding of the priorities, values, and specific cultural practices of the child's family because these will affect the child's performance of self-care tasks. For example, many parents report that independence in performing adaptive tasks has low priority in the morning when family members are rushing to get to school or to work on time. Cultural practices affect the child's performance of daily living skills and the family's acceptance of intervention techniques, and, as a result, expectations for independence with these tasks can vary significantly from one culture to the next. In addition, cultural influences affect the type of daily living skill tasks that the child is expected to perform (e.g., clothing that is expected to be donned or doffed, dining utensils that are expected to be used).

Assessment of Performance: Identifying Impairments and Functional Limitations

The therapist may first spend some time evaluating the functional impairments that affect the child's daily living skills. A sensorimotor evaluation allows the therapist to evaluate the child's ability to move around his or her environment and to maintain more static postures (e.g., sitting, standing). An evaluation of

Table 13.1. Skill acquisition in the typical development of daily living skills

		Functional Domain				
			Self-care			
Approximate Age	Motor	Feeding	Dressing	Hygiene	Social/play	School and prevocational skills
Birth to 3 months	Grasps with whole hand involuntarily	Anticipatory response to food stimulus				
3–6 months	Reaches bilaterally for toys and actively, purposefully grasps for toys	Holds bottle independently			Recognizes self in mirror, imitates facial expression, and holds mutual gaze	
6–9 months	Transfers object from hand to hand, reaches for toys with one hand, and uses index finger to point, explore toys	Feeds self cracker, drinks from cup, and finger feeds			Protests separation from familiar adults	
9–12 months	Holds block in each hand and brings together at midline, uses pincer grasp for tiny object, and lets go of toy on purpose	Holds handle of cup when drinking	Cooperates by extending arm and/or leg	Indicates discomfort with soiled diapers	Enjoys solitary play and reciprocates for tickling and peekaboo	Attempts to scribble with crayon and turns pages in book

Age						
1–2 years	Holds crayon using fisted grasp and stands and walks unsupported	Uses spoon to feed, spills, drinks from straw, and distinguishes edible from nonedible foods		Develops bowel/bladder control and partially washes hands	Uses gestures and words to indicate wants, turns doorknob to open door, imitates housework, and performs complex imitations	Imitates strokes with crayon and attends to simple story
2–3 years	Pedals tricycle and enjoys jumping and climbing	Uses napkin	Unties and removes shoes and fastens large front buttons	Turns water faucets on and off	Engages in parallel play (i.e., more interest in peers than in group activity), puts away jacket and toys, and displays stranger anxiety	Sorts items by shape and color, constructs simple designs with blocks, and understands concepts of size and space
3–4 years	Accelerates and decelerates when running and hops on one foot	Independently uses spoon and/or fork with little spillage and drinks from soda can or bottle	Manages snaps and front zipper, puts shoes on correct feet, and knows front from back of clothing	Arranges clothes to prepare for toileting, flushes toilet, blows nose into tissue, brushes/combs hair, and brushes teeth effectively	Plays cooperatively in group to attain group goal, shows interest in "making things," talks in sentences, places dirty clothes in hamper, and sets table with assistance	Recalls simple sequences (e.g., digits, sentences, motor sequences), and counts with one-to-one correspondence

(continued)

Table 13.1. *(continued)*

| Approximate Age | Functional Domain | | | | | |
| | Motor | Self-care | | | Social/play | School and prevocational skills |
		Feeding	Dressing	Hygiene		
5–6 years	Holds crayon using mature tripod grasp, skips, and performs somersault	Uses knife for cutting and/or spreading	Unfastens back buttons or zipper	Bathes or showers when reminded, covers nose during sneeze, cuts fingernails, and adjusts water temperature for bath	Engages in more complex group play (e.g., dramatic play, games), looks both ways before crossing street, initiates telephone calls to others, and follows game rules	Understands time concepts, describes similarities and differences, and shows developing verbal and reasoning skills
7–9 years			Ties bows	Styles own hair and washes ears	Identifies "best friend," engages in increased competition with peers, and shows marked increase in listening and cooperation	Knows value of coins and sweeps, mops, or vacuums floors
10–12 years			Ties necktie		Straightens room without reminders, shows sufficient development in language and cognitive abilities for social interaction	Uses stove or microwave, uses household cleaning agents appropriately, and is able to count change for purchase costing more than $1

fine motor control assists the therapist in predicting the child's ability to manipulate both toys and tools (e.g., writing instruments, eating utensils, groom-
ing equipment). Visual-perceptual testing is useful in identifying visual-motor
and visual-nonmotor skills as well as impairments that significantly affect function in all ADLs. Cognitive testing gives the therapist an understanding of the
child's level of comprehension, ability to attend to an activity, competence in
problem solving, and capability for memory. Table 13.2 presents examples of
tests that can be used to measure the performance components in combination
with a clinical assessment of these skills.

Assessment of Function: Identifying Disability

The actual assessment of self-care abilities includes observation of the child's
ability to perform specific tasks involved in self-feeding, in grooming/hygiene,
in dressing, in toileting, and in other relevant tasks. A family report is particularly important in helping the therapist to understand the specific way in which
the child typically performs the activity. For example, some children with diminished trunk control dress while in bed, whereas others prefer to be seated in
a wheelchair. It is important for the therapist to determine the types of equipment the child uses at home; in addition, it may be helpful for the therapist to
provide the child with adaptive equipment for use during the assessment process. The assessment of play skills includes identification of the toys or the activities that the child prefers or that seem to elicit the greatest response from
the child. The therapist also assesses the child's ability to manipulate objects
and to adapt to changes during play. The child's ability to interact and to cooperate with others during playtime also is evaluated during the assessment.

School and Prevocational Assessments: Putting Disability in Context

School performance assessment includes multiple areas of evaluation. An interview with the child's teacher can be extremely helpful in identifying the child's
strengths and needs with regard to function in a school environment. If the child
has not yet attended a school program, then developmental testing may be used
to assist with the determination of appropriate school or appropriate class placement. The school performance assessment also should include evaluations of
the child's motor proficiency with regard to functional mobility in the school
setting, visual-perceptual skills, ability to manage school materials, and self-
care abilities necessary for independent function in a school environment (e.g.,
dressing, self-feeding, toileting). The prevocational assessment addresses the
child's physical appearance and hygiene, hand dexterity, cognitive abilities (including the ability to learn and remember new tasks, maintain attention to task,
and adhere to a schedule), and ability to cooperate and work with others. Because the child's skills in performing household chores can be considered precursors to later vocational skills, it often is helpful for the therapist to obtain a
family report. In addition to histories provided by parents with regard to their

Table 13.2. Tests for assessment of functional limitations affecting activities of daily living

Test	Area of functional ability	Reference
Bruininks-Oseretsky Test of Motor Proficiency	Sensorimotor, fine motor	Bruininks, R.H. (1978). *Bruininks-Oseretsky Test of Motor Proficiency examiner's manual.* Circle Pines, MN: American Guidance Service.
DeGangi-Berk Test of Sensory Integration	Sensorimotor, fine motor, visual-perceptual	Berk, R.A., & DeGangi, G. (1983). *DeGangi-Berk Test of Sensory Integration manual.* Los Angeles: Western Psychological Services.
Developmental Test of Visual Motor Integration (VMI)	Fine motor, visual-perceptual	Beery, K.E. (1989). *The VMI, Developmental Test of Visual-Motor Integration: Administration, scoring and teaching manual.* Cleveland, OH: Modern Curriculum Press.
Hawaii Early Learning Profile (HELP) and HELP for Special Preschoolers	Sensorimotor, fine motor, cognitive/academic	Furuno, S., O'Reilly, K., Hosaka, C., Inatsuka, T.T., Allman, T.L., & Zeisloft, B. (1984). *Hawaii Early Learning Profile (HELP).* Palo Alto, CA: VORT Corporation. Santa Cruz County Office of Education. (1987). *HELP for Special Preschoolers.* Palo Alto, CA: VORT Corporation.
Jebsen Hand Function Test	Fine motor	Jebsen, R.H., Taylor, N., Trieschmann, R.B., Trottler, H.J., & Howard, L.A. (1969). An objective and standardized test of hand function. *Archives of Physical Medicine and Rehabilitation, 50,* 311–319. Taylor, N., Sand, P.L., & Jebsen, R.H. (1973). Evaluation of hand function in children. *Archives of Physical Medicine and Rehabilitation, 54,* 129–135.
Motor-Free Visual Perception Test	Visual-perceptual	Colarusso, R.P., & Hammill, D.D. (1972). *MVPT—Motor-Free Visual Perception Test manual.* Novato, CA: Academic Therapy Publications.

(continued)

Table 13.2. *(continued)*

Movement Assessment of Infants	Sensorimotor	Chandler, L.S., Andrews, M.S., & Swanson, M.W. (1980). *Movement Assessment of Infants.* (Available from Post Office Box 4631, Rolling Bay, Washington 98061.)
Peabody Developmental Motor Scales	Sensorimotor, fine motor	Folio, M.R., & Fewell, R.R. (1983). *Peabody Developmental Motor Scales.* Allen, TX: DLM Teaching Resources.
Peabody Individual Achievement Test–Revised (PIAT–R)	Cognitive/ academic	Markwardt, F.C., Jr. (1989). *Peabody Individual Achievement Test–Revised.* Circle Pines, MN: American Guidance Service.
Purdue Pegboard Test	Fine motor	Gardner, R.A., & Broman, M. (1979). The Purdue Pegboard: Normative data on 1334 schoolchildren. *Journal of Clinical Child Psychology, 1,* 156–162. Mathiowetz, V., Rogers, S.L., Dowe-Keval, M., Donahue, R., & Rennells, C. (1986). The Purdue Pegboard: Norms for 14- to 19-year olds. *American Journal of Occupational Therapy, 40*(3), 174–179. Tiffen, J. (1968). *Purdue Pegboard examiner manual.* Lafayette, IN: Lafayette Instrument Company.
Test of Visual-Perceptual Skills	Visual-perceptual	Gardner, M.F. (1988). *TVPS, Test of Visual-Perceptual Skills (non-motor) manual.* San Francisco: Health Publishing Company. Gardner, M.F. (1992). *TVPS–UL, Test of Visual-Perceptual Skills (non-motor) upper level manual.* Burlingame, CA: Psychological and Educational Publications.

child's behavior and task performance, therapist-made checklists or scales, other criterion-referenced tests, and standardized tests assist the therapist in collecting useful and often quantifiable information in terms of the child's skills related to ADLs (Radcliffe & Moss, 1996). There are a number of tests that specifically assess adaptive, play, school, and prevocational skills; many developmental tests contain subsections that are useful in assessing adaptive and other ADL skills. Examples of these tests are presented in Table 13.3.

Many of the tests listed in Table 13.3 can be used to measure changes in basic daily living skills; however, they may lack specificity for aspects of daily living that are culturally determined. More global functional independence measures such as the Pediatric Evaluation of Disability Inventory (PEDI) or the Functional Independence Measure for Children (see Table 13.3) may be used to measure change over an extended period of time or to incorporate the level of caregiver assistance and environmental modifications or equipment needed for self-care (Coster & Haley, 1992; State University of New York at Buffalo, 1993). Other important outcome measures to consider in terms of change in daily living skills include amount of time spent in completion of daily living skills, child and parent satisfaction with selected techniques and devices, and ability and motivation to incorporate strategies that are learned or rehearsed at home or in the clinic to relevant community settings. Once the assessment process is complete, the therapist formulates a plan for intervention to maximize independence in ADLs. This plan often includes the provision of recommendations and family training for activities that will be performed at home. In some situations, under the guidance of the therapist, direct treatment is necessary in order to help the child practice and refine the necessary prerequisite skills for independent performance in adaptive play, school, and prevocational activities.

TREATMENT OPTIONS AND STRATEGIES

Intervention to promote the acquisition and the development of daily living skills is based on the assessment of the child's underlying sensorimotor, cognitive, psychosocial, and perceptual impairments that affect or interfere with his or her function. The treatment approach may focus on remediation of the child's underlying impairment, training in compensatory techniques, or a combination of both. In order to facilitate learning of new skills, modalities of treatment may include neuromotor or biomechanical approaches to address sensorimotor control, environmental adaptation, provision of adaptive equipment, and cognitive teaching strategies. As previously discussed, family involvement in treatment is essential to management strategies because daily living skills are typically carried out within the context of the home and must fit into the culture of the family. Educational program staff also may need to be trained in techniques that will be carried over into the child's school environment.

Motor Skills Training

The therapist working with the child who has motor dysfunction needs to address the development of the motor components that are necessary for successful completion of functional skills. Specific areas for treatment may include facilitation of appropriate range of motion; muscle tone; strength; endurance;

Table 13.3. Tests for assessment of daily living skills

Test	Activities of daily living assessed by test	Reference
Gesell Developmental Schedules (1989 revisions)	Self-care, play/ social interaction, school/ academic	Knobloch, H., Stevens, F., & Malone, A.F. (1980). *Manual of developmental diagnosis.* New York: Harper & Row.
Gesell Preschool Test	Self-care, play/ social interaction, school/ academic	Ames, L.B., Gillespie, C., Haines, J., & Ilg, F. (1979). *The Gesell Institute's child from one to six: Evaluating the behavior of the preschool child.* New York: Harper & Row. Haines, J., Ames, L.B., & Gillespie, C. (1980). *The Gesell Preschool Test manual.* Rosemont, NJ: Modern Learning Press.
Jacob's Prevocational Skills Assessment	Prevocational	Jacobs, K. (1985). *Occupational therapy: Work-related programs and assessments.* Boston: Little, Brown.
Klein-Bell Activities of Daily Living Scale for Children	Self-care	Law, M., & Usher, P. (1988). Validation of the Klein-Bell Activities of Daily Living Scale for Children. *Canadian Journal of Occupational Therapy, 55*(2), 63–67.
Preschool Play Scale	Play/social interaction	Knox, S.H. (1974). A play scale. In M. Reilly (Ed.), *Play as exploratory learning* (pp. 247–266). Thousand Oaks, CA: Sage Publications.
Pediatric Evaluation of Disability Inventory (PEDI)	Self-care	Coster, W.J., & Haley, S.M. (1992). Conceptualization and measurement of disablement in infants and young children. *Infants and Young Children, 4*(4), 11–12. Haley, S.M., Coster, W.J., Ludlow, L.H., Haltiwanger, J.T., & Andrellos, P.J. (1992). *Pediatric Evaluation of Disability Inventory (PEDI): Development, standardization, and administration manual.* Boston: PEDI Research Group and New England Medical Center Hospital.

(continued)

Table 13.3. *(continued)*

Test	Activities of daily living assessed by test	Reference
Functional Independence Measure for Children (WeeFIM)	Self-care	Msall, M.E., DiGaudio, K.M., & Duffy, L.C. (1993). Use of functional assessment on children with developmental disabilities. *Physical Medicine and Rehabilitation Clinics of North America, 4*(3), 517–527.
		State University of New York at Buffalo. (1993). *Guide for the Uniform Data Set for Medical Rehabilitation for Children (WeeFIM), version 4.0*. Buffalo: Author.
Vineland Adaptive Behavior Scales	Self-care, play/social interaction	Sparrow, S.S., Balla, D.A., & Cicchetti, D.V. (1984). *Vineland Adaptive Behavior Scales: Survey form manual (interview ed.)*. Circle Pines, MN: American Guidance Service.

gross motor control; and fine motor control, including the promotion of grasp, release, and functional manipulation. The intervention techniques and the approach used may vary according to the therapist's theoretical background and training. For example, a therapist may use neurodevelopmental handling techniques to decrease undesired movements and to facilitate desired movement when assisting the child during a dressing activity. The therapist who uses more of a motor-learning approach, however, may engage the child in a simulated dressing activity such as placing rings on the child's arms and legs to simulate donning a shirt or pants. Intervention also may include the application of the principles of positioning (see Table 13.4) in order to provide the child with adequate postural stability for optimal function and to provide him or her with a safe environment for carrying out an ADL. For the child with minimal dysfunction, positioning may be as simple as providing him or her with a school chair that promotes a stable position with an extended trunk (i.e., the child's hips, knees, and ankles flexed to a 90-degree angle, with feet supported flat on the floor). In order to provide support for the trunk, the child with moderate involvement may learn dressing skills while seated in a corner or while lying on the floor to eliminate some of the need to work against gravity (see Figure 13.1). The child with more significant involvement may require more extensive positioning while performing or being assisted in adaptive tasks. This assistance may include positioning equipment such as adapted chairs, bath seats, or commodes (see Figures 13.2 and 13.3).

Table 13.4. Principles of positioning for activities of daily living

Functional area	Principle	Technique/equipment
Feeding	Provide stability through the trunk to enable a child to have optimal use of hands for self-feeding and a stable base on which to maintain the head in proper alignment for proper oral-motor function and digestion of food	Commercially available adapted chair, wheelchair, therapeutic holding techniques, inserts attached to adapt a standard chair, or tray attached to chair or wheelchair
Bathing	Provide a safe environment while in the tub or shower for a child and/or a caregiver as well as provide appropriate stability to optimize function	Tub/shower chair, reclined bath seat, commercially available baby bath rings, or bed bath
Grooming/ hygiene	Provide adequate support through the trunk to encourage optimal hand skills	Appropriate positioning (e.g., chair in front of sink) or appropriate placement/ setup of supplies
Toileting	Provide appropriate postural support and stability to enable a child to perform toileting needs in a safe manner	Adapted toilet seat, commode, or footstool to support feet
Dressing	Provide postural stability, inhibit the effect of abnormal tonal patterns, and eliminate the need to work against gravity	Chair (regular or adapted) or positioning on floor or in corner
School/play	Provide postural stability to enable a child to engage in classroom or play activities	Adapted seat or positioning on floor

Compensatory Strategies

Adaptive equipment also can be used to enhance function. Equipment may range from simple devices such as enlarged handles, which facilitate grasp for children who have weak hand muscles, or long-handled objects, which extend reach for children who have limited range of motion, to technological devices such as computers or environmental control systems for children with more extensive physical involvement. Several variables must be taken into consideration before

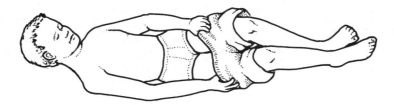

Figure 13.1.   Child dressing while lying on the floor to eliminate some of the need to work against gravity. (From Byarm, L.E. [1996]. Neurodevelopmental therapy. In L.A. Kurtz, P.W. Dowrick, S.E. Levy, & M.L. Batshaw [Eds.], *Children's Seashore House handbook of developmental disabilities: Resources for interdisciplinary care* [p. 258]. Rockville, MD: Aspen Publishers, Inc.; reprinted by permission.)

recommending specific self-care devices for the child. The device should be able to enhance function without being cumbersome. It should be easily accepted within the cultural values of the child's family and should not pose a financial burden. The device should be practical for the environment in which it will be used, and maintenance should be relatively easy. Studies have shown that often the simplest device is the one most consistently used by the majority of individuals (Johnson & Deitz, 1985). Table 13.5 presents examples of commonly used adaptive devices.

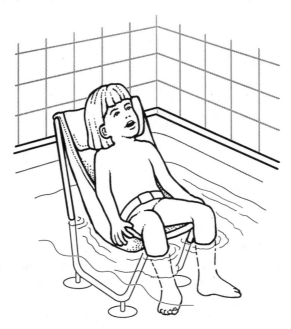

Figure 13.2.   Child supported in bath chair.

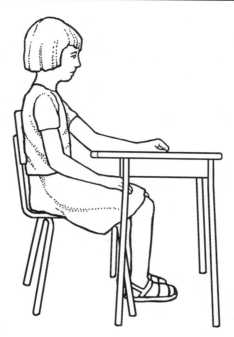

Figure 13.3. Appropriate seating for school participation.

Environmental adaptations also should be considered in the designing of treatment strategies. These adaptations may include simple rearrangement of furniture and adaptive equipment or more extensive architectural adaptations, including the installation of special devices (e.g., ramps; specialized tubs or showers; wheelchair-accessible kitchen counters, cabinets, and doorways). Environmental adaptations should address not only physical barriers but also perceptual or cognitive issues. For example, the amount or the type of sensory stimulation on the walls and the floors or the objects within the room can be modified to calm or to arouse the child and, as a result, affect his or her ability to attend to and successfully complete a task.

Splinting also is frequently used to enhance functional skills. Splints may be used to support weak joints or to inhibit the effects of spastic muscles by holding the child's hand in a functional position, which allows for improved grasp, manipulation, and release. Examples of common splints are illustrated in Figures 13.4–13.8. Splints designed for the simple purpose of preventing or correcting a deformity are often worn during periods of inactivity or sleep. This category of splint may include a resting hand splint (see Figure 13.4) or a ball abduction splint (see Figure 13.5). Splints that are designed to directly promote function are typically worn during functional activity and may include a wrist cock-up splint (see Figure 13.6), a soft thumb loop splint (see Figure 13.7), or

Table 13.5. Commonly used adaptive devices and techniques for activities of daily living

Problem area	Principle of adaptation	Functional skill area			
		Dressing	Hygiene	Feeding	Play/school
Limitations in reaching	Compensate with extended handles or eliminate need to reach	Dressing stick, long shoe horn, elastic shoelaces, or sock donner	Extended handled comb, brush, or sponge; or toilet aid	Electric feeder or long-handled spoon	Elevated or tilted work surface or reachers
Limitations in grasping	Eliminate need for grasp or build up handles to compensate for weak grasp	Zipper pull, button aid, or Velcro closures	Built-up handles on toothbrush, comb, and so forth; universal cuff; sponge or wash mitt; or wiping tongs	Universal cuff, utensils with built-up handles, or hand splint	Pencil grip, automatic page turner, card holder, or switch-activated toys
Limitations in assuming sitting or standing positions	Provide external support or eliminate the need for sitting or standing	Dress in supine or sidelying position or dress while seated in wheelchair	Tub or shower seat, grab bars, transfer board, toilet safety frames or rails, or high-back toilet supports/commodes	Appropriate seating	Appropriate seating or tray
Limitations in general strength	Use lightweight devices, use powered equipment, use gravity to assist with strength, or limit or eliminate the need to move against gravity	Dress in supine or sidelying position	Electric toothbrush	Plastic utensils or elevated table or tray	Lightweight toys or double set of school books to avoid carrying books home
Limitations in control of movement	Use weighted devices or friction surfaces to increase accuracy or use adaptive positioning to stabilize proximal body parts	Weighted handles on button aids or zipper pulls or Velcro closures	Soap on a rope or rubber-suction bath mat	Covered cup or nonslip mat	Computer or typewriter, nonslip mat or suction cup toys, or adapted toys

From Geyer, L., Okino, S., & Kurtz, L.A. (1996). Adaptive device and techniques for activities of daily living. In L.A. Kurtz, P.W. Dowrick, S.E. Levy, & M.L. Batshaw (Eds.), *Children's Seashore House handbook of developmental disabilities: Resources for interdisciplinary care* (pp. 449–458). Rockville, MD: Aspen Publishers, Inc.; adapted by permission.

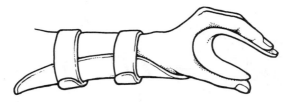

Figure 13.4. Resting hand splint. This splint maintains the spastic hand in a functional position to prevent deformity and may be used to provide low load stretch with limited range of motion. The optimal position for using a resting hand splint is with the wrist at 0–30 degrees of extension, the metacarpoplialangeal joints at 60–70 degrees of flexion, the interphalangeal joints in a neutral position, and the thumb in an opposition/abduction position. If used with a nondominant or nonfunctional hand, a child should have the splint on for 2 hours and then off for 2 hours during the day and should wear it continuously during sleep. If used with a functional hand, a child should wear the splint continuously during sleep or during periods of inactivity. Volar placement is most common with the splint, but dorsal placement may be helpful for spasticity. (From Blanchet, D., & McGee, S.M. [1996]. Principles of splint design and usage. In L.A. Kurtz, P.W. Dowrick, S.E. Levy, & M.L. Batshaw [Eds.], *Children's Seashore House handbook of developmental disabilities: Resources for interdisciplinary care* [p. 467]. Rockville, MD: Aspen Publishers, Inc.; reprinted by permission.)

an opponens splint (see Figure 13.8). Some splints may have a dual purpose; for example, a wrist cock-up splint may be used to maintain functional extension in a spastic wrist while providing appropriate support during functional activity.

Therapeutic Play

Facilitation and development of appropriate play skills is an important area of daily living skills that the therapist should address. The ability to engage in free play provides a forum for the child to explore his or her own abilities, experiment

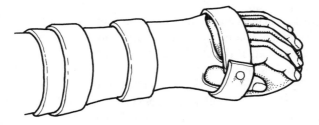

Figure 13.5. Ball abduction splint (spasticity reduction splint). This splint decreases spasticity when there is a reflex-inhibiting pattern of thumb and finger abduction. The optimal position for using a ball abduction splint is with thumb abduction and opposition (i.e., line of thumb strap goes across thumb web space). A child should wear the splint, if tolerable, at night for prolonged stretch and intermittently throughout the day. This splint is difficult for one person to mold on a very spastic hand. (From Blanchet, D., & McGee, S.M. [1996]. Principles of splint design and usage. In L.A. Kurtz, P.W. Dowrick, S.E. Levy, & M.L. Batshaw [Eds.], *Children's Seashore House handbook of developmental disabilities: Resources for interdisciplinary care* [p. 467]. Rockville, MD: Aspen Publishers, Inc.; reprinted by permission.)

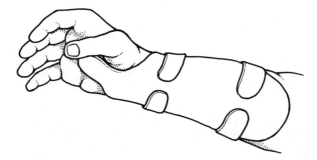

Figure 13.6. Wrist cock-up splint. This splint provides support to the wrist and the hand arches while allowing finger movement. The optimal position for using a wrist cock-up splint is with the wrist at 0–30 degrees of extension. A child should wear the splint as needed for function. A thumb piece may be added to the splint to position thumb in opposition if necessary. (From Blanchet, D., & McGee, S.M. [1996]. Principles of splint design and usage. In L.A. Kurtz, P.W. Dowrick, S.E. Levy, & M.L. Batshaw [Eds.], *Children's Seashore House handbook of developmental disabilities: Resources for interdisciplinary care* [p. 468]. Rockville, MD: Aspen Publishers, Inc.; reprinted by permission.)

with objects, learn cause-and-effect relationships, develop creativity, and cope with anxiety and frustration. Free play also provides a forum for practice of decision making and problem solving, both of which are early components of prevocational development (Clark & Allen, 1985). Children with disabilities have been found to spend less time than typically developing children in free play and more time in daily living activities. As a result, children with disabilities may develop secondary impairments of decreased motivation, lack of assertiveness, poorly developed social skills in structured situations, or decreased self-esteem (Missiuns & Pollack, 1991). Recommendations to enhance the development of play skills vary depending on the child's specific areas of limitation. Suggestions may be offered to guide a parent or a caregiver with purchasing toys that are commercially available and appropriate for the child's developmental levels and skills. The child with hemiplegia may benefit from toys that encourage bimanual hand use. The child with associated sensory involvement may benefit from toys that are rich in visual, tactile, vibratory, proprioceptive, or auditory feedback. If the child has more significant involvement, then simple cause-and-effect toys that require a light touch to activate may be appropriate. Adapted toys are available for children with motor involvement. Battery-operated toys may be activated via a switch. After careful assessment, the therapist determines the type of switch and the method of activation that is appropriate for the child. Computers with adapted hardware and special software also are useful in providing play opportunities for children with cerebral palsy (see Chapter 15 for a detailed discussion of assistive technology). Participation in occupational therapy (OT) groups is another method that should be considered when addressing therapeutic play. OT groups can provide an arena

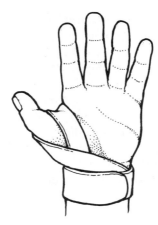

Figure 13.7. Soft thumb loop splint. This splint decreases thumb flexion and adduction in the spastic hand with the use of a reflex-inhibiting pattern, which allows use of hand for function. The optimal position for using a soft thumb loop splint is with thumb abduction and opposition (i.e., line of thumb strap goes across thumb web space). A child should wear this splint during functional activity. A child may need to use Neoprene, Neoplush, or other strapping material for additional support. (From Blanchet, D., & McGee, S.M. [1996]. Principles of splint design and usage. In L.A. Kurtz, P.W. Dowrick, S.E. Levy, & M.L. Batshaw [Eds.], *Children's Seashore House handbook of developmental disabilities: Resources for interdisciplinary care* [p. 467]. Rockville, MD: Aspen Publishers, Inc.; reprinted by permission.)

to facilitate many of the social aspects of play and to address many of the secondary disabilities previously discussed.

Educational and Prevocational Intervention

Facilitating independence in adaptive skills in the school setting encompasses many of the options and strategies previously discussed in this chapter. In order

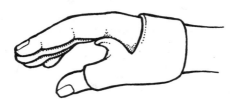

Figure 13.8. Short opponens splint. This splint supports a weak thumb in an abducted and opposed position to allow for function. The optimal position for using a short opponens splint is with the wrist at 0–30 degrees of extension (i.e., for long opponens), the thumb abducted and opposed, and the interphalangeal joint left free for function. A child should wear the splint during functional activity. (From Blanchet, D., & McGee, S.M. [1996]. Principles of splint design and usage. In L.A. Kurtz, P.W. Dowrick, S.E. Levy, & M.L. Batshaw [Eds.], *Children's Seashore House handbook of developmental disabilities: Resources for interdisciplinary care* [p. 467]. Rockville, MD: Aspen Publishers, Inc.; reprinted by permission.)

to attempt to facilitate carryover of as many of the adaptive skills that are used in both the home and the school setting, the occupational therapist should be in communication with the staff at the child's school. This carryover may include provision of adapted seating to enable the child to have a stable sitting posture to promote fine motor skills, the availability of special equipment such as a pencil grip to facilitate a weak grasp, or computer access to facilitate communication and instruction. Recommendations regarding where a child should be seated in the classroom to limit distractions or to compensate for perceptual weaknesses are often helpful. Development of a buddy system enlisting fellow students to assist one another in specified areas is another option that should be considered. Prevocational or vocational training is an area that should not be overlooked when working with the child who has cerebral palsy. As previously discussed, many of the prerequisites necessary in order to develop work roles and attitudes develop from the child's free-play experiences during early childhood. Opportunities to practice adaptive skills and to participate in daily household chores and responsibilities also contribute to the development of prevocational experiences, and children with disabilities frequently have limited exposure in these areas. Early prevocational intervention may focus on ADLs to promote problem solving and decision making, experimentation with work roles, and opportunities to practice appropriate social and perceptual/fine motor skills. Examples of these interventions include playing with construction toys, dramatic play, or caring for family or school pets. Opportunities to practice tasks and responsibilities such as participation in a cooking group, small fund-raising projects, or becoming a teacher's assistant can be employed. Development of work skills through leisure or craft activity also should be considered. Increased independence in self-maintenance skills (e.g., the ability to assume responsibility for personal care, school responsibilities, or community living skills) should be considered in later stages of development, as well. Other examples may include the ability to use a telephone book, order food in a restaurant, use public transportation, or complete personal hygiene tasks. When working with an adolescent, vocational intervention may include adaptations in the workplace or assistance with specific problems with task performance (Clark & Allen, 1985).

Case Study

An assessment of Willy's functional abilities was performed through a family interview. It was reported that Willy's cognitive and visual-perceptual skills were tested at his school and were found to be age

(continued)

Case Study–continued

appropriate. Willy demonstrated the ability to perform work that was expected of typically developing students in his grade level. The assessment did, however, reveal that sensorimotor and fine motor skills significantly affected Willy's ability to participate in ADLs. Willy and his family reported that they particularly wanted to know if Willy could be more independent with feeding, dressing, bathing, and schoolwork. Willy's motivation to become more independent with self-care activities was judged to be a significant strength. Clinical observations during task performance showed that Willy required maximum assistance for all bed mobility, transfers, and sitting. Because the severity of the athetoid movements in his right upper extremity did not allow for simple gross assistance with this hand, Willy was noted to use only his left upper extremity for all fine motor tasks. Willy's left elbow and wrist tended to assume a flexed pattern during all fine motor tasks. He was able to grossly grasp objects between his left fingers and palm, but he was unable to hold a writing instrument or a feeding utensil. Willy was able to isolate his left index finger in order to point and poke at objects. Occupational therapy sessions focused on the identification of adaptive equipment and techniques that could facilitate independence and ease adaptive and school activities. After several trial sessions, it was concluded that adaptive bathing and dressing equipment would not help Willy in becoming more independent with dressing or bathing. Thus, Willy's family was instructed to use optimal positioning strategies to ease the burden of Willy's care for these activities (an elevated reclining tub seat was found to be particularly helpful). A left wrist cock-up splint was constructed and appeared to give Willy better control in maintaining grasp of objects; his self-feeding skills significantly improved when he used the splint. In addition to the splint, a spoon with a built-up handle, an adaptive bowl with a built-up edge to assist with scooping, and a nonslip mat placed under the bowl were incorporated in Willy's daily living activities. These devices allowed Willy to feed himself thick foods that would stick to his spoon with only minimal assistance. Despite trials with various adaptive writing aids, Willy was not successful with a writing instrument. His keyboard skills were more functional, and with the use of the left wrist cock-up splint and a lap tray that stabilized his left elbow and forearm, his punch rate and accuracy significantly improved. In addition, it was found that when Willy stabilized his right forearm and right hand under the tray, his keyboard control improved even more.

SUMMARY

Children with cerebral palsy may require help with a variety of functional limitations that underlie their successful development of ADLs. In various performance stages of the child's life, therapy may need to shift focus to the remediation of specific limitations that impede development. However, it is critically important for treatment strategies to remain focused on the ultimate goal of remediation: promoting a transition to independent living, thus promoting self-esteem, enhancing the quality of life, and reducing the burden of care for both the child and his or her caregivers (Kibele, 1988; Magill & Hurlbut, 1986). It is not surprising that studies designed to identify the factors that contribute to vocational success in adults with cerebral palsy demonstrate that higher levels of independence in self-care skills, along with relative strengths in cognitive ability, functional mobility, social interaction skills, and educational level, result in a strong likelihood for successful employment and independent living (O'Grady, Nishimura, Kohn, & Bruvold, 1985).

REFERENCES

Ames, L.B., Gillespie, C., Haines, J., & Ilg, F. (1979). *The Gesell Institute's child from one to six: Evaluating the behavior of the preschool child.* New York: Harper & Row.

Beery, K.E. (1989). *The VMI, Developmental Test of Visual-Motor Integration: Administration, scoring and teaching manual.* Cleveland, OH: Modern Curriculum Press.

Berk, R.A., & DeGangi, G. (1983). *DeGangi-Berk Test of Sensory Integration manual.* Los Angeles: Western Psychological Services.

Blanchet, D., & McGee, S.M. (1996). Principles of splint design and usage. In L.A. Kurtz, P.W. Dowrick, S.E. Levy, & M.L. Batshaw (Eds.), *Children's Seashore House handbook of developmental disabilities: Resources for interdisciplinary care* (pp. 465–488). Rockville, MD: Aspen Publishers, Inc.

Bruininks, R.H. (1978). *Bruininks-Oseretsky Test of Motor Proficiency examiner's manual.* Circle Pines, MN: American Guidance Service.

Byarm, L.E. (1996). Neurodevelopmental therapy. In L.A. Kurtz, P.W. Dowrick, S.E. Levy, & M.L. Batshaw (Eds.), *Children's Seashore House handbook of developmental disabilities: Resources for interdisciplinary care* (pp. 249–259). Rockville, MD: Aspen Publishers, Inc.

Case-Smith, J. (1994). Self-care strategies for children with developmental deficits. In C. Christiansen (Ed.), *Ways of living: Self-care strategies for special needs* (pp. 101–156). Rockville, MD: American Occupational Therapy Association.

Chandler, L.S., Andrews, M.S., & Swanson, M.W. (1980). *Movement Assessment of Infants.* (Available from Post Office Box 4631, Rolling Bay, Washington 98061.)

Clark, P.N., & Allen, A.S. (1985). *Occupational therapy for children.* St. Louis: C.V. Mosby.

Colarusso, R.P., & Hammill, D.D. (1972). *MVPT–Motor-Free Visual Perception Test manual.* Novato, CA: Academic Therapy Publications.

Coster, W.J., & Haley, S.M. (1992). Conceptualization and measurement of disablement in infants and young children. *Infants and Young Children, 4*(4), 11–12.

Folio, M.R., & Fewell, R.R. (1983). *Peabody Developmental Motor Scales.* Allen, TX: DLM Teaching Resources.

Fraser, B.A., Hensinger, R.N., & Phelps, J.A. (1990). *Physical management of multiple handicaps: A professional's guide* (2nd ed.). Baltimore: Paul H. Brookes Publishing Co.

Furuno, S., O'Reilly, K., Hosaka, C., Inatsuka, T.T., Allman, T.L., & Zeisloft, B. (1984). *Hawaii Early Learning Profile (HELP).* Palo Alto, CA: VORT Corporation.

Gardner, M.F. (1988). *TVPS, Test of Visual-Perceptual Skills (non-motor) manual.* San Francisco: Health Publishing Company.

Gardner, M.F. (1992). *TVPS–UL, Test of Visual-Perceptual Skills (non-motor) upper level manual.* Burlingame, CA: Psychological and Educational Publications.

Gardner, R.A., & Broman, M. (1979). The Purdue Pegboard: Normative data on 1334 schoolchildren. *Journal of Clinical Child Psychology, 1,* 156–162.

Geyer, L., Okino, S., & Kurtz, L.A. (1996). Adaptive device and techniques for activities of daily living. In L.A. Kurtz, P.W. Dowrick, S.E. Levy, & M.L. Batshaw (Eds.), *Children's Seashore House handbook of developmental disabilities: Resources for interdisciplinary care* (pp. 449–458). Rockville, MD: Aspen Publishers, Inc.

Haines, J., Ames, L.B., & Gillespie, C. (1980). *The Gesell Preschool Test manual.* Rosemont, NJ: Modern Learning Press.

Haley, S.M., Coster, W.J., Ludlow, L.H., Haltiwanger, J.T., & Andrellos, P.J. (1992). *Pediatric Evaluation of Disability Inventory (PEDI): Development, standardization, and administration manual.* Boston: PEDI Research Group and New England Medical Center Hospital.

Hinojosa, J., & Anderson, J. (1991). Mothers' perceptions of home treatment programs for their preschool children with cerebral palsy. *American Journal of Occupational Therapy, 45*(3), 273–279.

Hinojosa, J., Anderson, J., & Ranum, G.W. (1988). Relationships between therapists and parents of children with cerebral palsy: A survey. *Occupational Therapy Journal of Research, 8,* 285–297.

Jacobs, K. (1985). *Occupational therapy: Work-related programs and assessments.* Boston: Little, Brown.

Jebsen, R.H., Taylor, N., Trieschmann, R.B., Trottler, H.J., & Howard, L.A. (1969). An objective and standardized test of hand function. *Archives of Physical Medicine and Rehabilitation, 50,* 311–319.

Johnson, C.B., & Deitz, J.C. (1985). Time use of mothers with preschool children: A pilot study. *American Journal of Occupational Therapy, 39*(9), 578–583.

Kibele, A. (1988). Occupational therapy's role in improving the quality of life for persons with cerebral palsy. *American Journal of Occupational Therapy, 43*(6), 371–377.

Knobloch, H., Stevens, F., & Malone, A.F. (1980). *Manual of developmental diagnosis.* New York: Harper & Row.

Knox, S.H. (1974). A play scale. In M. Reilly (Ed.), *Play as exploratory learning* (pp. 247–266). Thousand Oaks, CA: Sage Publications.

Kurtz, L.A., & Scull, S.A. (1993). Rehabilitation for developmental disabilities. *Pediatric Clinics of North America, 40*(3), 629–643.

Law, M., & Usher, P. (1988). Validation of the Klein-Bell Activities of Daily Living Scale for Children. *Canadian Journal of Occupational Therapy, 55*(2), 63–67.

Magill, J., & Hurlbut, N. (1986). The self-esteem of adolescents with cerebral palsy. *American Journal of Occupational Therapy, 40*(6), 402–407.

Markwardt, F.C., Jr. (1989). *Peabody Individual Achievement Test–Revised.* Circle Pines, MN: American Guidance Service.

Mathiowetz, V., Rogers, S.L., Dowe-Keval, M., Donahue, L., & Rennells, C. (1986). The Purdue Pegboard: Norms for 14- to 19-year olds. *American Journal of Occupational Therapy, 40*(3), 174–179.

Missiuns, C., & Pollack, N. (1991). Play deprivation in children with physical disabilities: The role of occupational therapy in preventing secondary disability. *American Journal of Occupational Therapy, 45*(10), 882–888.

Msall, M.E., DiGaudio, K.M., & Duffy, L.C. (1993). Use of functional assessment on children with developmental disabilities. *Physical Medicine and Rehabilitation Clinics of North America, 4*(3), 517–527.

O'Grady, R.S., Nishimura, D.M., Kohn, J.G., & Bruvold, W.H. (1985). Vocational predictions compared with present vocational status of 60 young adults with cerebral palsy. *Developmental Medicine and Child Neurology, 27,* 775–784.

Radcliffe, J., & Moss, E.M. (1996). Guidelines for use of tests in pediatrics. In L.A. Kurtz, P.W. Dowrick, S.E. Levy, & M.L. Batshaw (Eds.), *Children's Seashore House handbook of developmental disabilities: Resources for interdisciplinary care* (pp. 152–159). Rockville, MD: Aspen Publishers, Inc.

Santa Cruz County Office of Education. (1987). *HELP for Special Preschoolers.* Palo Alto, CA: VORT Corporation.

Sparrow, S.S., Balla, D.A., & Cicchetti, D.V. (1984). *Vineland Adaptive Behavior Scales: Survey form manual (interview ed.).* Circle Pines, MN: American Guidance Service.

State University of New York at Buffalo. (1993). *Guide for the Uniform Data Set for Medical Rehabilitation for Children (WeeFIM) (version 4.0).* Buffalo: Author.

Taylor, N., Sand, P.L., & Jebsen, R.H. (1973). Evaluation of hand function in children. *Archives of Physical Medicine and Rehabilitation, 54,* 129–135.

Tiffen, J. (1968). *Purdue Pegboard examiner manual.* Lafayette, IN: Lafayette Instrument Company.

CHAPTER 14

Promoting Function: Communication and Feeding

Cynthia B. Solot

The use of speech and language for communicating, learning, and regulating behavior is a critical developmental task and forms the basis for all social interactions. Children with cerebral palsy have significant neuromotor impairments that frequently affect their oral-motor system and, as a result, also affect their development of speech, language, and feeding skills. Brain lesions that underlie the motor limitations also may adversely influence mental development of these children. Cognitive impairments such as mental retardation and learning disabilities are common in children with cerebral palsy. Hearing or visual impairments, orthopedic anomalies, perceptual impairments, tactile-proprioceptive impairments, attentional difficulties, and other medical conditions (e.g., seizures, respiratory problems, gastroesophageal reflux [GER]) also are frequently associated with cerebral palsy and can compromise language development.

Environmental and psychosocial conditions have a decisive impact on language development; conversely, impairments of oral-motor function and communication may interrupt the typical processes of bonding and attachment. For example, parents may misunderstand a facial expression because of low muscle tone, misinterpret vocalizations because of increased laryngeal spasticity, or be unable to provide adequate nutrition when there are feeding problems. These problems can be devastating to both the parent and the child.

Promoting functional communication and feeding skills is best initiated as early as possible and is an ongoing process. Because the brain has greater plasticity at early ages, there are physiological reasons to stimulate the development of language, speech, and feeding from infancy. Early intervention also can prevent the development of nonfunctional patterns, which can be difficult to change. From the psychosocial standpoint, successful experiences early in life can enhance function as well as motivate children to continue the often arduous demands of multidisciplinary therapies.

In considering habilitation in children with cerebral palsy, it also is critical to remember that promoting function requires building skills as well as developing compensatory mechanisms to help the child function best within the limits of his or her physical and mental capabilities. Working beyond the child's capacity or working for too long on goals that the child cannot realistically achieve is counterproductive to optimal functioning (Hardy, 1983).

In this chapter, basic aspects of assessment and treatment of communication and feeding problems are reviewed and an illustrative case example is provided.

FEEDING

Feeding disorders in children with cerebral palsy are extremely common, vary widely in severity and in time of presentation, and relate to the degree of neuromotor impairment that is present. Similarly, the amount of adaptive equipment required and the need for medical or surgical management tend to be functions of the degree and the type of cerebral palsy that is present. Although feeding and language-related problems frequently occur together in the same child, it is important to keep in mind that speech production is not necessarily correlated with earlier oral-motor patterns (Love, Hagerman, & Taimi, 1980; Moore & Ruarck, 1996). Feeding and speech each have distinct coordinative demands and sequences. The following sections review oral-motor dysfunction as it relates to feeding; subsequent sections discuss the effect of oral-motor dysfunction on speech production and language.

Typical Development

The infant is prepared for feeding by the presence of reflexive behaviors (e.g., rooting) to open and direct the mouth to the food source. The suckle–swallow starts as a single reflex arc, which allows the child to take in food. Sucking requires the child to generate sufficient intraoral pressures with palatal closure at the back of the mouth and lip closure at the front of the mouth. The tongue must work in a controlled wave to withdraw fluid and then propel it to the back of the mouth for swallowing. This process must be coordinated with breathing, which is momentarily interrupted when swallowing occurs. As the child matures, the anatomy of the structures related to feeding (see Figure 11.6) change: The larynx descends in the neck, facilitating oral respirations; and the oral–pharyngeal space enlarges, allowing greater variety of movement. Neurological maturation permits integration of reflexes into voluntary movements that become increasingly complex. Oral–pharyngeal movements begin to occur independently of each other (e.g., the suck becomes independent of the swallow). The earliest tongue movements are in an anterior-posterior axis; with maturation, first vertical and then lateral tongue movements develop. Jaw movements become more varied, which, together with the eruption of teeth, permits the development of munching, biting, vertical, and rotary chewing patterns. Development of head control and postural stability allows for upright posture and the use of utensils in hand-to-mouth patterns. Developmental norms have been established for feeding sequences (Morris, 1992) (see Chapter 11).

Atypical Development

Given the complexity of the developmental processes leading to feeding behavior, it is easy to see how sensorimotor impairments can adversely affect feeding patterns. A few examples follow. Because coordination for sucking with swallowing does not emerge until 30–33 weeks' gestation, the child born prematurely may lack the suck–swallow reflex (Humphrey, 1967; Moore, 1988). The child with low muscle tone may have diminished reflexes. His or her oral structures may be too weak to move or to generate sufficient oral pressures for sucking, and his or her movements may be disorganized or uncoordinated. The child with spastic or more rigid musculature may have abnormal posturing and may not have sufficient range of movement to suck, swallow, bite, or chew. The child with dyskinetic types of cerebral palsy may have involuntary fluctuations in movement, and his or her reflexes may be hyperactive.

During feeding, tonal abnormalities may prevent lip closure, which results in the loss of food or fluid. At the other end of the oral cavity, inability of the soft palate to elevate and to retract can lead to regurgitation of food into the nasal cavity. If extension patterns result in tongue thrust, much of the food placed in the child's mouth may be expelled because the tongue may be unable to transport food posteriorly. Differentiated lateral and vertical movements may be limited or may not develop at all, which would result in difficulty chewing higher textures of food. Poor bolus control may result in food spilling into the pharynx before the child is ready to swallow, which may lead to choking and aspiration. Weakness in muscles, which is responsible for jaw elevation or extension, may preclude mouth closure, graded jaw movements, and chewing. Low truncal tone may extend the child's head into hyperextension, which reduces oral movements and coordination. Weakness in the pharyngeal, laryngeal, or esophageal structures can result in insufficient movements for swallowing.

Persistence of primitive reflex patterns can be inhibiting because the development of voluntary, independent, or mature movement patterns cannot proceed when the child's movement is dominated by reflex behavior. Because of abnormal mouth and tongue position, growth of the maxilla (i.e., upper jaw) may be impaired; this may lead to malformations of the dental arch and may affect feeding. Not only must each structure and muscle group work well alone but each also must work in a highly complex, coordinated fashion with all of the other components of the oral-motor system.

In severe cases in which the child cannot consume sufficient calories, supplemental or alternative feeding routes must be established. These might include nasogastric or gastrostomy tube feedings (see Chapter 11). It is preferable for oral feedings to occur together with tube feedings. If oral feeding is not possible, then it is critically important to provide an oral stimulation program to maintain oral skills. It is not uncommon for children to lose critical skills (e.g., sucking) when they are not used. After prolonged tube feedings without oral stimulation, children may develop sensitivity to touch around the mouth or the face and may have a very difficult time reestablishing oral feedings when tube feedings are no longer necessary.

Assessment

The major components in the evaluation of feeding include a thorough history obtained from caregivers and medical specialists; direct observation of nonnutritive oral-motor skills and feeding behaviors; observation of child–caregiver interactions in the feeding situation; and clinical trials by the clinician using a variety of positions, foods, and utensils. When clinically indicated, special studies such as videofluoroscopy to assess swallowing mechanisms may be necessary (see Chapter 11).

Useful historical information includes the child's typical feeding circumstances at home and at school (e.g., position during feeding, duration of feedings, volume, type of food consumed in a given period of time). It is important to know the child's preferred foods and food consistencies. The examiner also should assess the child's typical feeding behaviors when using his or her hands and utensils (e.g., a spoon, a cup, a straw). Patterns of biting, chewing, drinking (i.e., bottle and nipple type, cup, or straw), and swallowing should be explored. In order to ascertain if there is a risk for aspiration, it is critical to know the child's respiratory and phonatory characteristics during feeding; the clinician should determine whether there is emesis (i.e., vomiting), which is suggestive of GER, coughing, or choking and gagging, and, if so, under what conditions it is present. Behavioral characteristics and enjoyment of feeding also play a role in feeding success. Because certain medications can affect oral health, alertness, and appetite, it is important to be aware of any medications that the child takes. Knowledge of the child's growth history and any other contributing medical conditions is important in the assessment of feeding disorders.

Observation of feeding by the caregiver provides extremely useful information about the social milieu in which the child feeds, and it highlights the maladaptive patterns that may have developed relative to how food is presented, what type of food is provided, and the child's behavioral and motoric responses to the feeding situation. These observations provide a starting point for the clinician to develop helpful interventions as well as a framework in which information obtained in the history can be used.

As with any comprehensive evaluation, the clinician should proceed systematically with the evaluation of the child's posture, tone, reflexes, respiratory patterns, and position during feeding (e.g., held in arms, seated). The clinician also should determine the following: the best seating equipment; the resting position and the position of oral structures with movement; the use of adaptive equipment (including its appropriateness); the function with various food consistencies; and the performance with various feeding behaviors such as drinking, biting, and chewing.

Trials with different feeding methods help determine appropriate intervention strategies. Consultation with caregivers provides useful information about the interventions that are realistic within the child's environment. The diagnostician should be prepared to try a variety of positioning arrangements, food types (e.g., liquid, puréed, solid), utensils, and facilitative techniques. When indicated, medical studies such as those mentioned previously should be obtained prior to instituting a therapeutic program.

Therapy

Because feeding is such a complex process, intervention works best with a team approach. The input of physical therapists, occupational therapists, speech-language pathologists, nutritionists, physicians, social workers, educators, and the child's family is invaluable. Before embarking on a therapeutic program, it is crucial to have a thorough knowledge of the typical development of feeding and developmental sequences. As with any therapeutic program, goals will be best achieved if they are realistic to the child and his or her caregiver's needs and promote daily functional practice.

Feeding therapy evolves from careful evaluations of the child's nutritional needs, developmental level (motoric and behavioral), and physiological patterns. Once these aspects of function have been established, therapy is designed to provide adaptations to gradually advance the child from one step to the next. Research differentiates oral-motor therapy from feeding therapy (Morris, 1989). The former refers to the development of sensation and movement; the latter refers more specifically to oral feeding.

Many aspects of therapy for children with cerebral palsy can be considered either inhibitory or stimulatory/facilitative. Inhibition activities attempt to decrease the effects of hyperfunction; examples include decreasing the effects of abnormal posture and tone (e.g., extensor patterns, abnormal reflexes), decreasing involuntary movements, or limiting hypersensitivity. Stimulatory facilitative techniques attempt to strengthen movements and increase range, stability, type, quality, or coordination of movements. Management of tone—increased or decreased—is a key aspect of intervention.

One of the first and most important aspects of therapy is to establish proper positioning, which, in addition to the management of tone, allows for alignment of the trunk, the head, and the neck (see Figure 11.7). For infants, positioning may be provided in the caregiver's arms or may require adaptive seating. Most older children require some modification of their seating position for feeding purposes. Positioning must take into consideration mouth functioning as well as management of the child's airway and gastroesophageal needs.

In addition, the optimal texture of food that the child can eat must be determined. For example, liquid (thin or thick), puréed (smooth or with texture), or solid (chopped, minced, soft, or table food consistency) foods may be used. The properties of the food type (e.g., its viscosity or response to saliva and oral manipulation) affect the speed and the manner in which the child eats. Balancing nutritional needs with food type can often be challenging. For instance, if the child is fed more highly textured foods to advance oral-motor skills but does not consume enough calories because of the time and energy needed to eat, then oral-motor and feeding therapy goals are not appropriate. In this case, reducing texture for nutritional purposes and using more highly textured consistencies in therapy or for snacks may be more practical.

The amount of time spent in feeding is important. Feedings should take approximately 30 minutes. The risk for aspiration increases with feeding durations exceeding 40 minutes (Arvedson & Brodsky, 1993). Time spent feeding should not tax the child or the caregiver, take away opportunities for other activities, or result in energy expenditure that exceeds calories consumed.

After selecting appropriate utensils (e.g., type of bottle and nipple, cup, spoon), the therapist must apply the proper techniques for development and coordination of sucking, swallowing, biting, and chewing. For instance, when chewing, placement of solid food posteriorly and laterally on alternating sides of the mouth helps develop vertical jaw movements and tongue lateralization. When spoon feeding, pressure on the mid-portion of the child's tongue with the bowl of the spoon inhibits tongue protrusion, encouraging lip and cheek rounding and cleaning of the spoon with the upper lip rather than with the teeth or the palate. Manual support to stabilize the jaw, tongue base, and lips also can improve feeding efficiency. When hypersensitivities to touch occur, programs for desensitization must be established.

Feeding therapy must be introduced only after safety for oral feedings has been established. Clinical indicators for aspiration must be carefully evaluated, remembering that 50% of all aspiration is silent (see Chapter 11). When the infant is unable to eat by mouth and is provided with alternative forms of feeding, it is very important to maintain oral function with nonnutritive sucking; other forms of oral stimulation can be used in older children.

DROOLING

Drooling, or sialorrhea, is a very common problem in children with cerebral palsy because of a lack of coordinated control of the orofacial and head and neck muscles. In some cases, the degree of drooling is so excessive that it causes significant health and social problems. Constant wetness of the chin and perioral areas can lead to skin irritation, chapping, malodor, or secondary infection. Once these problems occur, the continuing drooling makes them extremely difficult to control.

The child who drools does not produce an excess amount of saliva. Instead, he or she is unable to control and swallow the saliva that is produced. The child may experience less frequent swallowing because of poor motor control, or he or she may have reduced sensory awareness of saliva, which typically stimulates a swallow.

Social problems associated with drooling are numerous. The child's clothing is constantly wet and must be changed frequently by the caregivers. Bibs and napkins are often used in an effort to keep the child's clothing as dry as possible. Dribbled saliva can soil communication aids such as books and computers as well as the clothing of the caregivers. Parents are usually aware of and concerned about this problem. Often, the child who has higher functioning capabilities may be aware of this problem, may be embarrassed by it, and may actually initiate the investigation into treatments available for the drooling.

Some investigators (Crysdale, 1994) advocate a team approach in the management of drooling. The members of the team may include a speech-language pathologist, an occupational therapist, a physical therapist, a psychologist, an otolaryngologist, a plastic surgeon, a developmental pediatrician, a neurologist, and a pediatric dentist. Input from these specialists and other individuals involved in caring for the child should be sought in the management of this difficult problem.

Although drooling may be reduced spontaneously as neuromuscular control improves with age, some children may require intervention of some type. Conservative management strategies should be attempted first (Johnson & Scott, 1993). These include the following: development of oral-motor skills and swallowing function through feeding therapy; oral-facilitation exercises; and production of stable, upright positioning of the head and trunk. Increasing awareness of saliva may help to encourage more frequent swallowing as well as the need to wipe the face.

Medical management is considered when more conservative approaches are not successful. Management of drooling with anticholinergic drugs can reduce the amount of saliva produced, but it also may result in undesirable side effects, such as dry mouth, restlessness, blurred vision, sedation, urinary retention, or constipation (Lew, Younis, & Lazar, 1991).

Surgical management of drooling should be considered when conservative measures have been unsuccessful in eliminating or satisfactorily reducing the severity of the problem. Referral for surgical management is rarely made before the child is 6 years of age.

One to one and a half liters of saliva are typically produced in a 24-hour period. Up to 70% of these secretions are produced by the two submandibular glands. Operations to treat drooling fall into two major categories: those intended to reduce the total amount of saliva produced and those designed to change the point of entry of saliva into the oral cavity/oropharynx so that swallowing of saliva is facilitated (Crysdale, 1994). Surgical procedures involve some or all of the following: excision of the submandibular glands, rerouting of the submandibular and/or parotid ducts, ligation of the parotid ducts, and excision of the sublingual glands. With all of these procedures, dramatic improvement in the child's symptoms and improvement in his or her social activities has been reported. Complications of surgical intervention are minor and include temporary cheek swelling and cyst formation. The salivary production after these procedures is often thicker than it was preoperatively, but this does not typically pose a problem for the child. Occasionally, additional fluids are required during eating.

Saliva has a protective function in maintaining dental hygiene and in preventing dental caries. Early investigators who performed treatment directed at reducing the amount of saliva were concerned with the possibility of increased dental caries secondary to decreased salivary flow around the teeth. Daily postoperative fluoride treatments were recommended in some of the earlier studies. However, even without special dental care, the number of dental caries has not increased in these individuals.

Upper airway obstruction secondary to large tonsils or adenoids may be a contributing factor to drooling in some children. Because the child with enlarged tonsils and enlarged adenoids is often unable to breathe through his or her nose, the mouth must be kept open to permit respirations, predisposing the child to drool. Tonsillectomy and adenoidectomy may be considered prior to discussing surgery on the salivary glands.

SPEECH, LANGUAGE, AND COMMUNICATION IN CHILDREN WITH CEREBRAL PALSY

The child with cerebral palsy is at risk for delays or specific impairments of speech, language, and communication. *Speech* may be defined as the perception and production of patterns of sound that serve as the physical representation of a symbolic system. *Language* is the symbolic system itself and may have multiple physical manifestations, including speech, writing, and gesture.

Communication refers to the use of language as a primary means of initiating and maintaining social interactions. The degree to which the child with cerebral palsy will have difficulty with speech, language, and communication is a function of the severity and the type of motor impairment (see Chapter 1). These difficulties also are strongly influenced by the presence of concomitant sensory and cognitive impairments. The following section addresses specific issues that affect speech production. Subsequent sections review issues related to language and communication.

Speech

Speech is a complex behavior that integrates a series of perceptual, cognitive, and motoric processes; these processes create recognizable and reproducible patterns of sound. Speech movements are a result of a dynamic interaction among the processes and the structures of respiration, phonation, resonation, and articulation. Just as typical speech represents a balanced synthesis of these processes, abnormal speech emerges in recognizable patterns of poorly orchestrated speech movements.

Dysarthria is the term used to describe movement disorders of neurological origin that are often seen in cerebral palsy and are often diagnosed as affecting speech production. Any or all of the component systems in speech may be affected in a number of ways. Abnormalities are noted in range, strength, precision, speed, tone, steadiness, and coordination of speech movement. *Apraxia* and *dyspraxia* refer to the disorders of voluntary movement and programming of speech movements that are greater than would be expected given the child's physical and linguistic capabilities. Typically, the speaker with dyspraxia, although having difficulty organizing and generating speech sounds, does not have a comparable deficit in the execution of nonspeech oral movements.

The components of speech movement (i.e., respiration, phonation, resonation, and articulation) are reviewed in the following sections. It is important to remember that for these movements to result in meaningful speech, they must occur within the context of linguistic knowledge. In other words, while language can and does occur in the absence of speech (e.g., through the use of communication boards and sign language [see Chapter 15]), meaningful speech cannot occur without language (e.g., babbling during infancy, which is an example of nonmeaningful speech).

Respiration   *Respiration* refers to the movements of breathing and provides the power source for speech. It is a complex process that involves neural integration and the interaction of many of the structures of the head, the neck, and the trunk. Patency of the nose, mouth, pharynx, larynx, and trachea is necessary to permit air entry into the lungs. In neonates, the high position of the larynx brings the epiglottis into close contact with the soft palate, thus making these individuals breathe through their noses. As the child grows, the larynx descends in the neck and allows the child to breathe through his or her mouth.

The typical respiratory cycle occurs approximately 20 times a minute, although faster rates are commonly seen in infants. Resting inspiration and expiration components are typically of equal duration. For speech purposes, it is necessary to generate sufficient pressure and to maintain and regulate that pressure by making the necessary muscular adjustments at each point within a speech utterance. For speech breathing, inspirations are quick and comprise 10% of the respiratory sequence (Orlikoff, 1992). In order to support speech, inspirations must be sufficient in volume and must be adequately controlled so that air is not exhaled prior to speech onset. Once speech has been initiated, chest and abdominal forces must work together so that exhalations are controlled with a steady, prolonged release of air. Depending on lexical demands, expiratory patterns show variability (to produce varied stress patterns or the number of syllables or word groups needed).

Abnormalities of neurological control can interfere with respirations if laryngeal opening is not coordinated with diaphragmatic descent or if diaphragmatic relaxation begins before a full breath has been taken. An obstruction in any part of the upper airway also can impede free air movement and impair respiratory efforts. Limitations in respiratory function depend on the severity and the type of cerebral palsy. For example, problems can be seen with spasticity because of immobility of truncal musculature. Hypotonicity also can result in insufficient volume or depth of respiration. Dyskinetic types of cerebral palsy that are characterized by involuntary movements can result in irregular respiratory cycles or in interruption of the respiratory sequence.

In children with cerebral palsy, the most frequently seen problems related to respiration include decreased breath volume, rapid rate, poor ability to generate or control taking a deep inhalation, poor control of exhalatory movements, and incoordination of multiple muscle groups (McDonald & Chance, 1964).

Children with problems in respiration sound strained or weak. They often produce fewer than typical syllables or words per breath. Their use of the breath stream may be inefficient, and they may begin speech in the middle of or at the end of an exhalation. There may be excessive pauses or long durations between utterances. There may be a breathy or a strained quality to their output. Pitch, range, and loudness may be reduced. Audible inspirations and discontinuous or uncontrolled speech or voice may occur as a result of these respiratory difficulties.

There are many quantitative measures for the assessment of respiration (Hardy, 1983; Orlikoff, 1992). However, most clinical settings do not have the instrumentation to perform this kind of physiological measurement nor is it necessarily superior to a good clinical evaluation. Instrumental measures (on any of the speech subsystems) can be very useful in supporting and clarifying clinical observations; they also may provide objective measures of progress and outcome.

A clinical evaluation including observation of natural speaking patterns and production during elicited procedures can provide the speech-language pathologist with a great deal of information about the functional capacity of the respiratory system. In both the infant and the older child, it is important to observe the respiratory musculature at rest as well as in motion. Children with cerebral palsy may demonstrate breathing patterns in which the upper chest is depressed during inhalation, which is known as *reversed breathing*. At rest, flared ribs and a depressed sternum or abdomen may be seen. If left untreated, this can result in reduction of the size of the rib cage and the volume of air that can be inhaled (Westlake & Rutherford, 1961). Abdominal or diaphragmatic breathing is the more desirable pattern of respiration. However, weakness in flexor muscles of the neck and shoulders can lead to excessive "belly breathing," which may decrease respiratory capacity and efficiency.

Changes in tone or postural instability can alter respiratory patterns. Therefore, it is important to observe the child in his or her usual position and to provide corrected positioning to observe the effect on ventilatory patterns. Recruitment of associated muscle groups and the degree of effort while performing respiratory maneuvers should be noted.

Specific speech measures may include the following: duration of exhalation while prolonging a vowel or a continuant consonant, production of a series of syllables or words, or counting as long as possible on one breath. It will be necessary to observe coordination of speech with breathing and note when speech begins in the breathing cycle. In addition to steadiness and control of speech on an exhalation, length of utterances and duration between utterances also must be observed. Children often enjoy activities involving singing that allow observations of breath control. A variety of activities, such as blowing bubbles or moving a ball in a tube, also may help to determine whether the child can generate sufficient respiratory strength.

Phonation   *Phonation* refers to the generation of sound on the breath stream by the vibration of the vocal cords. It provides voice, which is the carrying power for speech. The phonation process requires a complex interaction of the respiratory cycle and laryngeal function. During expiration, the laryngeal structures move slightly inward from the open (i.e., abducted) position seen during inspiration. For phonation to occur, the vocal cords are brought into the midline (i.e., adducted) position by the action of the laryngeal muscles. As the diaphragm and the chest cage relax, air is forced past the approximated vocal cords by the subglottic pressure that is developed during expiration. Loudness is determined by the velocity of the exhaled air column. Vocal pitch is modified by alterations in length, tension, and thickness of the vocal cords. Factors that prevent complete vocal cord adduction, such as vocal cord paralysis or the presence of a mass (e.g., vocal nodules), will cause the child's phonation to be hoarse or breathy.

Phonatory characteristics vary depending on the type and the severity of cerebral palsy. Problems occur most often with pitch, loudness, or quality of voice. *Pitch* refers to the fundamental frequency of speech sounds. A voice may be too high or too low; it may have limited range, or it may be unstable (i.e., poor maintenance of pitch). Intonation, one aspect of pitch, provides important information about the meaning of an utterance (e.g., the raising of pitch at the end of a sentence to indicate a question). *Loudness* refers to the amplitude of sound. Speech may be too loud or too soft. Voice quality may be hoarse or rough, wet sounding from an inability to clear saliva, breathy, weak, thin, or strained-strangled (Darley, Aronson, & Brown, 1975).

Both physiological and positional factors can affect phonation. For instance, throughout an utterance, adductor tension of the vocal folds can lead to difficulty with the initiation of phonation or with the maintenance of phonation. As air is being squeezed through a narrowed glottis, lack of vocal cord mobility with adductor tension can result in the voice having a very strained quality. Conversely, difficulty in adducting the vocal folds tends to create a quality of breathiness as the breath stream flows through an open glottal space. Dystonic movements or positional changes during speech can create excessive fluctuations in the perceived vocal characteristics. In addition, silent inspirations can become audible in the presence of coordination errors. Lack of efficiency of the breath stream reduces the child's ability to prolong phonation, which is a necessity for the production of multiple words per breath.

Last, the interdependency of speech subsystems is evident because the production of many speech sounds requires the rapid adduction (i.e., approximation) and abduction (i.e., release) of the vocal folds, a very complex maneuver using many of the intrinsic and extrinsic laryngeal muscles. Voiced consonant sounds require phonation. For example, the sound /b/ is voiced compared with its unvoiced cognate /p/. Other voiced and unvoiced sound pairs include /s/ and /z/, /g/ and /k/, /d/ and /t/, and /f/ and /v/.

As with respiration, quantitative measures of phonation are available to evaluate structural, physiological, aerodynamic, and acoustic features (Hardy, 1983; Orlikoff, 1992). Most clinicians employ perceptual evaluation of voice. This includes making judgments about the features of the voice used in habitual speech (e.g., loudness, pitch, quality, duration, steadiness). In addition, the child is asked to complete exercises in different conditions to assess the limits and capabilities of the mechanism for change. For example, the child may be asked to prolong an open vowel; count as high as possible on one breath; produce short, repetitive vowel sounds; sing as high or as low as possible; or speak as softly or as loudly as possible. A great deal of information can be obtained regarding the quality of phonation while listening to involuntary phonations in laughing or crying, particularly in young children who may not be able to complete more formal assessments.

Resonation   *Resonation* refers to the coupling of air in the oral and the nasal cavities that creates the perception of nasality. The amount of nasality is regulated primarily by the structures of the soft palate, the pharynx, and the upper airway with some contribution from the back of the tongue. Essentially, to close off the oral cavity from the nasal space, the soft palate must elevate and retract while the muscles of the pharynx constrict. Timing and coordination of movement also are essential in carrying out this complex activity. For the production of most consonant sounds during speech, velopharyngeal closure allows the buildup of intraoral air pressure and seals off the nasal space so that excess air does not enter the nose.

Velopharyngeal incompetence or insufficiency (VPI) can result in problems with hypernasal resonance, compensatory articulation errors, decreased volume, and hoarseness caused by the strain to the laryngeal muscles. Flaccid, spastic, or fluctuating musculature or an impairment of muscular coordination can result in VPI. On occasion, the presence of enlarged tonsils can interfere with velopharyngeal closing (Shprintzen, 1989). Head position also is a variable, and velopharyngeal closure is typically better with the head in a neutral or a flexed position. The effect of VPI may be quite distorting to the speech signal. It is important to differentiate between hypernasality (i.e., too much air in the nasal port) and hyponasality (i.e., too little air in the nasal port), which may be a result of an obstruction in the nasopharynx (e.g., enlarged adenoids, mucosal swelling during a cold).

Objective assessment of velopharyngeal function includes imaging techniques, aerodynamic measures, and acoustic measures (Hardy, 1983; Orlikoff, 1992). Perceptual rating scales are effective tools because they are the perception of hypernasality caused by VPI that is most critical. One can detect the flow of air typical of VPI by placing a mirror below the nostrils during the production of a series of words or syllables using pressure consonants (e.g., /p/, /k/, /t/, /s/). Audible nasal emission also may be perceived with this procedure. The ability to rapidly produce and release pressure can be evaluated by asking the child to repeat syllables or words with pressure consonants. Repetition of sentences or phrases that are heavily weighted with nonnasal sounds often highlights the presence of VPI.

Articulation   Articulation involves altering the stream of air with the structures of the tongue, the lips, the teeth, and the jaw to form the sounds of speech. Articulation is an exceedingly complex system of rapidly produced muscular maneuvers. One of the most important things learned from speech science is that speech is not composed of a series of distinct movements for each sound, but rather it is characterized by a process of coarticulation (i.e., overlapping movements). In other words, the production of each sound is affected by its neighboring sounds. For instance, in the word *book,* the shape of the tongue for the vowel and the retraction and elevation of the back of the tongue for the /k/ at the end of the word is already being formed during production of the initial "b." If the word were *bus,* the tongue shape at the /b/ would be different to accommodate the positions needed for the following vowel and consonant. This process may explain why some children can produce the specific sounds in words but may show speech deterioration in ongoing discourse.

Speech learning requires motor output as well as acoustic input and processing. Children with cerebral palsy may be adversely affected in both areas. However, for the purposes of this discussion, only the motor aspects are addressed.

During sound production, the mandible typically lowers and rises in a controlled, graded fashion within a very short range of movement. The lips open and close as well as round and retract. The tongue protrudes; its tip elevates and retroflexes. The back of the tongue elevates and retracts. Independence of the tongue from the other oral structures is necessary to produce precise movements. Children with cerebral palsy often have malformations of the upper dental arch that can affect sound production. The mandible may be unable to elevate (causing an open-mouth posture) because of muscular flaccidity; there may be mandibular hyperextension if oral movements are initiated more randomly, as in dyskinesia or with extensor thrust patterns. If the child has good tongue mobility, then the jaw restriction may affect production of specific mouth closure sounds (e.g., /b/, /p/) and rate of speech production but not overall intelligibility. However, if the jaw restriction is accompanied by a relatively immobile tongue, then the effect on speech intelligibility may be severe. The child's tongue may thrust involuntarily or may have a very restricted range, strength, coordination, and speed of movement. The child's lips may be limited in range and strength of movement. Sometimes it is difficult for children to approximate the lips or to approximate with enough pressure to form the resistance to the air stream necessary to form sounds. Regardless of the difficulties that the child may demonstrate, it seems that imprecision of speech sounds is almost always accompanied by prosodic disorders, which may be a hallmark of dysarthria in cerebral palsy (Hardy, 1983). Prosodic problems such as excess and equal stress, slow rate, prolonged intervals of phonemes, loudness variations (e.g., excess loudness, monoloudness), and reduced stress are common findings.

In assessing articulatory function, it is necessary to examine the position and the relationship of the child's oral structures at rest and in motion. Observation of the oral structures in nonspeech movements can confirm neuromotor involvement or the capacity of the child's system to develop compensatory movements; however, these types of observations should not be used to make assumptions about the severity of articulation (Hardy, 1983). Similarly, judgments about speech should not be made from observing vegetative function. Research also notes that the limitations in the uses of diadokokinetic (i.e., rapid, alternating movements) rate testing in cerebral palsy have been observed (Hardy, 1983).

With the caveats mentioned in this chapter in mind, some of the more useful approaches to assessment are briefly described in the following section.

Although there are quantitative measures available for the evaluation of speech, most clinicians employ perceptual evaluation. It has been argued that the ultimate test of the acceptability of speech is based on its intelligibility to listeners (Wertz & Rosenbek, 1992). Therefore, one of the first and most important aspects of a speech assessment is to listen to the child converse and to determine intelligibility and severity in functional communication. From this, systematic appraisal of speech may proceed. There are a variety of rating scales and articulation tests available. The articulation tests are designed for typically developing children, but they can be adapted to obtain a speech-sound inventory for children with cerebral palsy; the clinician should identify patterns in the child's place and manner of speech-sound production. For younger children, real objects often must be substituted for pictures. For other children, pictures must be enlarged, boldly colored, or placed squarely within their field of vision.

It is very important to observe speech patterns at the phrase and the sentence levels and to observe the effects of increased physiological demand on the speech system. It is preferable to have a spontaneous sample of speech rather than an imitative sample because an elicitation may not represent the child's own repertoire. Other important features to be evaluated include effects of altering trunk and head position, response to trial therapy procedures, degree of effort involved in speaking, variations throughout an utterance, and prosodic features.

Speech Therapy

Perhaps the most important task in developing an effective program of therapy is to determine the physical and the developmental capabilities of the child and to set achievable goals that are obtainable within the child's limitations; this will contribute most to the child's overall communicative effectiveness. For many children, it will be necessary to develop acoustically acceptable compensatory speech efforts. Some children may need a combination of oral speech and augmentative systems of communication (see Chapter 15). For children with severe impairments, oral speech may not be possible. Regardless of the particular child's situation, a good therapy program should be created from a systematic assessment of each of the speech subsystems. When targets that are determined to be remediable and important to improving functional communication are identified, goals must be integrated into a coherent program. Because of the interdependency of one speech subsystem with another, it is preferable to integrate goals rather than to work on one subsystem at a time. In addition, success is more likely when goals are implemented in speech contexts rather than in nonspeech contexts.

One of the first considerations in speech therapy should be to develop postural stability through proper positioning and inhibition of abnormal reflex patterns. This often requires the use of adaptive equipment or special handling. For example, if the child is dominated by extension patterns, then his or her mouth will open and the neck and trunk will not be in position to allow for adequate respiration, phonation, and articulation. Placing the child in flexion; supporting his or her head, neck, and shoulders in a neutral position; and bringing the body to midline establish the opportunity for the child to perceive desired positions and better enable the child to produce more functional movement. Positioning to allow face-to-face contact between speaker and listener also is of critical importance for communication purposes.

In order to promote optimal movement, it is necessary for the infant or the child to be relaxed. Therefore, relaxation activities are often helpful during therapy. The principle of relaxation also should guide the therapist to prevent working at a level that is too difficult for the child; overexertion can produce strain, overflow movements, and increased primitive reflex activity. Some other important guidelines in developing therapeutic techniques have been outlined. These include working from vegetative to voluntary movement, working from gross to specific movement, progressing from passive to resistive motion, and developing tolerance for handling new movements (Westlake & Rutherford, 1961). In older children, development of self-monitoring skills and strategies to adjust movements aids functional use of therapeutic maneuvers. The therapist also must develop activities that are within the child's cognitive-linguistic level and are in motivating, play-based formats.

Many activities can improve function in each subsystem, beginning in infancy and continuing throughout adulthood. In the respiratory system, some examples of activities include developing rapid inhalation followed by longer, controlled exhalation; beginning an utterance at the peak of the exhalation; and coordinating speech with exhalation. Pairing phonation with exhalation should begin with simple, open vowel sounds and progress through single syllables to polysyllables, phrases, and sentences with increasing demand on quality of phonation and articulation. Adjusting the number of syllables spoken most naturally per breath (within the child's respiratory capacity) can be one of the most practical aids to spoken intelligibility. Teaching placement of grammatically natural pauses also is very useful.

The laryngeal system is one of the more difficult systems to manage in children with cerebral palsy. Hardy (1983) suggested that improved vocal quality can be achieved within a relatively restricted range of pitch and loudness level and within a reduction of tension on initiation of phonation.

Regimens to treat VPI include speech therapy, prosthetics, and surgery. Speech therapy to improve resonance is of limited value unless it has been demonstrated that some velopharyngeal closure is possible (McWilliams, Morris, & Shelton, 1990). Practice with voiceless consonants can be helpful to children with mild VPI. When the degree of VPI is significant, there are two other choices for intervention. In cases of significant neuromuscular aerodynamic insufficiency, the preferred method is the creation of a prosthetic device that lifts the palate to provide closure of the velopharyngeal port. This procedure requires successive fittings of the appliance to achieve the desired size and position. It requires a cooperative child and the presence of teeth on which the appliance can be anchored. Children with hypotonicity typically do better with this approach than do children with spasticity because the presence of a hyperactive gag response and strong muscular forces can stress the appliance in children with spasticity (Dworkin, 1991). The second method to improve resonance is a surgical correction of the VPI (e.g., posterior pharyngeal flap, sphincter pharyngoplasty). Because these procedures employ the child's own tissue and must work in concert with existing musculature, some degree of motion in the child's velopharyngeal mechanism is needed to achieve best results.

Work to improve articulation can begin very early with encouragement of sound play and babbling in infants. The therapist can shape the child's automatic vocalizations through play, movement, and imitation. Later, the phonological system can be developed. Specific activities can be employed to improve articulatory accuracy for both vowel and consonant sounds. The type of instruction used depends on the child. For example, some children respond well to auditory and modeling cues, whereas other children respond to visual or tactile cues. The level of verbal instruction also must be suited to the individual child. Selection of sounds targeted for stimulation depends on the age of the child and his or her physical capabilities. Sounds are learned with a gradual approximation toward the target. Consideration must be given to the sound's place of production (e.g., tongue tip to area behind the upper teeth for /t/, /d/, and /l/; lips together for /m/ and /b/; back of the tongue up to the soft palate for /k/ and /g/) as well as its manner of production (e.g., voicing the sound in /g/ versus its voiceless cognate /k/; stopping the air stream, then releasing it for /p/, /k/, and /t/; partially occluding the air stream for /f/, /v/, /s/, and /z/). With some motor impairments, it is best to practice at the syllable or word level rather than in isolated contexts. Sometimes, just having the oral structures approximate their required position will allow an acoustically acceptable sound to occur and assist the listener to "read" the child's intent by watching the child's mouth.

Altering prosodic features can be difficult; if prosodic goals are limited and carefully selected, however, then they may prove very useful. For example, reducing the child's speaking rate may help him or her to have more time to position the articulatory structures. It can be helpful to teach the child to increase pause time and frequency. Increased syllable durations also are recognized to benefit speech. Working on patterns of stress, intonation, and rhythm may be more difficult (Hardy, 1983).

It is important to help the child to achieve as much independence in communication efforts as possible. Sometimes, in very severe cases of dysarthria, even the most rudimentary speech productions can only be understood by those familiar to the child. In such circumstances, time spent developing oral speech can significantly add to the child's functioning, especially when combined with alternative systems that can be used to expand, supplement, and assist in developing communicative competence.

Language and Communication

Language is a system of symbols used to communicate. There is a receptive (i.e., comprehension) component as well as an expressive (i.e., output) component. The domains that constitute language include the systems of phonology (i.e., sound system), syntax (i.e., grammar), semantics (i.e., meaning), and pragmatics (i.e., social aspects). There are both verbal and nonverbal systems of language. There are nonsymbolic means of communication (e.g., pointing, reaching), symbolic means (e.g., pointing to the mouth to indicate hunger, words), and conventionalized forms of communication (e.g., head shake, wave, words).

The typical development of language proceeds along well-defined sequences within each domain. For example, first words typically emerge at 1 year of age. Phrases appear at 18 months of age with incremental increases in the development of vocabulary, sentence structure, concepts, and narrative skills as the child matures.

The ability to interpret environmental experiences and to affect events begins in infancy. Limitations in cognitive, linguistic, sensory, and motor behavior can have serious early consequences on the child's development. For example, researchers found that early cry behaviors of children with developmental disabilities differ from cries of typically developing children and that cries of children at risk are perceived differently from those of typically developing children (Lester & Zeskind, 1979). This can result in reduced parental response to the behavior and, ultimately, reduce the behavior itself. Smiling and laughing also may be more difficult for the child with developmental disabilities because of respiratory and phonatory constraints and impairment in motion of the facial muscles; their attempts to communicate (e.g., smiles) may be less recognizable and less easily interpreted (Dunst, 1985). This can create a troubling scenario in which the child's efforts are not reinforced, leading to passivity and reduced communicative effort and opportunity.

Another important aspect of early language development is that parents ascribe intentionality to the child's behaviors, leading the child toward conventionalized forms of language. If parent–child interactions are limited, this process is interrupted. Parents who try to stimulate their child may find an unresponsive infant quite discouraging or may find it difficult to read their child's intent when communications are attempted. For effective communication to occur, there must be intent, initiation, and reciprocity.

Children with cerebral palsy may have fewer opportunities for peer interaction, which serves as a valuable source of language experience. The greater the motor disability, the less opportunity the child has for active, physical exploration and manipulation of the environment, which are critical requirements in the formation of concepts (Bloom & Lahey, 1978).

Language delay is commonly seen in children with cerebral palsy for a number of reasons. The brain lesions underlying cerebral palsy also may involve the neurological structures responsible for the processing of language. Specific language-learning disorders may be present. Mental retardation is a common cause of language delay in children with cerebral palsy. However, it is possible for children with mental retardation to have additional superimposed language disorders that are more significant than would be expected from their level of intellectual functioning alone. Another important cause of language delay is hearing loss. In addition, associated conditions adversely affect language learning and language use, including seizures, attention deficits, visual impairments, and other complicating medical conditions.

Language Assessment

When evaluating the language of the child with cerebral palsy, it is important to consider the child's social and affective circumstances within his or her communicative environment, his or her opportunities and experiences with communication, and his or her specific receptive and expressive language skills. In order to do this, the clinician must obtain a history from the child's parents and teachers, observe the child with other individuals, interact and play with the child, and conduct formal tests.

Some important questions to ask during an assessment are

- Does the child have communicative intent?
- Is the child an effective communicator by whatever means are employed?
- What is the child's language level?
- Are language skills consistent or inconsistent with the child's sensory skills and cognitive levels?
- In what ways is the child responsive to stimulation?

There are standardized scales and tests of language development applicable to all age groups (see Table 14.1). Because the experiences of children with cerebral palsy are different from those of typically developing children, they may require adaptations in test administration. Children with visual impairments often need to have enlarged test plates. Verbal directions may need to be changed to accommodate the child's motor skills and to maintain the test item's integrity (e.g., one-step command, two-step command). Adapted positioning during this portion of the evaluation is important to allow the child to manipulate and to view materials.

The evaluation of infants typically focuses on linguistic precursors, such as auditory awareness, eye gaze, comprehension, use of gestures, cognitive skills of cause and effect, and object permanence. As the child begins to use words, then his or her vocabulary, concepts, sentence length, and grammatical complexity are evaluated. Use of more complex language (e.g., narrative or

Table 14.1. Standardized scales and tests of language development

Infant

The Rosetti Infant-Toddler Language Scale (Rosetti, 1990)
The Infant Scale of Communicative Intent (Sacks & Young, 1982)
Carolina Curriculum for Infants and Toddlers with Special Needs (Johnson-Martin, Jens, Attermeier, & Hacker, 1991)

Preschool

Peabody Picture Vocabulary Test–III (Dunn & Dunn, 1997)
Expressive Vocabulary Test (Williams, 1997)
Preschool Language Scale–3 (Zimmerman, Steina, & Pond, 1992)
Clinical Evaluation of Language Fundamentals–Preschool (Wiig, Secord, & Semel, 1992)
The Word Test–Revised (Huisingh, Barrett, Zachman, Blagden, & Orman, 1990)
The Non-Speech Test (Huer, 1988)

School-Age

Peabody Picture Vocabulary Test–III (Dunn & Dunn, 1997)
Expressive Vocabulary Test (Williams, 1997)
Clinical Evaluation of Language Fundamentals–3 (Semel, Wiig, & Secord, 1995)
The Word Test (Zachman, Huisingh, Barrett, Orman, & Blagden, 1989)

descriptive skills, inferential skills, abstract language) is assessed at a later stage. At all ages, the child's functional comprehension and use of language in a social context are considered. For example, how does the child interact with others and use language to express needs, relate ideas, and answer questions? The child's linguistic processing skills also are assessed at each stage of the evaluation. For example, does the child need input to be repeated or provided more slowly?

Language Therapy

Perhaps the most important objective of language therapy is to focus on the overall goal of establishing functional communication. Accepting the child's output, even if it is in unconventional forms, helps the child to gain a sense of control over his or her world and gives him or her a feeling of success as a communicator. Once this is established, the child can be stimulated (within the limits of his or her capacity) to develop more language. Knowing the child's level of cognitive and language functioning helps guide therapy toward success and permits realistic expectations in terms of the rate and the style of learning that is possible.

In addition to helping the therapist establish effective communication interactions with the child's family, his or her caregivers, and his or her teachers, therapy should be directed toward improving specific skills in the child. At the preverbal level, goals might be developed to establish face-to-face contact so that eye gaze and reciprocal babbling can occur. Gestures should be encouraged whenever possible because they are a very effective means of obtaining needs. Highly motivating games such as peekaboo or rolling a ball back and forth can lay a foundation for the turn taking, which is the basis of conversation. When the child signals an intent with his or her eyes, vocalizations, or gestures, that intent should be recognized and responded to appropriately. Later, as the child develops confidence and skill, more constraints can be placed on him or her. For instance, once it can be established that the child wants something in particular (e.g., a drink), he or she can be asked to choose the type of drink. The child can make a choice with eye gaze, by pointing, or with a word. If the child is verbal, then he or she can be asked to expand on an utterance. Once the child has developed symbolic knowledge, in addition to increasing phrase structure, goals can be established to increase his or her fund of vocabulary and concepts. For children with cerebral palsy, it is particularly important to examine their environments to find stimuli that are available and relevant to their everyday needs.

Case Study

Willy is verbal and conversational, although his speech is severely dysarthric. Willy's family members find his speech to be fairly intelligible when he speaks slowly in shorter utterances or when the subject of his conversation is known. Unfortunately, for those who do not know Willy, intelligibility is poor. Psychological testing revealed that Willy's cognitive level is average but that he has a learning disability with poor reading skills. In addition, his nutritional status was poor. When Willy was evaluated, his family wanted to know how his speech skills could be improved. The family also wanted Willy to be more independent with feeding, and they wanted to determine whether drooling could be reduced.

The feeding evaluation revealed that Willy had adequate oral-motor skills to handle all food consistencies. There was no clinical sign of aspiration. His seating, however, was not appropriate, and he was referred to a seating clinic to improve trunk and head position during feeding. However, because of poor manual control, Willy was largely dependent for feeding. Overall growth was minimal but proportional. When nutritional supplements were provided at least twice a day, he began to gain weight. Occupational therapy provided adaptive equipment to foster independence with a spoon.

(continued)

Case Study–continued

Willy's speech was slow and imprecise, and his voice sounded strained-strangled. Pitch and loudness levels were low, and pauses were prolonged and often at inappropriate places in a phrase. Inhalations were sometimes audible.

Speech therapy for Willy was directed toward developing compensatory articulation to allow for independent oral communication with familiar people. For example, although Willy could not produce most sibilant sounds (e.g., /s/, /z/, /sh/, /ch/, /dg/), he learned to produce a /th/ sound as an acoustic alternative. Because of the high frequency of occurrence of these sounds in English, this helped to improve his overall intelligibility. Willy also learned to use an /n/ (i.e., tongue-tip elevation sound) for the stop consonants /t/ and /d/ and to produce mouth shapes for vowels that were closer to their targets. His phrasing was improved somewhat by reducing the phrase length per breath and by developing more linguistic pause placement.

Despite these improvements, Willy's speech remained difficult for strangers to understand. In order to develop a supplemental communication system for settings in which his speech was ineffective, Willy was referred for an augmentative communication evaluation (see Chapter 15).

With regard to his drooling, Willy's pediatrician recommended a trial of therapy with glycopyrrolate, an anticholinergic medication. On review of the results of this trial, consideration will be given to surgical interventions to control drooling.

SUMMARY

Promoting feeding and communicative competence in the child with cerebral palsy can be a challenging, although rewarding, pursuit. It is important to recognize that "typical" functioning of the speech, language, and feeding systems may not be possible and should not be held up as the only standard for determining what constitutes a satisfactory outcome. Optimal function is the goal. Because each child with cerebral palsy presents a unique profile of motor, cognitive, socioemotional, linguistic, and familial characteristics, comprehensive evaluation of the child must occur (and should be ongoing during treatment phases) before goals are established.

When developing treatment programs, the larger goal of communicative effectiveness must be kept in mind. For some children, conventional forms of communication and traditional forms of therapy will suffice to produce satisfactory outcomes; for other children, alternative methods of feeding and communication must be employed. The therapist must develop successful individualized therapy programs that grow with the child and help families and educators to accept and use a variety of feeding and communication modalities. With patience, compassion, and an open mind, there is much we can do for each child and much each child can teach us.

REFERENCES

Arvedson, J., & Brodsky, L. (Eds.). (1993). *Pediatric swallowing and feeding.* San Diego, CA: Singular.

Bloom, L., & Lahey, M. (1978). *Language development and language disorders.* New York: John Wiley & Sons.

Crysdale, W. (1994). Drooling. In G. Gates (Ed.), *Current therapy in otolaryngology: Head and neck surgery* (pp. 213–218). St. Louis: C.V. Mosby.

Darley, F., Aronson, A., & Brown, J. (1975). *Motor speech disorders.* Philadelphia: W.B. Saunders.

Dunn, L., & Dunn, L. (1997). *Peabody Picture Vocabulary Test–III.* Circle Pines, MN: American Guidance Service.

Dunst, C. (1985). Communicative competence and deficits: Effects on early social interactions. In E. McDonald & D. Gallagher (Eds.), *Facilitating social-emotional development in multiply handicapped children* (pp. 93–140). Philadelphia: Michael C. Prestegord & Co.

Dworkin, J.P. (1991). *Motor speech disorders: A treatment guide.* St. Louis: Mosby Year Book.

Hardy, J. (1983). *Cerebral palsy.* Upper Saddle River, NJ: Prentice-Hall.

Huer, M.B. (1988). *The Non-Speech Test for Receptive/Expressive Language.* Fullerton, CA: Don Johnston Developmental Equipment.

Huisingh, R., Barrett, M., Zachman, L., Blagden, C., & Orman, J. (1990). *The Word Test–Revised.* East Moline, IL: Lingui Systems.

Humphrey, T. (1967). Reflex activity in the oral and facial area of the human fetus. In J.F. Bosma (Ed.), *Second symposium on oral sensation and perception* (pp. 195–233). Springfield, IL: Charles C Thomas.

Johnson, H., & Scott, A. (1993). *A practical approach to saliva control.* Tuscon, AZ: Communication Skill Builders.

Johnson-Martin, N.M., Jens, K.G., Attermeier, S.M., & Hacker, B.J. (1991). *The Carolina curriculum for infants and toddlers with special needs* (2nd ed.). Baltimore: Paul H. Brookes Publishing Co.

Lester, B., & Zeskind, P. (1979). The organization and assessment of crying in the infant at-risk. In T. Field (Ed.), *Infants born at risk* (pp. 121–144). Jamaica, NY: SP Medical & Scientific Books.

Lew, K.M., Younis, R.T., & Lazar, R.H. (1991). The current management of sialorrhea. *Ear, Nose, and Throat Journal, 70,* 99–105.

Love, R.J., Hagerman, E., & Taimi, E.G. (1980). Speech performance, dysphagia and oral reflexes in cerebral palsy. *Journal of Speech and Hearing Disorders, 40*(1), 59–75.

McDonald, E., & Chance, B., Jr. (1964). *Cerebral palsy.* Upper Saddle River, NJ: Prentice-Hall.

McWilliams, B.J., Morris, H., & Shelton, R. (Eds.). (1990). *Cleft palate speech.* Philadelphia: B.C. Decker.

Moore, C., & Ruarck, J. (1996). Does speech emerge from earlier appearing oral motor behaviors? *Journal of Speech and Hearing Research, 39,* 1034–1047.

Moore, L. (1988). *The developing human: Clinically oriented embryology* (4th ed.). Philadelphia: W.B. Saunders.

Morris, S. (1989). Development of oral-motor skills in the neurologically impaired child receiving non-oral feedings. *Dysphagia, 3,* 135–154.

Morris, S. (1992). *The normal acquisition of feeding skills: Implications for assessment and treatment.* Central Islip, NY: Therapeutic Media.

Orlikoff, R. (1992). The use of instrumental measures in the assessment and treatment of motor speech disorders. *Seminars in Speech and Language, 13,* 25–38.

Rosetti, L. (1990). *Infant-Toddler Language Scale.* East Moline, IL: Lingui Systems.

Sacks, G., & Young, E. (1982). An Assessment tool: The Infant Scale of Communicative Intent. *Update Pediatrics, 7,* 1–5.

Semel, E., Wiig, E., & Secord, W. (1995). *Clinical Evaluation of Language Fundamentals* (3rd ed.). San Antonio, TX: The Psychological Corporation.

Shprintzen, R. (1989). Nasopharyngoscopy. In K. Bzoch (Ed.), *Communicative disorders related to cleft-up and palate* (3rd ed., pp. 216–229). Boston: Little, Brown.

Wertz, R., & Rosenbek, J. (1992). Where the ear fits: A perceptual evaluation of motor speech disorders. *Seminars in Speech and Language, 13,* 39–54.

Westlake, H., & Rutherford, D. (1961). *Speech therapy for the cerebral palsied.* Chicago: National Easter Seal Society for Crippled Children and Adults.

Wiig, E., Secord, W., & Semel, E. (1992). *Clinical Evaluation of Language Fundamentals–Preschool.* San Antonio, TX: The Psychological Corporation.

Williams, K. (1997). *Expressive Vocabulary Test.* Circle Pines, MN: American Guidance Service.

Zachman, L., Huisingh, R., Barrett, M., Orman, J., & Blagden, C. (1989). *The Word Test.* East Moline, IL: Lingui Systems.

Zimmerman, I., Steina, V., & Pond, R. (1992). *Pre-School Language Scale–3.* San Antonio, TX: The Psychological Corporation.

CHAPTER 15

Assistive Technology

Jennifer Rauck Burstein,
Mary Lisa Wright-Drechsel, and Audrey Wood

The 20th century has witnessed a transformation in U.S. society from an industrial base to a technological base. Technology has transformed every aspect of American life and has taken on a special significance for individuals who have disabilities such as cerebral palsy. For typically developing individuals, technology creates opportunities to work and live more efficiently. For individuals with disabilities, technology creates opportunities for greater functional independence and for increased participation in the goods of society. In other words, technology can help individuals with disabilities overcome some of the disadvantages they experience relative to the rest of society.

This observation has received legislative endorsement through laws such as the Technology-Related Assistance for Individuals with Disabilities Amendments of 1994 (PL 103-218) (see Chapter 19). This law defines assistive technology as

Any item, piece of equipment or product system, whether acquired commercially off the shelf, modified, or customized, that is used to increase, maintain, or improve the functional capabilities of individuals with disabilities. (p. 54)

Assistive technology also is defined by PL 103-218 as a set of services that includes evaluation, selection or adaptation, and training. In addition, the law describes the purpose of assistive technology as helping individuals with disabilities to have greater control of their lives; to participate more fully at home, at work, in school, and in other social settings; to interact more with individuals without disabilities; and to enjoy the same opportunities in life as do individuals without disabilities.

In order to ensure the rights of individuals with disabilities, PL 103-218 emphasizes the concrete manifestations of assistive technology in the form of devices and services. In practice, assistive technology is a tool for the enhancement of function and, as such, becomes an extension of the processes of habilitation and rehabilitation (it is seen as a means to a functional goal and not as an end in itself).

IMPLICATIONS FOR CHILDREN WITH CEREBRAL PALSY

Children with cerebral palsy manifest impairments of sensory, motor, and cognitive function, and these impairments can affect the child's ability to participate in activities involving communication, mobility, environmental mastery, recreation, and activities of daily living (ADLs) (see Chapters 12, 13, and 14). Assistive technology can enhance functioning in any of these skill areas and is prescribed to address specific impairments in an effort to ameliorate disabilities and to prevent handicaps. For example, the child with a mild motor impairment may require one-hand computer access to supplement written communication skills. By contrast, the child with more severe impairments, such as spastic quadriplegia, may need a computer technology system with integrated devices to enhance function and independence; an augmentative communication system may be provided to facilitate successful communication, a power wheelchair to enhance mobility, an environmental control unit to ensure access to electrical appliances and devices.

SKILL APPLICATION

As an extension of the process of habilitation and rehabilitation, assistive technology targets specific skill areas. These areas include communication, mobility, environmental mastery, learning, and recreation.

Communication

Assistive technology provides a means for individuals who have poor communication abilities to "augment" their verbal and written expression. The American Speech-Language-Hearing Association provides the following definition of augmentative and alternative communication (AAC):

> An area of clinical practice that attempts to compensate (either temporarily or permanently) for the impairment and disability patterns of individuals with severe

expressive communication disorders (i.e., the severely speech-language and writing impaired). (1989, p. 107)

A variety of AAC devices can be used by children with cerebral palsy whose gestural, verbal, and written communication does not meet all of their communication needs. These devices range from "low-tech" picture communication boards to "high-tech" computers with synthesized speech output. The features of AAC devices include symbols, displays, selection techniques, and output modes.

Symbols   AAC devices incorporate different types of symbols. Beukelman and Mirenda (1992) classified symbol systems as tangible/tactile, representational, abstract, or orthographic. Tangible or tactile symbols include objects, miniature objects, partial objects, and textured symbols. A textured symbol is defined as "a paired association between a texture and an object or activity" (Murray-Branch, Udvari-Solner, & Bailey, 1991). Representational symbols are photographs, colored pictures, or line drawings. There are a number of commercially available line drawing symbol sets (e.g., Picture Communication Symbols, Rebus Symbols, Picsyms, Blissymbolics). Abstract symbol systems include symbol sets in which the symbol form does not suggest its meaning (Beukelman & Mirenda, 1992). Two examples of abstract symbol systems are Yerkish Lexigrams and Non-Speech Language Initiation Program. Orthographic symbols are based on letters, such as Morse code, braille, and phonemic symbols. An individual's symbol set could include any one of these symbol types or a combination of several symbol types.

Displays   Displays on AAC devices are either fixed or dynamic. On a fixed display, the symbols and the arrangement of symbols remain constant. Conversely, on a dynamic display, the symbols or the arrangement of the symbols may change with each selection (see Figure 15.1). For example, from a choice of topics, the child may point to a symbol on a computer screen that represents "toys." The computer then would offer the child a number of specific toys from which to choose. After the child selects the toy desired, the screen may change again to offer general topics.

Selection Techniques   Children select items on an AAC device through either direct selection or scanning. Direct selection is used when the child directly indicates items on the AAC device. This can be accomplished with physical contact by a body part or an adaptive device (e.g., head pointer, hand splint), with a light pointer, or through voice recognition technology or eye gaze. Selection through scanning involves a time element (Vanderheiden, 1988). The child is presented with items or groups of items in a sequence and then indicates his or her choice when the desired item is presented. Examples of types of scanning include 1) linear scanning, in which one item is presented at a time; 2) row/column scanning, in which the child selects the row that contains the item and then selects the specific location of the item; and 3) block scanning, in which

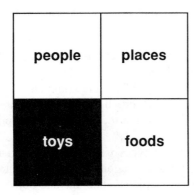
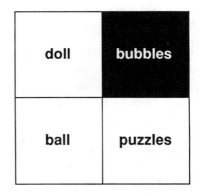

Figure 15.1. AAC device with dynamic display. First, the child selects a category from the first screen. (In this situation, the child chooses "toys.") Then the screen changes to offer four options within the "toys" category. The child then selects a toy of his or her choice. (In this situation, the child chooses "bubbles.")

sequentially smaller blocks of items are presented. Various switches can be utilized to make the selection with the different scanning techniques. Selection methods used with scanning include automatic, inverse, and step scanning (Beukelman & Mirenda, 1992). With automatic scanning, the child waits as the device (or an individual) scans the items and then he or she makes the selection at the appropriate time. With inverse scanning, the child holds down the switch to scan the items and then releases the switch to make a selection. With step scanning, the child activates the switch to move an indicator to the desired item or group of items; when the desired item is highlighted, he or she waits for a specified period of time, and the device interprets the lack of input as acceptance of the highlighted item. The items scanned can be presented visually (as symbols) or auditorily (as sounds).

Whether the child makes selections with direct selection or with scanning, message encoding also can be employed. Message encoding is used to increase the rate of communication and to provide a large vocabulary set with a limited number of access sites. With encoding, the child selects a sequence of symbols in order to convey a single message (see Figure 15.2). Each sequence is the "code" for a particular message. The symbols sequenced can be letters, numbers, pictures, colors, or a combination of these symbols. (Morse code is a familiar type of encoding.) Message prediction is a type of encoding in which subsequent selections are limited based on the initial selection. This is used to facilitate both recall and the speed of communication.

Output Modes Output modes are described as either intrinsic or extrinsic. Intrinsic output requires the communication partner to observe each selection as it is being made and to synthesize the complete message. For example, as an

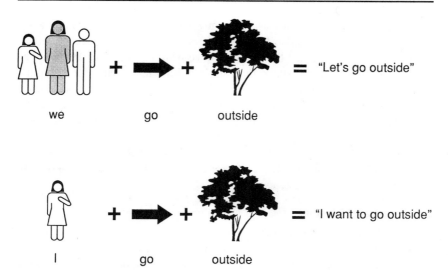

Figure 15.2. Message encoding. The child selects different sequences of symbols in order to produce a particular message.

individual is pointing to letters on a nonelectronic alphabet board, the communication partner must observe each letter as it is being selected and put the letters together. Ongoing feedback is important with intrinsic output to ensure that each communication partner knows what the other partner has received. The individual not using the board may need to say each letter aloud as it is selected and then say the spelled word to confirm that he or she has interpreted the message correctly. This process of conversational construction is described by Higginbotham (1986). Extrinsic output transforms an individual's selections into visual or auditory information. Examples include synthesized and digitized speech, print, and electronic displays (e.g., Light Emitting Diode, Liquid Crystal Display, computer screen).

Mobility

Locomotion and other sensorimotor skills rapidly develop during the first 3 years of the child's life. These skills are the primary means for learning socialization, independence, and competence. Through movement, the child is first able to interact with his or her environment as well as have an impact on it. In order to move or maintain positions, the child with cerebral palsy has to contend with abnormal tone, reflexive patterns, limitations in range of motion (ROM), sensory impairments, and uncoordinated motor patterns. The use of assistive or adapted devices can facilitate the child's function in static positions by utilizing equipment such as prone or supine standers, adapted seating systems, and sidelyers. There also are many devices that can be used to facilitate the child's mobility skills. The primary goal of a mobility device is to effectively and efficiently assist the child to move from one place to another. The device chosen will be specific to the child's abilities and needs. For the young child who has good upper-extremity function, walkers, canes, adapted bicycles, or scooters may be used. For the older child who has adequate upper-extremity function, crutches and wheelchairs may be the best option. For the child who does not have functional use of his or her upper extremities or who has limitations in strength and endurance, power cars, carts, or wheelchairs may best suit his or her needs. (Refer to Chapter 12 for a more in-depth description of both positioning and mobility devices.)

Environmental Mastery

Assistive technology can facilitate or enhance the child's ability to gain access to, move within, and explore his or her environment. It can provide the child with a means to control the features of the environment or to actually use the objects and devices that occupy the environment. The abilities to gain access to, control, and use space are all components of environmental mastery. Three general application areas in this realm include modifications to physical space, adaptive devices or products, and environmental control systems. Physical modifications can range from furniture arrangements or height adaptations to structural changes such as ramps, elevators, or automatic doors. Adaptive devices can range from generic products such as battery-operated scissors to adaptive products such as reachers or extension handles. Environmental control units (ECUs) or systems involve an activation method and a control unit that picks up the activation signal and sends it to targeted appliances or devices. ECUs are varied and diverse to match the multidimensional aspects of the environment. They are generally categorized by the type of transmission or the signal code that they send to a receiver or a control unit (e.g., infrared systems that emit a light signal, radio frequency systems that send radio waves, ultrasound systems that emit sound waves, house wiring that sends digital signals over electrical wiring). These systems can be coordinated or integrated with a power wheelchair or a computer system.

Learning

The multidimensional nature of learning, including sensory processing, sensorimotor components, and cognitive requirements, can present special challenges (e.g., written expression) to the child with cerebral palsy. Assistive technology with adapted aids or modified techniques, with generic aids, or with computer systems can facilitate the child's learning experiences and written communication skills. Handwriting aids and modifications include stamp pad letters, letter stencils, pencil grips, and worksheets. Generic aids include typewriters, calculators, tape recorders, and word processors. For the child with multiple sensory, motor, and cognitive needs, computer systems with multiple input modes, a variety of software, and numerous output modes can better address learning or writing issues. Multiple input modes include mice, trackballs, switches, and alternative keyboards. Software can enhance visual, auditory, and tactile aspects of input and output modes, or it can modify information into other formats with specific options or features that are either preprogrammed or programmable (i.e., allowing for customization). Output modes include printers, monitors or screens, braille devices, and auditory output devices.

Recreation

For the child with cerebral palsy, play experiences can be challenging on both a motor and a sensory level. As the typically developing child develops, he or she builds on early play experiences that can grow or expand to include organized team sports, individualized athletics, or leisure pursuits. Play also is an avenue for social interaction with peers. For the child with cerebral palsy, assistive technology in the form of adapted toys, computer systems, or adapted sports equipment can provide opportunities for these types of play experiences. In order to facilitate grasp and manipulation, many toys can be adapted with large-size knobs or loops (see Figure 15.3). To facilitate activation, battery-operated toys are easily adapted for use with a variety of switches. Computer systems with a variety of software enable the child with cerebral palsy to play various board or arcade games, create videos, play or compose music, or draw and create works of art. A variety of sports equipment, ranging from adapted or three-wheel bikes to adapted skis, also is available to children with cerebral palsy.

ASSESSMENT OF FUNCTION

An assistive technology assessment is an ongoing process that requires a team approach. At the center of the team is the child and his or her family. The goals of the family determine the focus of the assessment. Other team members involved in the assessment vary depending on the child's needs and may include teachers, speech-language pathologists, occupational therapists, physical therapists, psychologists, audiologists, vision specialists, classroom aides, nurses, physicians, and social workers. When evaluating the child's need for assistive technology, it is imperative to include team members who have knowledge of the assistive technology as well as experience in the assessment process. Assistive technology teams may be available through school districts, area hospitals, or therapy clinics. Some children's school teams may include individuals with expertise in evaluating assistive technology. However, an outside evaluation team frequently needs to be brought in to meet the child's technology needs and to expand the resources available to the child.

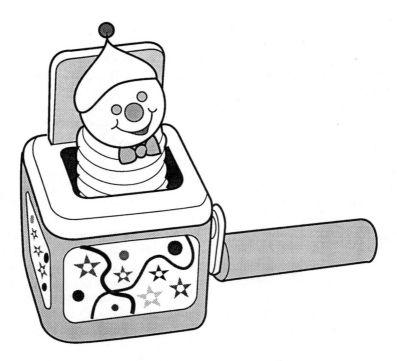

Figure 15.3. An adapted toy. The child uses a large knob on the toy to facilitate grasp and manipulation.

Phases of Assessment

The assistive technology assessment process can be divided into four steps, or phases.

 Information Gathering   The initial phase of an assistive technology assessment involves gathering information regarding the child's needs and capabilities. A needs assessment focuses on the skills or functions that the child wants and needs in order to perform in various settings. This information can be gathered through an interview or a questionnaire that is completed with the child and his or her family. The outcome of the needs assessment will be a set of goals that the child and his or her family want to accomplish with the use of assistive technology. The child's capabilities assessment is a comprehensive view of the child's skills in the areas of sensory, cognitive, speech and language, and musculoskeletal/neuromotor function.

 Sensory   Sensory registration and processing of auditory, visual, tactile, vestibular, proprioceptive, and kinesthetic information play an integral part in how the child perceives and in turn interacts with his or her environment on both a cognitive and a motor level. Impairments in sensory processing and registration are common in children who are diagnosed with cerebral palsy. It is important to have information on the status of sensory systems (e.g., vision, hearing) from both ophthalmology and audiology reports. Clinical assessments of visual-motor function, visual perception, and functional vision also are pertinent to the technology assessment. In terms of the devices' features (from the type of input methods to the type of output modes), sensory information from these sources can better identify the specific needs of the child. It also guides the team in the selection of technology devices that may help augment the registration or the processing of sensory information or may compensate for any sensory impairments.

Cognition   Cognition refers to the child's overall developmental level of functioning. At a basic level, the child's awareness of the environment and his or her responses to it are assessed. An understanding of cause-and-effect relationships (e.g., touching a switch turns on a radio) is critical for the child to benefit from assistive technology. If the child is unable to comprehend this relationship, the team's goals may need to focus on concept training. The child's ability to follow directions—from simple one-step directions to more complex multistep directions—also is assessed. The child's individualized education program can provide information regarding his or her academic and literacy levels.

Speech and Language   A speech-language pathologist can provide information regarding the child's functional communication status (i.e., the child's language comprehension and expression). In addition, the child's ability to use speech for purposeful communication is assessed. Many children with cerebral palsy have severe expressive communication impairments (see Chapter 13). Some children may be able to produce a small number of words or phrases that are intelligible only to people who know them well. If the child is unable to use speech to meet all of his or her communication needs, an assistive technology evaluation for augmentative communication is warranted.

Musculoskeletal/Neuromotor   Children with cerebral palsy typically have motor impairments that can result in movement dysfunction; however, each child will demonstrate individual differences in his or her limitations and capabilities. An in-depth neuromotor and musculoskeletal evaluation should be completed prior to an assistive technology evaluation. Essential areas for evaluation include ROM, postural alignment, muscle tone, balance and postural responses, muscle strength, motor control, and developmental/functional skill level (see Chapter 12). Reports from and interaction with an orthopedic surgeon and physical therapist or occupational therapist can provide this type of information regarding the child's musculoskeletal status, and this will shape and refine the assessment for the use of equipment and devices.

Environmental Assessment   An environmental assessment is completed in order to gain specific information regarding the various settings in which the child needs to achieve the functional goals that were specified during the evaluation process. Because technology used in one setting may be inappropriate in another, the assessment considers both physical aspects of the environment and the role expectations of the child within each setting. For example, a power wheelchair may be the most appropriate means of mobility for the child in school or in the community, but it may take up too much space in a small apartment. Or, an electronic communication device may be the child's primary expressive mode of communication, but it would be dangerous to use while he or she is bathing. There are settings in which secondary "low-tech" devices are needed when the primary device cannot be used. An environmental assessment is used to identify these various needs.

Clinical Observations   The focus of the secondary phase of the assessment process is to synthesize, analyze, and confirm the data collected in the initial phase. This phase provides the chance to gather any additional information from the child and his or her family and to observe the child's responses to various environmental stimuli. This process can involve screening of any of the skills previously discussed in this chapter, actual handling of the child, and examining the child's positioning equipment or any other assistive technologies that he or she uses. This phase is an essential stepping stone from information gathering to the hands-on phase of the assessment process because it allows professionals to make educated guesses in terms of positioning, equipment, and setups that will be necessary during a full hands-on assessment.

Hands-On Assessment   During the hands-on assessment phase of the evaluation process, many of the child's skills are observed and evaluated simultaneously in a series of functional activities. The focus of the assessment is guided by goals identified during the initial phase of the assessment process. Whether the skills involve communication, mobility, environmental mastery, learning, or recreation, the issues of access are an integral part of the assessment phase. Access in the context of assistive technology refers to the child's ability to control or to operate a device. Access also may involve multiple modes of input. Thus, the team considers not only how the child will physically access the system but also the type of information that must be entered into the system.

Functional Assessment for Access and AAC System Use

Two aspects of an assistive technology assessment that warrant further discussion are access evaluation and the AAC evaluation.

Access Evaluation   Although the evaluation of functional movement patterns in relation to access is not a sequential process, the components of motor movement need to be individually examined. These components include isolated movement patterns, tonal/reflex patterns, joint ROM, sensorimotor processing, environmental demands, and endurance. Movement and the ability to perform isolated movements are always issues for the child with cerebral palsy. Movement patterns tend to be poorly isolated and the child is often dominated by muscle groups that work in flexor or extensor patterns. In order to translate these patterns into successful access, many movement patterns may need to be examined and critiqued in order to make a match between the child and the access method. The movement of upper extremities is a good starting place for any evaluation of access. Functional use of the upper extremities is an early manifestation of voluntary motor control and forms the basis for eye–hand coordination (i.e., visual-motor integration). Activation of the upper extremities may occur as coarse, whole-arm patterns or as more finely tuned, isolated responses of the hands and the digits. If upper- or lower-extremity patterns are not functional for access, more proximal areas are explored, such as the head, the neck, or the trunk. The use of proximal patterns can compromise truncal stability and position, but it may be worth the risk if a movement pattern can activate a device.

Tonal and reflexive patterns vary greatly among children with cerebral palsy. Each pattern can present special challenges for access. Even when the child reaches a device, low muscle tone or hypotonia generally affects strength or force of movement patterns, and he or she may lack the strength to maintain a position on the device or may not have the power to activate the device in the first place. Spasticity patterns generally present as fixing (i.e., stiffening a group of muscles in order to maintain posture) or overflow patterns that make the process of getting on and off a device problematic. Reflex patterns are often associated with spasticity and further complicate functional movement. Mixed tonal patterns present with fluctuations of tone, which make movement patterns inconsistent and repeated patterns difficult. All tonal patterns affect the process of intentional movement, from initiating a movement, activating the device, holding a position or a posture, and returning to a resting position.

ROM limitations and contractures are common in children with cerebral palsy. Limits in ROM directly affect the positioning of the child and the positioning of a device, and, thus, device placement will always be contingent on the child's available range. Placement should be comfortably within that range.

There is a continuous flow of sensory information that occurs as a child moves through and interacts with his or her environment. Sensorimotor processing may be defined in terms of this feedforward and feedback process, which allows the central nervous system to register input, synthesize information, and produce motor responses. Because cerebral palsy is primarily a movement disorder, the perception of proprioceptive, kinesthetic, or tactile information can be impaired or distorted. This type of information is vital to both body awareness and awareness of body position in space. Choosing access methods that enhance or compensate for these specific impairments can improve motor response. Figure 15.4 illustrates a variety of devices available for enabling switch activation. Textured surfaces, keyguards, joystick templates, and visual or auditory feedback are just a few examples of means to further define a space or of compensatory measures that tap an alternate sensory mode for switch activation. Auditory and visual impairments also are commonly associated with cerebral

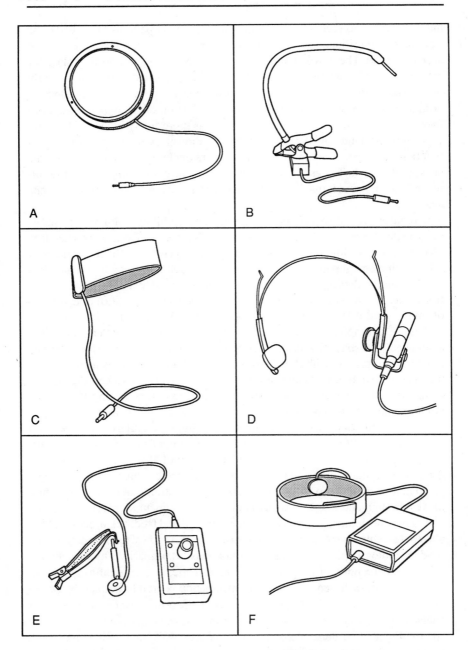

Figure 15.4. Devices for switch activation. The child activates the switches through a variety of methods: A) physical contact, B) air pressure, C) motion, D) light, E) sound, and F) muscle tension.

palsy (see Chapter 1). There are specific devices that are geared to meet the needs of people who have visual or auditory impairments, and these devices also may be appropriate for the child with cerebral palsy. More subtle visual impairments such as visual-perceptual or visual-motor impairments can be addressed using visual enhancements (e.g., increasing the size of pictures or letters, employing contrasting color schemes, using paired auditory and visual feedback). Enhancing auditory information can be accomplished with volume controls, with earphones, or with the pairing of visual and auditory feedback.

Endurance and fatigue are very significant factors for the child with cerebral palsy. If the motoric demand is too high, the child will expend all of his or her energy on accessing a device, leaving little reserve energy to focus on the cognitive demands of the task. Modes of access are not exercises or attempts to increase ROM. A good match between the child's motoric capabilities and his or her mode of access is the method that is the easiest for him or her to achieve. Ease of access is a principle that needs to be emphasized in every hands-on assessment.

AAC Evaluation   An assessment for an AAC system begins with an access evaluation (see the section on "Functional Assessment for Access and AAC System Use" in this chapter). Once potential access methods have been identified, the child is evaluated for the individual features of a communication system (i.e., symbols, displays, selection techniques, and output modes). The child's level of abstract association, sensory skills, and literacy help to determine the type of symbols needed for communication. The child with a visual impairment may benefit from tactile or textured communication symbols. Objects or photographs can be used with children who demonstrate limited abstract association. Children who are developing literacy skills need to have orthographic symbols available.

The arrangement of symbols on the AAC device display is influenced by the number of choices the child is capable of handling at one time and whether a static or a dynamic display is necessary. A dynamic display is beneficial if the child can gain access to only a limited number of choices but has the cognitive ability to encode. For example, if the child's display contains four symbols and the selection of each of these symbols leads to a new display with four additional symbols, the system can hold 16 purposeful messages. Additional levels can be added to increase the number of messages. However, at each stage the child may choose from only four symbols at a time. A static display is beneficial when the child is able to select from a large number of choices. A static display also is appropriate when the child's perceptual skills limit his or her ability to handle changing displays.

In order to use encoding, the child must be able either to shift between levels on a dynamic display or to apply multiple meanings to a single symbol. For example, there are only two signals or symbols in Morse code. How these two signals are sequenced determines the message conveyed. With picture symbols, the child needs to be able to use the same symbol in a variety of sequences. A symbol representing GO can be combined with symbols for "store," "walk," or "home." The combination of these symbols reflects telegraphic speech (e.g., GO STORE, GO HOME). In order to further expand the number of messages available, the child needs to be able to apply multiple meanings to a single symbol. If the symbol for GO is a green arrow pointing to the right, the symbol can represent GO, GREEN, and RIGHT. When the child is capable of gaining access to an AAC device with more than 100 selections and can sequence three or more symbols, thousands of messages can be programmed into his or her device. Some AAC devices have preprogrammed software available for individuals with this level of capability. Once the child has demonstrated the ability to use encoding with a large number of choices, evaluation for particular software may be necessary.

The output mode(s) needed by an AAC user is determined by the environment in which he or she needs to communicate and his or her ability to comprehend the output. Speech output is most desirable but may not be appropriate for the child who has a severe hearing impairment. Although synthetic (i.e., computerized) speech tends to offer superior quality, it is more expensive than recorded (i.e., digitized) speech. Recorded speech may be preferred because of its qualities of human voice. Printed output, whether on paper or on a screen, allows the communication partner to read the message. Output on a screen is frequently accompanied by speech output and allows the communication partner to read the message if he or she did not hear it. Print on paper allows the AAC user to compose a message in advance and then share it with a communication partner at a later time. In this scenario, the communication partners would be limited to those who have literacy skills.

Assessment Outcomes

Information from each assessment phase is compiled. Results of the assessment indicate whether the child can benefit from assistive technology to accomplish the goals set forth by the team. Recommendations may be made for teaching skills that will allow the child to use more sophisticated technology in the future. The features of the device(s) for which the child has demonstrated a need are described, and then particular devices that meet the child's needs are listed. In many cases, one particular device may appear most appropriate and, therefore, may be recommended. In other cases, there may be more than one device that would meet the child's needs. In this case, members of the team may pick a preferred device. Input from the child and the child's family is crucial when looking at preference. In addition, the team needs to consider how the device will be integrated with the child's existing system and with his or her future technological needs. When there is an indication that the child may not use the device(s) for its intended purpose, a trial period is recommended. The goals and the length of the trial period should be predetermined. When the child has demonstrated the ability to use the technology for its intended purpose, purchase of the equipment is usually recommended.

OBTAINING AND FUNDING ASSISTIVE TECHNOLOGY

Once the need for specific equipment is determined, the process of obtaining and funding begins. With input from all of the members of the team, information from the assessment is used to develop a prescription in which all equipment needs and costs are listed. The cost of equipment must include the purchase and/or rental cost and the expense of training the child, the child's family, and other team members.

The next step is to identify funding sources: What sources are available and who represents potential future sources? Eligibility criteria for these funding sources must be investigated and matched to the child's needs. The types of assistive technology covered also must be noted. The information gathered is used to develop a funding plan. Funding from a variety of sources may be necessary because each resource may provide only a limited dollar amount that can be applied toward equipment. Possible sources of funding can include medical insurance, public assistance, early intervention programs, public education money, vocational rehabilitation agencies, private organizations and foundations, service organizations, or community-based services. Educational programs will only pay for equipment and services that are determined to be educationally relevant. If the equipment is necessary for the child to benefit appropriately from his or her educational program, then the school district is responsible for obtaining it.

Insurance companies require that equipment be deemed "medically necessary" before they assume financial responsibility for its acquisition. A written report from the assistive technology assessment needs to be submitted with a doctor's prescription. Documentation of the child's needs, his or her performance during the assessment process, and how he or she will benefit from the use of assistive technology devices must be stressed. In addition, photographs and a videotape may be helpful in demonstrating the need for and potential benefits of the device for the child.

CUSTOMIZATION AND TRAINING

The process of providing technology for improving the functional skills of children with cerebral palsy is ongoing and does not end with the acquisition of devices. Once assistive technology devices have been obtained, follow-up services are required. The amount of follow-up that is required depends on the customization and the training needed to achieve the functional goals of the child and his or her family. Many devices require customization to the child's particular needs. The child, his or her family, and others interacting with him or her need to be trained in the use and the care of the devices. Customization and training are integral parts of the process of providing technology and are critical in facilitating optimal use and preventing device abandonment. The development of a long-range plan is necessary in order to identify the roles and the responsibilities of the different team members.

CASE STUDY

With the completion of a needs and capabilities assessment, the following goals were identified for improving Willy's functional skills:

1. Determine appropriate augmentative communication modes for expressive communication. Although Willy spoke in complete sentences, his speech intelligibility was poor as a result of severe dysarthria. Familiar listeners frequently had difficulty understanding what he said.
2. Develop means for producing written text. As a result of significant fine motor impairments, Willy was unable to print. He required a means to produce text for written expression and to complete academic work.
3. Develop independent means of mobility. Although Willy had a manual wheelchair, he was dependent on others to push it. He did not have the coordination or the strength to propel the wheelchair himself.

Information obtained from an environmental assessment supported the need for "high-tech" options to meet Willy's goals. Willy's back-up systems for mobility (i.e., manual wheelchair) and communication (i.e., speech) were already in place. Willy was totally dependent on technology for producing written text.

From an access evaluation, it was determined that Willy's access was most successful when he was positioned in his seating system with his left forearm stabilized on his tray and his right forearm stabilized under his tray. It also was determined that he required a left wrist splint.

An augmentative communication evaluation revealed that Willy could use a membrane keyboard with 128 keys. He depressed the keys with his left index finger and could identify small colored pictures representing many parts of speech (e.g., nouns, verbs, adjectives, prepositions). He

(continued)

Case Study–continued

could sequence symbols to access preprogrammed messages and was able to type out simple sentences. It was determined that Willy could use a complex augmentative communication device with a 128-location keyboard, picture symbols, and the alphabet; he also could benefit from a software program that provided him with a large vocabulary set and the ability to customize (i.e., store messages particular to his interests and needs). In addition, text-to-speech capability (i.e., being able to type a word or sentence and having it produced through the speech output) was necessary. A wheelchair mount was recommended so that Willy's communication device could travel with him. Willy's AAC system was purchased for him with public assistance funding.

Willy was able to produce written text through traditional word processing on a computer system. He used a mini keyboard with a frequency-of-use letter array. He could access the keyboard with his left index finger in a one-hand typing method. Willy's keypunch accuracy was good and his typing speed was fair, averaging 10 words per minute. This rate was acceptable for his level of literacy and the amount of written work he was required to complete for school. Willy had access to a computer system with a mini keyboard at school. Homework was completed in alternative formats, including tape recording and checklists. Future plans included the acquisition of a computer system for him to use at home.

Despite his athetoid movements, Willy demonstrated the desire and the ability to operate a power wheelchair. It was necessary for him to sit in a supportive system to stabilize his trunk and lower extremities. Once well positioned in the chair, he was able to operate a joystick that had mounting adjustments for his left upper extremity. A tray was needed for increased support and stability. As a result of his athetoid movements, Willy required parameter adjustability to allow for better control and responsiveness. (See Chapter 12 for a more detailed discussion of parameter adjustability.)

SUMMARY

Assistive technology refers to a variety of equipment and services that are available to help maintain, increase, or improve the functional capabilities of individuals with disabilities. For the child with cerebral palsy, assistive technology can have a significant effect on his or her ability to participate in activities involving communication, mobility, environmental mastery, learning, recreation, and ADLs. Equipment and services are tailored to the needs of the individual child, and periodic reassessment is required to ensure that the child continues to receive the full, intended benefit of the intervention. The assessment process is interdisciplinary and family centered and seeks to delineate the child's specific sensory, motor, and cognitive capabilities and to define assistive technology needs as they occur in specific, real-life settings.

Assistive technology may be "low-tech" and relatively inexpensive or "high-tech" and carry a prohibitive price tag. A number of different funding mechanisms are available to assist in the procurement of funds for assistive technology, and obtaining access to such funding should ideally be a part of the interdisciplinary planning process.

REFERENCES

American Speech-Language-Hearing Association. (1989). Competencies for speech-language pathologists providing services in augmentative communication. *Asha, 31,* 107–110.

Beukelman, D.R., & Mirenda, P. (1992). *Augmentative and alternative communication: Management of severe communication disorders in children and adults.* Baltimore: Paul H. Brookes Publishing Co.

Higginbotham, D.J. (1986). Message formulation augmentative communication systems: Studies in social communication and interaction. *Dissertation Abstracts, 47,* 1588. (University microfilms No. DA 8601104).

Murray-Branch, J., Udvari-Solner, A., & Bailey, B. (1991). Textured communication systems for individuals with severe intellectual and dual sensory impairments. *Language, Speech, and Hearing Services in Schools, 22,* 260–268.

Technology-Related Assistance for Individuals with Disabilities Amendments of 1994, PL 103-218, 29 U.S.C. §§ 2201 *et seq.*

Vanderheiden, G. (1988). Overview of the basic selection techniques for augmentative communication: Present and future. In L. Bernstein (Ed.), *The vocally impaired: Clinical practice and research* (pp. 265–294). New York: Grune & Stratton.

RECOMMENDED READINGS

Bernstein, L. (Ed.). (1988). *The vocally impaired: Clinical practice and research.* New York: Grune & Stratton.

Blackstone, S. (Ed.). (1986). *Augmentative communication: An introduction.* Rockville, MD: American Speech-Language-Hearing Association.

Butler, C. (1986). Effects of powered mobility on self-initiated behaviors of very young children with locomotor disability. *Developmental Medicine and Child Neurology, 28,* 325–332.

Carlson, S., & Ramsey, C. (1995). Assistive technology. In S. Campbell (Ed.), *Physical therapy for children* (pp. 621–659). Philadelphia: W.B. Saunders.

Cook, A., & Hussey, S. (1995). *Assistive technologies: Principles and practice.* St. Louis: C.V. Mosby.

Franks, C., Palisano, R., & Darbee, J. (1991). The effect of walking with an assistive device and using a wheelchair on school performance in students with myelomeningocele. *Physical Therapy, 71,* 570–579.

Jaffe, K. (1987). *Childhood powered mobility: Developmental, technical, and clinical perspectives.* Washington, DC: Rehabilitation Engineering Society of America.

Johnson, M.J., Baumgart, D., Helmstetter, E., & Curry, C.A. (1996). *Augmenting basic communication in natural contexts.* Baltimore: Paul H. Brookes Publishing Co.

Kurtz, L.A., Dowrick, P.W., Levy, S.E., & Batshaw, M.L. (1996). Children's Seashore House handbook of developmental disabilities: Resources for interdisciplinary care. Rockville, MD: Aspen Publishers, Inc.

Landers, A. (1994). The ABLEDATA database of assistive technology. *Exceptional Parent, 24*(3), 56.

Mann, W., & Lane, J. (1991). *Assistive technology for persons with disabilities: The role of the occupational therapist.* Rockville, MD: American Occupational Therapy Association.

Struck, M. (1996). Computer access: A link to classroom learning. *OT Practice, 1*(8), 18.

CHAPTER 16

Orthotic Management

James Walker and Meg Stanger

The orthotic management of children with cerebral palsy continues to be both exciting and challenging as a result of the increasing range of available treatment options, the merging of biomechanical and neurophysiological principles, and the integration of parents' and professionals' ideas about improving the functioning of children with neurological involvement. As of 1998, the application of orthotic designs and materials is more diverse than the historical approach of using metal braces with orthopedic shoes. The purposes and types of orthotic devices used with children with cerebral palsy vary among facilities and geographic regions. This diversity has led to differing opinions regarding the use of orthotic devices and highlights the need for improved scientific research to determine the effectiveness of using different orthoses for children with cerebral palsy.

CONSIDERATIONS FOR THE USE
OF ORTHOTIC DEVICES IN PEDIATRICS

Orthotic management, including prescription, fabrication, fine-tuning adjustments, long-term use, and follow-up care, of children differs in many important respects from that of adults. Medical professionals involved in the orthotic management of children with cerebral palsy must take into consideration that a child's musculoskeletal system is growing and developing. In order to understand the purpose and efficacy of orthotic intervention with children, these professionals must have a thorough understanding of the growth and the development of the musculoskeletal system as well as a thorough understanding of the influence of normal and abnormal physiological and biomechanical forces on that system. Orthotic management of children with cerebral palsy ideally involves a team of experts, including the child's parents and a number of professionals. Depending on the facility, the team may include a primary physician, a pediatric orthopedist, a pediatric neurologist, a physical therapist, an occupational therapist, and an orthotist (see Chapter 3 for a discussion of the interdisciplinary approach to treating cerebral palsy). Each team member possesses different skills that he or she can contribute to the decision-making process; however, it is important to remember that someone on the team must be knowledgeable in the growth and development of the immature musculoskeletal system. The child's parents are key members of the team and are integral to any decision-making process.

This chapter briefly discusses the interplay between a child's immature musculoskeletal system and internal and external mechanical forces acting on the musculoskeletal system; the mechanical forces created by an orthosis; and the nomenclature for identifying various orthotic devices, types of orthotic design, and goals of orthotic intervention. The chapter also intertwines various reviews of literature relating to the use of orthotic devices for children with cerebral palsy.

GROWTH AND DEVELOPMENT
OF THE MUSCULOSKELETAL SYSTEM

A child's musculoskeletal system is growing and changing from the cartilaginous model in fetal development to a fully ossified skeleton that is present by the end of puberty. For these reasons, a child's skeleton is more susceptible than is an adult's to both internal and external mechanical forces. Internal forces, such as those produced by the pull of muscles on bones or those produced by the external forces of weight bearing, alter the shape and angle of bones in the immature musculoskeletal system (see Chapters 6 and 7 for a detailed discussion of musculoskeletal development and assessment).

With central nervous system (CNS) damage (e.g., that seen in children with cerebral palsy), alterations in the direction and the strength of muscle pull and weight bearing may occur. These alterations result in abnormal forces on the immature musculoskeletal system and may produce secondary deformities that alter biomechanical alignment of the skeleton. Deformities of the musculoskeletal system can lead to impairments; functional limitations; and, eventually, disability. The altered CNS control of the musculoskeletal system of children with cerebral palsy is associated with impairments of motor control. In addition to abnormal biomechanical alignment deformities, children with cerebral palsy may exhibit inaccurate sequencing and timing of muscle activation, alterations in the normal agonist–antagonist interplay, insufficient force production, and insufficient balance strategies (Damiano, Vaughan, & Abel, 1995; Fetters, 1991; Olney & Wright, 1994). Literature suggests that orthotic devices that are properly designed and aligned will help a child with cerebral palsy overcome some of these difficulties (Baker, Giuliani, Sparling, & Schenkman, 1993; Harris & Riffle, 1986; Lough & Soderberg, 1991; Mossberg, Linton, & Friske, 1990; Ounpuu, Bell, Davis, & DeLuca, 1993).

KINETICS

A basic understanding of the forces acting on the body is necessary to comprehend the purpose and rationale for using an orthotic device and to understand how orthoses affect movement, overall function, and efficiency of gait. Ultimately, both internal and external forces affect movement and the overall function of the child.

The tensile forces generated by the pull of muscles have both a magnitude and a direction. Torque refers to a rotary component produced by these tensile forces. *Torque,* or moment, is defined as the measure of the tendency of a force to produce rotation about a point or an axis. Torque increases as the distance from the joint axis to the line of force is increased (Soderberg, 1986). This concept is important when establishing the length of the shaft or the footplate portion of an orthosis and is discussed in further detail in this chapter with regard to specific orthotic devices.

As a result of gravity, a child's body weight exerts a vertical force downward when he or she is standing or walking. There is an equal and opposite ground-to-foot force, or *ground reaction force* (GRF; Meadows, 1995). GRFs act on the body only when the child's foot is in contact with the ground. The GRF consists of three components during the stance phase of a single step (Rodgers & Cavanaugh, 1984; see Figure 16.1):

1. Vertical
2. Horizontal in an anterior–posterior direction
3. Horizontal in a lateral–medial direction

The GRF is balanced by an internal force generated at the muscles at each joint. When a child is standing in anatomical alignment, minimal force is required by the muscles to maintain this alignment. Normal gait and stance that maintain the GRF line close to the alignment of the joints require less force generation from the child's muscles and may be more energy efficient (Meadows, 1995). Pathological gait or standing postures such as crouched standing posture increase the GRFs. Therefore, the child's muscles must generate increased forces for stability (see Figure 16.2). The magnitude and the direction of the GRF line can be positively influenced by appropriate orthotic design.

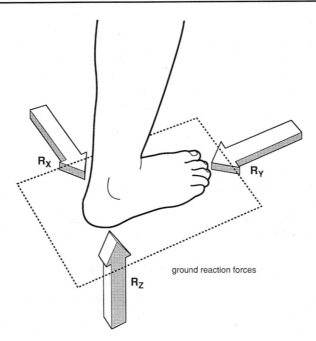

R_X

R_Y

ground reaction forces

R_Z

Figure 16.1. The direction of the ground reaction force exerted on the body surface in response to the body exerted on the ground. R_z represents the vertical force, R_y represents the anterior–posterior force, and R_x represents the lateral-medial force.

Effective design of orthotic devices incorporates principles of GRF control and joint stabilization through three-point pressure control (3PP; see Figure 16.3). GRF control is the technique by which an orthosis maintains the GRF line close to the anatomical joints of the child, and 3PP is a technique that helps to achieve joint stabilization. Control is achieved by locating one point of pressure above the axis of rotation, a second point of pressure below the axis of rotation, and a third opposing point of pressure at or near the axis of rotation. The longer the lever arm, the greater the control. If these points of pressure are distributed within a small area, attention must be given to the possibility of discomfort and the potential for skin breakdown. Pressure can be distributed throughout a larger area by increasing the surface area that is in contact with the skin and by increasing the length, the height, the width, or the circumference of the orthosis.

Orthotic devices also use the concept of an open or closed kinematic chain. The human body can be thought of as a large number of skeletal levers that are linked together by joints and activated by muscles. The linking together of several levers is referred to as a *kinematic chain*. The distal end of the kinematic chain is free in an open kinematic chain; the distal end is fixed in a closed kinematic chain (Deusinger, 1984). Sitting over the edge of a table with the legs dangling is an example of an open kinematic chain, whereas standing is an

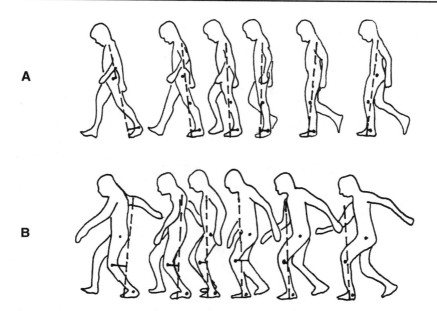

Figure 16.2. Ground reaction force (GRF; see dashed line) for two children. A) The GRF line remains close to the joint axis of the hip and knee in the typically developing 7 year old. B) The GRF line is displaced from the joint axis for the child with spastic diplegia. Displacement of the GRF line results in increased force generation and increased energy.

example of a closed kinematic chain. In closed kinematic chain activities, forces or motions that are distally applied have a proximal effect throughout the kinematic chain, which is caused by the linking of the segments. For example, an abnormal hindfoot position during stance will affect the structures of the knee and the hip. Walking is an example of an activity that involves alternating closed and open kinematic chain activities.

Many of the orthotic devices that are used to assist children with cerebral palsy aim to improve the child's ambulation skills. The accurate prescription of an orthotic device also requires an intimate understanding of the various phases of the gait cycle. Orthotic devices may significantly affect stance phase of a child's gait; however, they also may influence the swing phase. The stance phase consists of three components (i.e., rockers) (see Figure 16.4). The first rocker is heel strike to foot flat; the second rocker refers to having the foot flat as the tibia rolls forward, producing ankle dorsiflexion; and the third rocker, or the last component of stance phase, refers to heel-off to toe-off.

In summary, the key elements for members of an interdisciplinary team to consider when prescribing and determining the effectiveness of an orthosis for a child with cerebral palsy include

• An in-depth knowledge of the musculoskeletal development of children

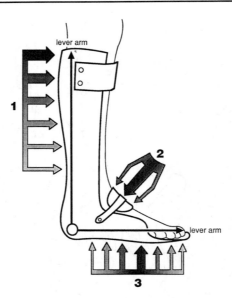

Figure 16.3. Three-point pressure control system over ankle plantarflexion. The arrows indicate the magnitude and location of the pressure.

- An understanding of the effects of internally and externally applied forces on an immature musculoskeletal system
- An understanding of how internal and external forces may be altered when using an orthotic device
- An understanding of the potential beneficial and detrimental influences that may be produced by an orthosis

An orthosis must also be evaluated for the effects that it may have on the joint(s) that it contacts and the effects it may have on the joints in the kinematic chain above and below the orthosis. Members of the interdisciplinary team involved in the prescription of an orthosis must have an in-depth understanding of the child's gait cycle and how the specific orthotic device and its components will affect this cycle. Prescribing an orthosis is complicated and requires the expertise of various members of the team.

NOMENCLATURE

There is some confusion and overlap surrounding the terms orthosis and splint. The same principles of alignment, goals, and action for effectiveness apply to both terms. An *orthosis* is defined as a device to straighten or correct a deformity, or disability, of the lower or upper extremities or the spine, whereas a *splint* is defined as a device used for the fixation, union, or protection of an

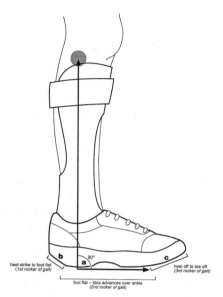

Figure 16.4. Combining the shoe, the orthosis, and the rockers of gait. A) The "combination angle" of footwear-heel height plus the orthotic device foot shaft angle creates the effective ground reaction force pattern. B) A cushioned or sach heel can improve the first rocker of gait by minimizing the "fulcrum" effect. C) A beveled or rockered toe can smooth the third rocker of gait by reducing unwanted ground reaction force, or knee extension moment.

injured part of the body (Thomas, 1977). However, new applications of the term splint often are used by rehabilitation professionals. For the sake of clarity, this chapter uses the following definitions:

- **Orthosis** A custom-made or custom-fit device designed to support and improve the function of the lower extremity, the upper extremity, or the spine. Orthoses are often fabricated from a plaster model by an orthotist, and they incorporate the use of high-temperature plastic materials. Orthoses are more durable and versatile than splints and may be more appropriate for an active child or an older child. In general, orthoses offer more options for joints and variable motion joints than splints (Cusick, 1990, 1995).
- **Splint** A device fabricated from a low-temperature plastic. Splints are often fabricated by a therapist or an orthotist as diagnostic tools or interim devices. Splints take less time than orthoses to fabricate, are directly molded on a child, and may be used as an alternative to more expensive orthoses for a small child who is growing rapidly or for a child whose function and alignment may be changing rapidly as a result of a recent injury or surgical intervention. Splints are often used for short-term intervention, as a trial before fabricating an orthosis, and for smaller children (Cusick, 1990, 1995).

Orthotic devices are identified by the anatomical joints that they are designed to support. An orthotic device usually contacts or encompasses the limb all the way up to the joint(s) and includes the joint as well as the shaft portion of the limb before the next proximal joint. For example, an ankle-foot orthosis (AFO) contacts the ankle and foot as well as a portion of the lower leg up to the knee; however, it does not include the knee. The following list is a categorization of common orthotic devices and the specific orthoses that may be included within each of these categories. (The orthotic devices are listed from most distal to most proximal and from those that offer the least to the most support.)

1. **Foot orthosis (FO)** A device that contacts all or a portion of the sole of the foot with very low or nonexistent medial and lateral trim lines or high trim lines that extend to the malleoli (i.e., bony structure on either side of the ankle joint). Different types of FOs include the following:

   Heel cup or heel seat: A device that aims to hold the calcaneus (i.e., heel bone) and overlying soft tissues firmly; trim lines are below the malleoli, and the medial trim line is often higher (see Figure 16.5A). This orthotic device often does not extend to the child's toes and is cut proximal to the metatarsal heads.

   University of California Biomechanics Laboratory (UCBL): An orthotic device that is molded to grip the calcaneus firmly with a higher medial trim line (see Figure 16.5B). The plantar surface is molded to support the child's longitudinal arch and extends to just proximal to the heads of the metatarsal bones (Carlson & Bergland, 1979).

   Supramalleolar orthosis (SMO): A device that extends proximally to above the malleoli but has low anterior and posterior trim lines (see Figure 16.5C). This orthotic device often extends to the child's toes.

2. **Dynamic ankle-foot orthosis (DAFO)** This orthotic device is fabricated from a thin flexible plastic and wraps around the child's foot to provide a total contact fit and to hold the child's heel and forefoot in optimal biomechanical position (see Figure 16.5D). DAFOs can be fabricated in a multitude of styles and, therefore, cannot be categorized simply as an FO or an AFO.

3. **Ankle-foot orthosis** A device that includes contact and support of the child's foot as well as his or her ankle and extends up the shaft of the lower leg; however, it does not include the child's knee. Different types of AFOs include the following:

   Solid AFO: Device that allows no motion at the ankle joint. The shaft contacts the posterior portion of the child's lower leg (see Figure 16.6B).

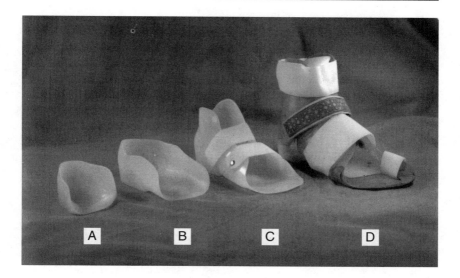

Figure16.5. Foot orthoses in order of increasing control. A) Heel cup. B) UCBL. C) Supra-malleolar orthosis. D) Dynamic ankle-foot orthosis.

Floor reaction orthosis: A solid AFO with a rigid anterior section of the shaft. The shaft contacts the anterior portion of the child's lower leg and promotes knee extension (see Figure 16.6D).

Articulated AFO (see Figure 16.6C): A device that offers variable degrees of motion at the child's ankle with a hinge or variable motion ankle joint. A leaf spring offers motion with the type of material used, the thinning of the material, or the design of the orthosis to create a flexion point within the material (see Figure 16.6A).

4. **Knee-ankle-foot orthosis (KAFO)** A device that includes contact and support of the child's foot and ankle as well as his or her knee and extends to the proximal aspect of the child's thigh.
5. **Hip-knee-ankle-foot orthosis (HKAFO)** A device that includes contact and support of the child's knee, foot, ankle, and hip. A pelvic band is typically used to connect the right and left legs of the orthosis.
6. **Thoracolumbosacral orthosis (TLSO)** A device that offers complete coverage of the child's trunk. Also known as "body jacket," a TLSO can have either a posterior or an anterior opening and can be fabricated from rigid or from soft materials.

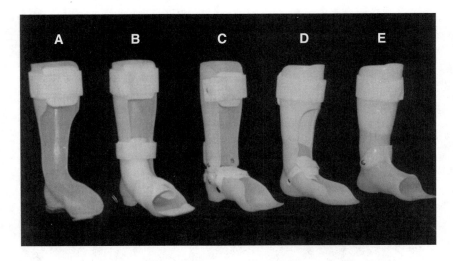

Figure 16.6. Types of ankle-foot orthoses (AFO). A) Posterior leaf spring. B) Solid AFO. C) Articulated AFO. D) Anterior floor reaction orthosis (FRO). E) Articulated FRO.

MATERIALS

Various types of materials provide the general structure of an orthosis and give the device strength, form, and flexibility. Proper material selection enhances the function of the orthotic device. The following is a list of the materials that are frequently used:

- **High-temperature thermoplastic materials:** These plastics range from flexible polyethylenes to semirigid copolymers and very rigid natural polypropylene. These materials come in sheets and require molding temperatures in excess of 300 degrees Fahrenheit. They are molded on a cast model of the child's limb or foot and not directly on the child.
- **Low-temperature thermoplastic materials:** These splinting materials are heated in warm water to a malleable state and then molded directly on the child. Examples of low-temperature materials are Aquaplast and Orthoplast.
- **Foam:** There are a wide variety of density foams (from soft to firm) that are used with children to cushion areas of increased pressure and bony structures. Firm foams are used for extrinsic posting.

COMPONENTS

The individual features of an orthosis that provide specialized function play a significant part in the functioning of most orthotic devices (see Figure 16.7).

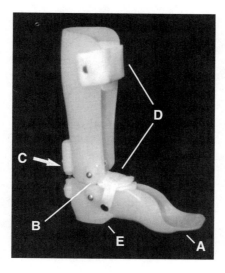

Figure 16.7. Sample components of ankle-foot orthosis. A) Toeplate, B) ankle joint, C) joint range motion limiter, D) straps at the calf and the ankle, E) extrinsic heel stabilizing post.

1. **Trim lines** Trim lines are the borders that define the height, the length, the width, and the circumference of an orthosis. Trim lines must accurately reflect the intended 3PP and the GRF controls. For example, a child who presents with severe forefoot valgus will require an increase in length and height of the lateral forefoot control trim line to compliment the medial trim line and improve 3PP control.

2. **Footplate** There are two separate definitions of the term *footplate*.
   - The portion of the orthosis in contact with the child's foot. This may include the plantar and dorsal surfaces and the medial and lateral walls of the orthosis.
   - A premolded and/or customized plate that is used to preposition foot structures, including the toe elevations, the peroneal arch, the metatarsal arch, the longitudinal arch, and the forefoot. The footplate is placed in contact with the foot at the time of casting and incorporated into the negative impression (see Figure 16.8).

3. **Toeplate** The portion of the footplate that extends from the metatarsal heads to the end of the toes. Toeplates are used to properly align and support the child's toes in functional relationship to his or her foot. A toeplate with elevation is useful in controlling a strong toe grasp or clawing of the toes.

4. **Joints** A mechanical joint is inserted in the fabrication process of an orthosis that coincides with the child's anatomical joint position and permits motion to occur at that anatomical joint. Mechanical joints usually have a

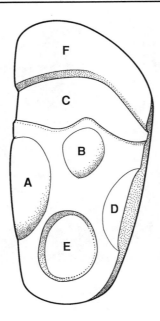

Figure 16.8. Specialized footplate that is used when casting an orthosis to ensure the strategic location of foot control. A) Longitudinal arch, B) Metatarsal arch, C) Metatarsal head depression, D) Peroneal arch, E) Heel cup, F) Toe positioning plate.

single axis, which allows for motion in only one plane. Motion at a mechanical joint may be adjustable, depending on the commercially available joint inserted in the orthosis.

5. **Strapping** Sections of material or Velcro that attach the orthosis to the child's limb, provide additional stability, and/or complete a 3PP control pattern. The materials used to construct the straps and the position of the straps can greatly enhance the alignment of the child's foot and limb and promote or limit his or her motion.

FABRICATION OF CUSTOM ORTHOSES

This section explains the fabrication process for the orthoses, proper positioning of the child during the fabrication process, and the adjustments made to the orthosis to reduce or increase the effect of GRFs and to improve the child's alignment and function.

Negative Impression

An orthosis begins with an accurately formed negative impression that is made directly on the child's limb with plaster or fiberglass. Positioning the child is vital to achieving an accurate plaster mold; to ensure optimal alignment, careful consideration must be given to the child's individual foot structures. Prone positioning provides maximum visibility for alignment of the child's hindfoot, his or her midfoot, and the sole and the arches of the foot. When prone positioning is not possible for a variety of reasons (e.g., strong extensor tone in prone positioning, anxiety and fear experienced by the child), a stable sitting position can be used for obtaining the plaster mold. When seated, the child's hip and knee should be flexed to minimize the influence of extensor tone on the position of the foot. To assist in obtaining proper positioning and alignment, available personnel, including the child's parents, should always be involved. Distraction techniques and toys will allay the child's anxiety and promote ease of positioning and alignment (see Figure 16.9).

Positive Model

A positive model is created when liquid plaster is used to fill the hollow of a negative impression. After the plaster dries, the negative wrap is removed to expose the positive model. The plaster model then can be modified to enhance the intrinsic fit and the alignment of the definitive orthosis. At this point, sheet plastic is heated to a moldable temperature and applied to the positive plaster model. Vacuum (i.e., the mechanically suctioned removal of the air) is applied to ensure a precise duplication of the positive model. Further extrinsic modifications may be added to the definitive orthosis or footwear.

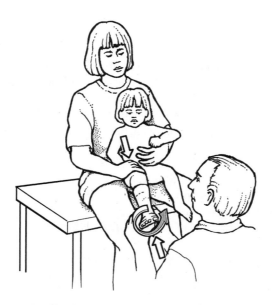

Figure 16.9. Technique for casting younger children. Position the child securely between the parent's legs; and flex the hip, knee, and ankle. The parent can provide a useful third hand to stabilize the child's leg while the orthotist positions the foot and ankle.

Intrinsic Modification

Intrinsic modifications are present within the structure of the orthosis and are incorporated during the fabrication process. Modifications to the positive plaster model, such as a buildup (i.e., an addition) of plaster to relieve a bony structure (e.g., the malleoli) or plaster removal to increase the depth of the metatarsal arch area, result in permanent intrinsic design.

Extrinsic Modification

Extrinsic modifications are added to an orthosis. These modifications, often referred to as posting (see next section on "Posting"), are in addition to the structural intrinsic design and are often applied to further enhance alignment. For example, the medial-lateral stability of a UCBL is increased by adding an external extrinsic post to the heel of the orthosis. An extrinsic modification also may be added to an orthosis internally. An example of an extrinsic modification added internally is a firm foam wedge on the footplate surface under the first and second metatarsal heads to accommodate a fixed varus forefoot position. Extrinsic modifications can often be removed or repositioned.

Posting

Posting is a strategy to fine-tune the direction of the GRFs, to enhance alignment, and to accommodate fixed deformities through the application of extrinsic materials (i.e., hard or soft foam) to specific locations of an orthosis.

ORTHOTIC DEVICES

In 1994, the International Society for Prosthetics and Orthotics (ISPO) held a consensus conference to examine the published evidence pertaining to the use of orthotic devices and to attempt to determine how and when orthoses should be used for children with cerebral palsy (Condie, 1995). The conference planning committee formulated the following list of "Aims or Objectives for Orthotic Treatment":

- To prevent and/or correct deformity
- To provide a base of support
- To facilitate training in skills
- To improve the efficiency of gait (Condie, 1995, p. 1)

Although this list of aims of orthotic treatment is very similar to the lists developed by Cusick (1990) and Knutson and Clark (1991), this chapter uses the list formulated by the ISPO to examine the use of orthotic devices.

At the conclusion of the ISPO Consensus Conference, a list of 29 conclusions and recommendations was formulated (see Appendix at the end of this chapter). These conclusions and recommendations are the foundation for the knowledge in the field of orthotic management of children with cerebral palsy. This list should serve as a basis for reference, for critical thinking, and for the future research of clinicians who work with children who have cerebral palsy and in orthotic management of cerebral palsy.

FOOTWEAR

The importance of the selection and modification of footwear, shoes, or sneakers for children with cerebral palsy must be emphasized. Footwear selection affects the child's motion in the sagittal, frontal, and transverse planes and may enhance the child's GRFs. The effective position of the orthosis in combination with the footwear sets the stage for stability in the stance phase of gait. One of the conclusions of the ISPO Consensus Conference was that footwear modifications—alone or in conjunction with orthoses—may produce beneficial effects, such as promoting more normal external joint movements, which may prevent overactivity of certain muscle groups (Condie, 1995).

The ISPO Consensus Conference also defined the design criteria for footwear that should be used with orthoses and that may assist families during the selection process. The criteria include the following:

1. A nonslip sole on the shoe for stance phase mobility
2. A wide toe box and opening throat for adequate orthotic forefoot space
3. A secure anterior closure to maintain the foot in the orthosis
4. A sturdy upper construction to prevent movement of the orthosis within the shoe during ambulation
5. Removable insoles
6. Footwear that can be stretched to significantly increase space for an orthosis (Weber, 1995)

Footwear will affect the child during the first rocker of gait. A firm or hard heel, coupled with a solid or a 90-degree plantar stop AFO, will act as a fulcrum to accelerate knee flexion and reduce the child's control of early stance. A low, soft, or cushioned heel, by contrast, will absorb the GRFs during the first rocker. This absorption of the GRFs will reduce the knee flexion moment and slow the first rocker, thereby increasing the child's control (see Figure 16.4).

Stability at the orthosis/shoe interface is required at mid-stance, or second rocker, to minimize unwanted motion and to effectively transmit intrinsic and extrinsic shoe modifications to the orthosis. The effect of the heel height of the shoe in combination with the orthosis (i.e., the combination angle) must be calculated. For example, a solid AFO set in 0-degree dorsiflexion gains 2–3 degrees of effective dorsiflexion when combined with a shoe of moderate heel height. The extra degrees of dorsiflexion will increase the knee flexion moment throughout stance phase. Clinically, variations in the footwear–orthosis "combination angle" (see Figure 16.4) can affect the overall flexion or the extension position of the child's knee.

Extrinsic shoe modifications to improve the third rocker of gait for children wearing a solid AFO are performed by tapering the sole of the shoe from the metatarsal heads forward to the end of the shoe. The rockering of a shoe when using any solid AFO will mechanically enhance forward momentum by increasing the speed of progression from heel-off to toe-off (Cusick, 1990). This is accomplished through the elimination of unwanted GRFs, or reduced knee extension moment.

DISCUSSION OF INDIVIDUAL ORTHOTIC DEVICES

The discussion for each category of orthotic device includes design characteristics, indications and contraindications for the use of the orthosis, actions of the orthosis during swing and stance phases of gait, and any research evidence to support or refute the use of orthotic devices for children with cerebral palsy.

Foot Orthoses

Foot orthoses act primarily in the frontal and transverse planes of motion during the stance phase of gait and aim to stabilize and align the hindfoot, midfoot, and/or forefoot. It is theorized that foot orthoses provide improved proximal joint alignment via the closed kinematic chain (Cusick, 1990; Embry, Yates, & Mott, 1990; Hylton, 1989; Small, 1995). Minimal control of plantarflexion or dorsiflexion is offered because the anterior and posterior trim lines below the ankle do not establish the necessary 3PP control to restrict motion.

This category of devices addresses abnormal pronation and supination. Pronation is the most common transverse plane deformity of the foot and the ankle in children with spastic diplegia (Gage, 1991). Abnormal pronation renders the foot less propulsive, shortens stride length, decreases the knee extension moment, reduces the stability of the foot as a base of support, increases energy consumption, and promotes progression of the deformity. Children with hemiplegia often walk with a varus or a supinated foot. A supinated position of the foot also interferes with propulsion at toe-off, thereby resulting in secondary deformities of the foot and the ankle and decreasing the efficiency of gait. Foot orthoses, ranging from minimal to maximal control, address the severity of the pronation or supination deformity.

Indications   Foot orthotics, including SMOs and other ankle height devices, work well with children who are able to ambulate independently but exhibit mild to moderate symptoms, such as the following:

- Medial/lateral instability of the subtalar joint
- Mid-foot instability, resulting in the forefoot being valgus or varus

- Mild to moderate spasticity
- Need for reduction of hypertonic foot reflex activity (Hylton, 1989)

Contraindications Foot orthoses generally are not recommended if the following parameters exist:

1. Lack of voluntary ankle dorsiflexion control
2. Moderate to severe spasticity
3. Fixed equinus toe drag during swing
4. Compromised proximal joint function and alignment
5. Inability to achieve heel strike
6. Inability to ambulate (Cusick, 1995)

Actions In order to discuss the swing and stance phases of gait, the four phases of the gait cycle are presented.

1. **Swing phase** Most FOs that have trim lines below the malleoli do not augment the swing phase of gait. FOs are unable to assist with foot clearance if the child exhibits weak ankle dorsiflexors or an equinus foot position during swing. An SMO design may afford limited plantarflexion control with the addition of a low-level posterior plantar resist strap or a higher posterior trim line. These additions may assist in pre-positioning the child's foot for initial contact.
2. **First rocker** Ankle plantarflexion at heel strike, leading to foot flat, is generally unrestricted with FOs.
3. **Second rocker** FOs maintain optimal alignment for improved stance stability and lever arm efficiency. Forward progression (i.e., ankle dorsiflexion) of the tibia over the foot is not restricted.
4. **Third rocker** Improved alignment during the second rocker stabilizes the child's foot for a more efficient push-off during the third rocker.

When an orthotic design extends to the child's toes, the orthotic toe plate and the shoe should be flexible or rockered in order to simulate toe extension and thereby reduce unwanted GRFs from the second and third rockers of gait (Lin, 1995).

Research Evidence Using a single-subject design, researchers evaluated the effects of an inhibitive AFO on the standing balance of a child with spastic quadriplegia (Harris & Riffle, 1986). An inhibitive AFO appears to be similar in design and height to a supramalleolar orthosis and appears to be the precursor to dynamic AFOs. Improved symmetry in stance and a longer duration of independent standing was observed when the child was wearing an orthosis compared with when the child was not wearing the orthosis.

Taylor and Harris (1986) described a case study that examined the effects of inhibitive AFOs on the functional motor performance of a child with spastic diplegia. Standing balance, ball-catching activities, and the fine-motor portion of the Peabody Developmental Scale were evaluated first with the child wearing inhibitive AFOs and later with the inhibitive AFOs removed. No quantitative differences were noted—with or without the inhibitive AFOs—with the standing balance and ball-catching activities. The child's score on the Peabody Developmental Scale was within the normal limits in two or three areas when the orthosis was worn and below 1 standard deviation from the mean in all three areas when the orthosis was not worn.

Yamamoto (1992) compared two types of SMOs (one with a solid back and one with a U-cut back) with the gait parameters of three children with cerebral palsy. Results of the study varied for stride length, for velocity, and for ankle-joint angles. Improvements were noted with heel strike and with position of the knee at initial contact with the solid-back SMO compared with the U-cut back SMO.

Dynamic Ankle-Foot Orthosis

As described previously, DAFOs are very thin, flexible, supramalleolar, total-contact orthoses with a custom contoured soleplate that supports and stabilizes the dynamic arches of the foot (Hylton, 1989). Cascade Prosthetics and Orthotics Co. (1996) defined the DAFO as an orthotic device that centers on a thin, flexible plastic that has a total contact fit shell to hold the child's heel and forefoot in correct biomechanical position. Although DAFOs appear to have been similar to a supramalleolar orthosis, with the addition of a contoured soleplate and a wraparound foot design, the DAFO concept has been incorporated into many styles of lower-extremity orthoses. There is also confusion in the literature regarding the terms *inhibitive AFO* and *dynamic AFO*. There appears to be a close similarity between their designs and their aims for control; however, DAFOs incorporate design principles that differ from other orthoses of similar style, height, and aim for control.

The thin, flexible material used in the fabrication of DAFOs allows for a small amount of natural triplanar motion to occur at the child's foot and the ankle. The rigid materials used with more standard orthotic devices allow less flexibility for small or no degrees of motion. Mechanical joints used in an articulated AFO permit motion in only one plane. The flexibility of the DAFO may simulate the complexity of the child's natural motions at the foot and the ankle, which occur in more than one plane of motion. The total contact fit of a DAFO may also help to increase proprioceptive feedback to the child.

Design Characteristics   The DAFO features six unique characteristics that may be beneficial for supporting the child with cerebral palsy:

1. A thin flexible shell that wraps around the child's foot, providing a total contact fit

2. Alignment of the child's subtalar joint in neutral position, with the forefoot aligned in relation to the hindfoot
3. Support for the natural arches of the child's foot
4. Support for under the child's toes, enabling his or her toes to meet the horizontal plane.
5. An instep strap to maintain total contact of the foot and to secure the child's forefoot position
6. Various heights, which are dependent on the design and the goal of the specific orthosis (The height of DAFOs cited in literature is most commonly the same height as a SMO [i.e., to mid-calf].)

Indications and Contraindications   Various styles of DAFOs are fabricated to meet the particular needs of each child. The style of DAFO chosen for the child should be considered just as any other style of orthotic device is considered. The specific alignment considerations and the level of functional standing or ambulation will determine the style that best meets the needs of each particular child.

Actions   In 1989, Hylton proposed that DAFOs have at least three positive effects: 1) the total contact flexible fit should be more easily tolerated by the child, and skin breakdown problems should be negligible; 2) the stability and proprioceptive feedback should assist the child with balance and postural control; and 3) the custom-contoured footboard should provide support to the child's natural arches and contours of the foot.

Research Evidence   Subjective clinical research on DAFOs shows that the device provides ease of positioning in wheelchairs and standers; improvements in postural and tone control, in balance when standing, and in weight bearing for the child with hemiplegia; as well as increased use of the involved arm for the child with hemiplegia (Hylton, 1989). However, it is important to remember that these findings are subjective and need to be substantiated by clinical research.

Solid Ankle-Foot Orthosis

The thermoplastic solid AFO introduced in the late 1960s offered a clear advantage over the traditional hightop shoe with metal uprights. The ability to customize fabrication promoted individualized alignment and support of the foot and the ankle. As a partial result of this advance, biomechanical and neurophysiological approaches have been incorporated into the orthotic management of children with cerebral palsy.

Design Characteristics   The truly rigid solid AFO was at one time a standard prescription for children with cerebral palsy. However, the trend in the 1990s is toward allowing increased joint mobility to improve the gait efficiency and function of children with cerebral palsy. The following features should be present in all solid AFOs:

1. The plastic should be of appropriate strength and design to prevent it from distorting when loaded, or weight bearing.
2. Footplate control modifications (previously discussed in the section on FO) should be incorporated.
3. The footwear should complement the AFO design.
4. The toe plate should range from flexible to rigid, depending on the desired effect.
5. The solid AFO should extend from just below the fibular head (avoiding pressure over the peroneal nerve) to the metatarsal heads or the end of the toes.
6. The ankle strap or other straps should be used to complete the 3PP control or maintain position.
7. The trim line patterns should reflect appropriate varus or valgus control of the hindfoot, mid-foot, and forefoot.

Indications and Contraindications A solid AFO may be used for children who are nonambulatory to prevent contracture of the plantarflexor muscles in children with significant spasticity; to provide foot and ankle stability, enabling the child to use a standing device; or to provide postoperative management after surgical lengthening of the Achilles tendon or fusions of joints of the foot. A solid AFO may be used for children who are ambulatory 1) to control the muscle tone imbalances of the foot and ankle, which are seen when the child ambulates; 2) to facilitate heel contact during gait for children who walk with their feet plantarflexed; 3) to control a mild crouched gait pattern; 4) to provide control for moderate to severe varus or valgus muscle imbalances or deformities; or 5) to provide support when limited ankle dorsiflexion range of motion (ROM) results in mid-foot collapse and pronation while weight bearing. The use of a solid AFO is generally contraindicated if the addition of motion at the child's ankle will improve function or improve the efficiency of his or her gait or transfers.

Actions During each phase of the gait cycle, the specific actions or functions of the solid AFO can be highlighted. The following is a list of the functions during the swing phase and during the first, second, and third rocker.

- Swing phase: Pre-positions the child's foot for ground clearance and heel strike
- First rocker: Initial contact should occur with a heel strike, or it may pass directly to foot flat. The fixed ankle eliminates plantarflexion action that stabilizes and decelerates heel strike to foot flat. The result is a rapid knee flexion moment or "fulcrum effect" that can be reduced by softening the heel (sach) of the shoes to absorb torque.
- Second rocker: The solid AFO provides a stable foundation for single limb weight bearing with 3PP control of the foot and ankle. However, ankle dorsiflexion (i.e., foreword progression of the tibia) is blocked, thereby influencing

the GRFs on the knee and increasing the knee extension moment as the body progresses forward. Choosing and fine tuning the AFO–footwear combination angle can assist with smoothing the gait and producing a more efficient gait pattern. For example, an AFO set in 5–7 degrees of dorsiflexion promotes knee flexion during stance. This flexion moment counteracts knee hyperextension and promotes a smooth forward progression from mid-stance to toe-off (Weber, 1995). An AFO set in 0–4 degrees of dorsiflexion provides a beneficial knee extension moment that may be needed to reduce a knee-flexed gait (Weber, 1995). Children who exhibit hip and knee flexion contractures will require an increased compensatory dorsiflexion angle to promote balance.

- Third rocker: Minimizing the prolonged knee extension moment that is produced by a lack of dorsiflexion is necessary for a child to have smooth forward progression and maximum propulsion. A solid AFO set in a slight dorsiflexion of 2–3 degrees improves the second and third rocker of gait. Shoe and toe plate modifications also can assist the child with minimizing the knee extension moment.

Research Evidence In 1990, researchers evaluated the energy expenditure in children with spastic diplegia while the children walked at self-selected speeds with and without their prescribed AFOs (Mossberg et. al, 1990). The study did not differentiate between solid or articulated AFOs. The investigators found that the children expended less energy when walking with their prescribed AFOs as compared with walking without the AFOs. However, the differences between the walking trials were not statistically significant. Further investigation specifying the type of AFO may provide valuable information regarding the energy expenditure and the use of orthotic devices.

Floor Reaction Orthosis

Most lower-extremity orthotic devices that make contact with the ground employ GRFs in order to be effective. However, the floor reaction orthosis (FRO) (see Figure 16.6D) is specifically designed to serve this purpose. The concept of the FRO, or ground reaction orthosis, was introduced in 1969 as an alternative to the KAFO. It was designed for the management of postpolio paralysis to stabilize the knee in extension during stance (Saltiel, 1969). The floor reaction principle has been applied to the management of children with cerebral palsy to assist children who walk with a moderately to severely crouched or a knee flexion posture. The primary cause of a crouched gait pattern is weakness of the ankle plantarflexors (either primary or secondary) with associated hamstring tightness and/or weak quadriceps (Harrington, Lin, & Gage, 1984; Sutherland & Cooper, 1978; Sutherland, Cooper, & Daniel, 1980). Increased work of the muscle in inefficient biomechanical alignment results in a gait pattern that uses greater energy consumption (Perry, 1992). The use of KAFOs to counteract this crouched gait pattern was the approach used prior to FROs; however, they generally failed because of their bulkiness, their inefficient joint excursion, and their high energy cost. FROs can be an effective alternative.

Design Characteristics   The FRO has a plastic solid ankle design with a rigid anterior compartment at the level of the tibial tubercle. The orthosis is usually set in plantarflexion and acts to produce an extension moment at the knee. The FRO has five unique characteristics:

1. Posterior entry
2. Rigid anterior panel just below the tibial tubercle
3. Rigid or articulated ankle with dorsiflexion stop
4. Toe plate extending the lever arm to the end of the toes (may range from flexible to rigid) to increase knee extension moment
5. Proximal strap to complete 3PP (Additional straps may be used if necessary to maintain position.)

Careful consideration should always be given to the AFO–footwear combination. It is recommended that some dorsiflexion angle be used be incorporated to enhance efficient forward progression (Harrington et al., 1984).

Indications and Contraindications   The FRO is an effective orthotic device for assisting children with cerebral palsy to improve their gait efficiency if the child presents with either or with both of the following characteristics: 1) weakness of the ankle plantarflexion and/or quadriceps muscle groups or 2) crouched stance and gait. FROs are most effective when used with children who present with the previously discussed impairments. FROs are not effective and are contraindicated for children who present with hip and knee flexion contractures greater than 10 degrees and for children who are nonambulatory or who ambulate with their knees extended and ankles dorsiflexed.

Actions   The solid FRO provides a strong knee extension moment and support to the tibia during the second rocker. This support reduces the energy requirement of the quadriceps muscles to control the knee and assists with promoting knee extension if the child walks with a crouched gait pattern. An articulated version of the FRO (see Figure 16.6E) allows plantarflexion ROM but does not permit dorsiflexion motion. The plantarflexion motion provides a smoother, more controlled first rocker and facilitates active push-off with plantarflexion muscles during the third rocker.

Research Evidence   The staff at Newington Children's Hospital (Hartford, Connecticut) found that often it was necessary to modify the foot–shaft angle from a 0-degree setting of dorsiflexion to a 5-degree setting of dorsiflexion for children wearing bilateral FROs. This modification decreased the knee extension moment and promoted smoother transition from the second to the third rocker of gait (Harrington et al., 1984).

Articulated Ankle-Foot Orthosis

The articulated AFO is the most versatile orthotic available for the management of lower-extremity alignment concerns in ambulatory children with cerebral palsy. An articulated AFO offers the intimate fit that a child needs to control his or her hindfoot, mid foot, and forefoot (see section on "Foot Orthosis" in this chapter). A variety of joints are available to customize control of ankle motion and its consequent impact on the knee' functioning (see Figure 16.10).

There are some orthotic designs that provide the benefit of anatomical joint motion through flexible resistance and without the use of mechanical joints. This technique employs the use of more naturally flexible materials, such as polyethylene, compressible padding, or simple thinning or trimming of the material to permit motion. The relative position of the trim line behind the malleoli in the posterior leaf spring orthosis creates a flexion point allowing ankle dorsiflexion during the second and third rockers and limits plantarflexion for foot clearance during the swing phase (Lin, 1995). Dynamic AFOs employ thin, flexible material and soft pads that allow mild pronation and supination within a total contact orthosis (Hylton, 1989), and a flexible toe plate allows flexion and extension of the metatarsal phalangeal joints. A specific style DAFO permits ankle dorsiflexion or forward progression of the third tibia through the use of a shorter shaft component and no anterior shaft strap.

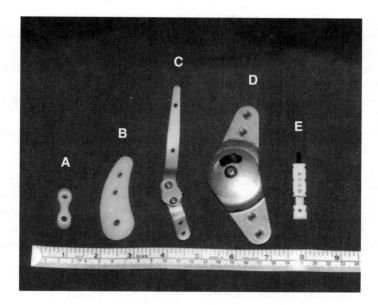

Figure 16.10. Various pediatric ankle joint options. A) Tamarac Flexor Joint, a free motion joint; B) Oklahoma Ankle Joint, a free motion joint; C) Kid-Dee-Lite, an adjustable range of motion (ROM) joint; D) Camber Axis Hinge, an adjustable ROM joint; E) Motion Control Limiter, which is used in combination with free motion joints.

Design Characteristics   Most articulated AFOs for ambulatory children have a neutral plantarflexion stop that allows for dorsiflexion beyond neutral position but prevents plantarflexion. This is to help prevent plantarflexion contractures and allows for a more functional gait. With improvements in pediatric componetry, an articulated AFO can be set up with any variation of free or limited ankle motion; flexible resistance stops can also be incorporated. In addition, a variety of mechanical joints with variable motion options are commercially available. These options allow team members to "fine-tune" the range of ankle dorsiflexion and plantarflexion.

With the use of gait analysis, research has found that subtle changes in the angle of an AFO, either with ROM settings at the ankle or with footwear, will shift the GRF line. A small increase in ankle dorsiflexion and its consequent posterior shift of the GRF line was shown to reduce the hip flexor moment, thereby reducing the demand on the hip extensor muscles. This fine-tuning may improve the quality and the efficiency of the child's walking pattern. The following features must be considered when fabricating a typical articulated AFO:

- Plastic of appropriate strength and design to prevent it from distorting when loaded
- Firm control of the child's hindfoot, mid-foot, and forefoot (as described in the "Foot Orthosis" section in this chapter)
- Toe plate ranging from flexible to rigid, depending on the desired effect
- Mechanical axis corresponding as closely as possible to the axis of the child's ankle
- Extension from just below the fibular head, covering the posterior portion of the lower leg, to the metatarsal heads or the end of the toes
- Ankle strap, a proximal strap, or other straps that are necessary to complete 3PP control or maintain position
- The footwear should complement the AFO to create the desired footwear–AFO combination angle

Indications and Contraindications   Variable amounts of ankle motion will allow a more functional and efficient gait pattern. Children who are active and are able to use stairs, able to rise up and down from the floor, and able to rise to standing from a chair will benefit from an articulated AFO, as opposed to a solid AFO. The following characteristics are indications that a child would benefit from the articulated AFO:

1. Passive ankle dorsiflexion ROM of 5–10 degrees (Cusick, 1990; Weber, 1995)
2. Presence of toe drag during swing phase
3. Absence of heel strike or the presence of toe walking

The importance of available passive ankle dorsiflexion to at least 5–10 degrees above neutral position must be stressed. If the child cannot achieve 5–10 degrees of dorsiflexion, the weight-bearing moment is transferred to his or her mid-foot. As a result, compensatory subtalar joint pronation with collapse and excessive pronation of the mid-foot will substitute for the lack of talocrural dorsiflexion motion. The excessive pronation may lead to pressure and skin breakdown, especially at the head of the navicular. Therefore, sufficient ankle dorsiflexion must be achieved prior to the use of an articulated AFO. Serial casting and/or surgical lengthening may be necessary for the child to achieve sufficient dorsiflexion range prior to fitting of an articulated AFO.

The following characteristics are contraindications that a child would not benefit from the use of an articulated AFO:

1. Fixed plantarflexion contracture that prevents the child from achieving at least 5–10 degrees of passive dorsiflexion
2. Significant weakness of plantarflexor muscles (see section on "FRO")
3. Knee flexion contractures

Actions   During each phase of the gait cycle, the articulated AFO can be broken down into specific actions or functions. Listed below are the functions during the swing phase and during the first, second, and third rocker:

- Swing phase: Pre-positions the foot for ground clearance, heel strike, or initial contact
- First rocker: Initial contact should occur with a heel strike. Limited plantarflexion will still cause some "fulcrum effect." Increasing range at the ankle joint when permissible and a soft sach heel will benefit the user's control.
- Second rocker: The child's increased ankle dorsiflexion range allows for a more natural advancement of the tibia over the foot, resulting in a natural stretch of the Achilles tendon and promoting a smooth progression of the body's mass over the supporting limb. Additional GRFs used to control the knee are available when limited ankle ROM parameters are employed.
- Third rocker: The standard 90-degree plantarflexion stop reduces push-off efficiency by blocking the propulsive action of the plantarflexion range that is typically available. The toe plate can be flexible or rigid to enhance the desired effect.

In terms of assisting a child with spastic diplegia who ambulates independently in a moderate crouched posture, several options are available. Using articulated AFOs, a dorsiflexion stop set at 5 degrees will use GRFs at mid-stance to counteract the child's knee flexion moment and promote the child's knee extension. A plantarflexion stop set at 10 degrees of plantarflexion will permit plantarflexion to aid in deceleration of the child's leg during first rocker and allows for improved push-off efficiency at the third rocker and strengthening of the plantarflexor muscles.

In terms of assisting a child with hemiplegia who ambulates with ankle plantarflexion throughout the stance phase and exhibits knee hyperextension at mid-stance on the involved side, full passive dorsiflexion motion is available at the child's ankle. One option for assisting this child is to set the plantarflexion stop of the articulated AFO at 5 degrees of dorsiflexion, which will promote knee flexion at mid-stance and limit any plantarflexion motion. As a result, the ankle dorsiflexion motion would be unlimited because a dorsiflexion stop has not been used.

Research Evidence In a kinematic case study of a 4 1/2-year-old child with spastic diplegia, researchers compared the use of articulated AFOs with the use of rigid AFOs during gait (Middleton, Hurley, & McIlwain, 1988). The child's gait resembled a typical pattern of ankle motion during stance when wearing the articulated AFO.

In another study using three-dimensional gait analysis, researchers studied the effect of a posterior leaf spring orthosis on ankle motions and power in 20 children with cerebral palsy (Ounpuu et al., 1993). The study found a significant increase in ankle dorsiflexion motion during swing phase when the children wore orthoses. Differences in the children's generation of power were not found.

In 1993, researchers compared the effects of hinged AFOs with fixed AFOs on a sit-to-stand task for 10 children with cerebral palsy (Baker et al., 1993). The study found statistically significant increases in trunk lean angles when the children wore fixed AFOs when rising from sit-to-stand position. The researchers suggested that the type of AFO may influence movement strategies when functional tasks are being performed.

Another study compared the use of no orthosis (i.e., the children wore shoes) with the use of fixed AFOs and hinged AFOs on kinematic and electromyographic changes in 15 children with spastic diplegia (Lough & Soderberg, 1991). Greater ankle dorsiflexion at mid-stance and a faster walking velocity were recorded when the children wore both types of hinged AFOs as compared with when the children wore shoes.

ADDITIONAL ORTHOTIC DEVICES

Although KAFOs and HKAFOs were used extensively in the 1950s and 1960s when bracing for children with cerebral palsy was common practice, KAFOs rarely have been prescribed since the 1970s for children who ambulate, except for children who exhibit knee instability or other atypical impairments. FROs have generally replaced KAFOs as the orthotic device of choice to manage a moderately to severely crouched gait. Design characteristics of KAFOs include an ankle joint that can be either solid or articulated; a knee joint that can include a wide variety of mechanical joints to limit or allow motion; thigh cuffs, which extend to 1 inch distal to the perineum; and a metal upright that secures the thigh cuff, knee joint, and ankle portion of the orthosis together. KAFOs use 3PP control to provide stability to the knee joint or improve knee extension by locking the knee joints.

Knee Orthoses

Knee orthoses generally are not prescribed as full-time ambulatory devices. They range in complexity from a knee immobilizer to the adjustable spring tension Ultraflex knee orthosis. Knee orthoses use the 3PP control principle to maintain knee extension or knee flexion. Knee orthoses are usually for specific circumstances; for example, postoperative management for ROM or to support weakened muscles, to maximize knee extension during standing or gait until appropriate antigravity control is achieved, or to limit knee hyperextension during gait. The use of knee orthoses is limited because control of the knee often can be achieved with AFOs and with the concept of the closed kinematic chain. In general, knee orthoses, knee immobilizers, and long-leg casts are used as supplemental tools to maintain ROM at night or restrict motion while the child is working on a specific task during therapy.

Hip Orthoses

There are strategies that emphasize distal joint stabilization to improve proximal joint control via the closed kinematic chain. As a result of this treatment philosophy and improved surgical management, the use of orthotics that include the hip, the knee, and the ankle joint simultaneously has virtually been eliminated. Hip orthoses are generally used to increase or maintain functional ROM at the hips and to position hips at risk for subluxation or dislocation in children who are not ambulatory. Hip orthoses can range from a simple abduction wedge placed between the child's legs to a custom-made orthosis that includes a pelvic band, hip joints, and thigh cuffs to position the child's hips in abduction. Hip orthoses or hip abduction wedges may be used at night by children who do not ambulate or as a method of maintaining or increasing hip abduction and/or hip extension ROM or positioning hips that are at risk for subluxation. Researchers found improved hip motion with no observed radiological improvements in seven children with cerebral palsy after a 16-month follow-up study of the use of hip orthoses at night (Nakamura & Ohamu, 1980).

An ambulatory hip orthosis is available but is not commonly used. The purpose of an ambulatory hip orthosis is to decrease hip adduction during gait and to position the hips for improved ROM or limit further hip subluxation. The Rancho Hip brace and the Camp brace are two examples of hip orthoses that may be used by children who ambulate with an adducted gait pattern. The ambulatory hip orthosis has been replaced by surgical procedures and pharmacological agents to control hip adductor tone.

Thoracolumbosacral Orthoses (TLSO)

Spinal deformity in children with cerebral palsy can manifest itself in the form of scoliosis and/or abnormal lordosis or kyphosis as a result of structural or muscle tone abnormalities. There is little evidence to support the use of orthotic devices to alter the natural history of scoliosis in children with cerebral palsy. However, spinal orthotic devices have several legitimate applications for children with cerebral palsy:

- To slow the progression of scoliosis, abnormal kyphosis, or lordosis as an alternative to surgery or as an attempt to delay surgery and allow as much skeletal growth as possible
- To improve positioning for increased function, such as head control or upper-extremity use, and appearance
- To improve the alignment of the pelvis, creating a stable foundation for sitting
- To address the long-term needs of the child who is not a surgical candidate for spinal correction or fusion
- To provide preoperative management while other medical conditions, such as nutritional status, improve
- To provide postoperative protection

Although TLSOs (see Figure 16.11) can be fabricated from measurements of children with flexible, more spinal symmetrical deformities, TLSOs usually are fabricated from a carefully molded plaster impression of the child's trunk. TLSOs traditionally have been fabricated from a rigid polypropylene shell. These were often rejected as a result of the child's discomfort; however, an increasing number of more flexible and softer orthoses are used with reports of increased compliance.

Research has found an average in brace improvement of 15 degrees among 55 children with neuromuscular scoliosis (average curvature was 42 degrees) while wearing the Boston Soft Body Jacket (Letts, Rathbone, Yamashita, Nichol, & Keeler, 1992). This study reported improved tolerance, improved postural positioning, and a marked improvement in the child's sitting stability. The use of a TLSO may slow the progression of a curve, but most curves will continue to increase in severity with time (Green, 1991).

CONCLUSION

The individual needs of children with cerebral palsy must be considered in order to determine the orthotic design that will benefit each child. In addition, the

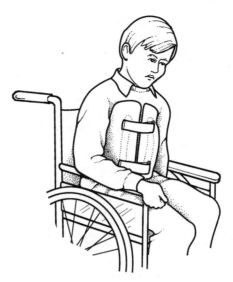

Figure 16.11.   A thoracolumbosacral orthosis (i.e., "body jacket") is a useful tool for improved seating posture and trunk control in the presence of scoliosis and increased kyphosis.

benefits and limitations that the orthotic device will provide for the child must also be considered. In order to meet the needs of each child, the team involved in the prescription, fabrication, and training in the use of a new orthotic device must have an understanding of the materials used in fabrication, the principles of orthotic design, and the goals for use of an orthotic device. In addition, each professional must maintain and improve his or her level of knowledge and remain well read in the literature and scientific research.

The orthotic management of children with cerebral palsy is challenging. Adding to this challenge is a lack of scientific research to validate the use of various orthotic devices. These studies are starting to be conducted and will continue to contribute to the overall management of cerebral palsy. The literature and studies need to describe, however, the type of orthotic device used, the settings for the joints of the orthotic device (when applicable), and the design features of the orthosis. The reports also should provide a detailed description of the child's musculoskeletal alignment and his or her possible secondary deformities. Without this information, a comparison of various orthotic devices is difficult to ascertain.

Long-term studies of the use of orthotic devices also need to be performed. Clinical claims are made that an orthotic device will prevent secondary deformities that may impair function or the efficiency of gait at skeletal maturity. These claims need to be substantiated through long-term follow-up studies of children as they progress to adulthood. The variety of orthotic designs and the materials available provide the practitioner, the child, and the child's family with a wide variety of choices. To provide effective safe intervention, professionals need to begin to validate the various orthoses and designs available to the child with cerebral palsy.

REFERENCES

Baker, M.J., Giuliani, C.A., Sparling, J., & Schenkman, M.L. (1993). Effects of ankle-foot orthoses on a sit-to-stand task in children with cerebral palsy [Abstract]. *Pediatric Physical Therapy, 5,* 193.

Carlson, J.M., & Bergland, G. (1979). An effective orthotic design for controlling the unstable subtalar joint. *Orthotics and Prosthetics, 33,* 39–49.

Condie, D.N. (1995). Conclusions and recommendations. In D.N. Condie, & C.B. Meadows (Eds.), *Report of a Consensus Conference on the Lower Limb Orthotic Management of Cerebral Palsy* (pp. 1–20). Copenhagen, Denmark: International Society for Prosthetics and Orthotics.

Cusick, B.D. (1990). *Progressive casting and splinting for lower extremity deformities in children with neuromotor dysfunction.* Tucson, AZ: Therapy Skill Builders.

Cusick, B.D. (1995). An overview of components and concepts involved in orthotic prescription for children with cerebral palsy. In D.N. Condie (Ed.), *Report of a Consensus Conference on the Lower Limb Orthotic Management of Cerebral Palsy* (pp. 94–122). Copenhagen, Denmark: International Society of Prosthetics and Orthotics.

Damiano, D.L., Vaughan, C.L., & Abel, M.F. (1995). Muscle response to heavy resistance exercise in children with spastic cerebral palsy. *Developmental Medicine and Child Neurology, 37,* 731–739.

Deusinger, R.H. (1984). Biomechanics in clinical practice. *Physical Therapy, 64,* 1860–1866.

Embry, D.G., Yates, L., & Mott, D.H. (1990). Effects of neuro-developmental treatment and orthoses on knee flexion during gait: A single-subject design. *Physical Therapy, 70,* 626–637.

Fetters, L. (1991). Cerebral palsy: Contemporary treatment concepts. In M.J. Lister (Ed.), *Contemporary management of motor control problems, proceedings of the II Step Conference* (pp. 219–224). Alexandria, VA: American Physical Therapy Association.

Gage, J. (1991). *Gait analysis in cerebral palsy.* Oxford, England: MacKeith Press.

Green, N.E. (1991). Cerebral palsy. In S.T. Canale & J.H. Beaty (Eds.), *Operative pediatric orthopedics* (pp. 611–681). St. Louis: Mosby-Year Book.

Harrington, E.D., Lin, R.S., & Gage, J.R. (1984, Spring). Use of the anterior floor reaction orthosis in patients with cerebral palsy. *Orthotics and Prosthetics,* 32–34.

Harris, S.R., & Riffle, K. (1986). Effects of inhibitive ankle-foot-orthosis on standing balance in a child with cerebral palsy. *Physical Therapy, 66,* 663–667.

Hylton, N.M. (1989). Postural and functional impact of dynamic AFOs and FOs in a pediatric population. *Journal of Prosthetics and Orthotics, 2,* 40–53.

Knutson, L.M., & Clark, D.E. (1991). Orthotic devices for ambulation in children with cerebral palsy and myelomeningocele. *Physical Therapy, 71,* 947–960.

Letts, M., Rathbone, D., Yamashita, T., Nichol, B., & Keeler, A. (1992). Soft Boston orthosis in management of neuromuscular scoliosis: A preliminary report. *Journal of Pediatric Orthopedics, 12,* 470–474.

Lin, R.S. (1995). Orthotic management of the cerebral palsied child. In D.N. Condie (Ed.), *Report of a Consensus Conference on the Lower Limb Orthotic Management of Cerebral Palsy* (pp. 137–139). Copenhagen, Denmark: International Society of Prosthetics and Orthotics.

Lough, L.M., & Soderberg, G.J. (1991). The effects of fixed and hinged ankle foot orthoses on gait myoelectric activity and standing joint alignment in children with cerebral palsy. *Physcial Therapy, 71* (Suppl.), 57–58.

Meadows, C.B. (1995). The scientific basis of treatment: III. To improve the dynamic efficiency of gait. In D.N. Condie (Ed.), *Report of a Consensus Conference on the Lower Limb Orthotic Management of Cerebral Palsy* (pp. 57–65). Copenhagen, Denmark: International Society for Prosthetics and Orthotics.

Middleton, E.A., Hurley, G.R.B., & McIlwain, J.S. (1988). The role of rigid and hinged polypropylene ankle-foot orthosis in the management of cerebral palsy: A case study. *Prosthetics Orthotics International, 12,* 129–135.

Mossberg, K.A., Linton, K.A., & Friske, K. (1990). Ankle-foot orthosis: Effect on energy expenditure of gait in spastic diplegic children. *Archives of Physical Medicine and Rehabilitation, 71,* 490–494.

Nakamura, T., & Ohamu, M. (1980). Hip abduction splint at night for scissor leg of cerebral palsy patients. *Journal of Orthotics and Prosthetics, 34,* 13–18.

Olney, S.J., & Wright, M.J. (1994). Cerebral palsy. In S.K. Campbell (Ed.), *Physical therapy for children* (pp. 489–524). Philadelphia: W.B. Saunders.

Ounpuu, S., Bell, K.J., Davis, R.B., & DeLuca, P.A. (1993). An evaluation of the posterior leaf spring orthosis using gait analysis [Abstract]. *Developmental Medicine and Child Neurology, 35*(Suppl. 69), 8.

Perry, J. (1992). *Gait analysis: Normal and pathological function.* New York: McGraw-Hill.

Rodgers, M.M., & Cavanaugh, P.R. (1984). Glossary of biomechanical terms, concepts and units. *Physical Therapy, 64,* 1886–1902.

Sackett, D.L. (1986). Rules of evidence and clinical recommendations on the use of antithrombotic agents. *Chest, 39,* 25–35.

Saltiel, J. (1969). A one-piece laminated knee-locking short leg brace. *Orthotics and Prosthetics, 23,* 68–75.

Small, G.J. (1995). The orthotic management of the foot in cerebral palsy. In D.N. Condie (Ed.), *Report of a Consensus Conference on the Lower Limb Orthotic Management of Cerebral Palsy* (pp. 123–126). Copenhagen, Denmark: International Society of Prosthetics and Orthotics.

Soderberg, G.L. (1986). *Kinesiology: Application to pathological motion.* Baltimore: Williams & Wilkins.

Sutherland, D.H., & Cooper, L. (1978). The pathomechanics of progressive crouch gait in spastic diplegia. *Orthopedic Clinics of North America, 9,* 143–154.

Sutherland, D.H., Cooper, L., & Daniel, D. (1980). The role of the ankle plantar flexors in normal walking. *Journal of Bone and Joint Surgery, 62A,* 354–363.

Taylor, C.L., & Harris, S.R. (1986). Effects of ankle-foot orthosis on functional motor performance in a child with spastic diplegia. *American Journal of Occupational Therapy, 40,* 492–494.

Thomas, C. (1977). *Taber's cyclopedic medical dictionary* (13th ed.). Philadelphia: F.A. Davis.

Weber, D. (1995). Gait related orthotic prescription criteria for children with cerebral palsy. In D.N. Condie (Ed.), *Report of a Consensus Conference on the Lower Limb Orthotic Management of Cerebral Palsy* (pp. 145–174). Copenhagen, Denmark: International Society for Prosthetics and Orthotics.

Yamamoto, K.T. (1992). Comparison of two types of supramalleolar ankle-foot orthosis on the gait parameters of children with cerebral palsy [Abstract]. *Pediatric Physical Therapy, 4,* 196.

APPENDIX

Conclusions and Recommendations from the 1994 ISPO Consensus Conference

The 1994 International Society for Prosthetics and Orthotics (ISPO) Consensus Conference, held at Duke University in Durham, North Carolina, accepted the initial proposition that lower limb orthoses may be used with individuals who have cerebral palsy to achieve four goals: 1) preventing and/or correcting deformity, 2) providing a base of support, 3) facilitating training in skills, and 4) improving the dynamic efficiency of gait.

The following is a list of the 29 conclusions and recommendations that the ISPO compiled from the conference (Condie, 1995):

1. The existing body of literature on the effects of orthotic intervention in cerebral palsy is, for the most part, seriously, scientifically, and experimentally flawed with very few studies graded above Sackett's Level V (Sackett, 1986).
2. The available scientific evidence on the causes of deformity suggests that muscle growth is reduced in the presence of spasticity, and this may lead to

From Condie, D.N. (1995). Conclusions and recommendations. In D.N. Condie, & C.B. Meadows (Eds.), *Report of a Consensus Conference on Lower Limb Orthotic Management of Cerebral Palsy* (pp. 1–20). Coppenhagen, Denmark: International Society of Prosthetics and Orthotics; adapted by permission.

the development of deformities. "Static" positioning, as it is applied in most existing orthotic designs, is probably less effective than the "dynamic" application of force in preventing or correcting such deformities.

Deformities, which are a result of abnormal *muscle* growth, may be complemented by skeletal or joint deformities resulting from abnormal *bone* growth, especially in the growing child who has open epiphyses.

3. The development of more effective orthotic designs for preventing or correcting such deformities will depend on further basic research to determine the optimum level and rate of application of the preventative or corrective forces.

4. The basic premise that distal stabilization of the lower limb joints leads to improved proximal control is supported. The immediate biomechanical effect of such action may readily be observed; however, the longer-term motor learning effect needs to be demonstrated.

5. The principle that good foot and leg position provides valuable feedback is also supported; however, the use of such information depends on the existence of an adequate control strategy.

6. It is recognized that appropriate orthotic designs, by controlling the position of the joints they encompass, may alter the biomechanical demands placed on more proximal joints when walking. In general, this change results in more normal external joint moments and may also avoid overactivity of certain muscle groups. Whether these orthoses also produce a motor learning effect still needs to be demonstrated.

7. It was noted that footwear modifications, alone or in conjunction with orthoses, may produce similar beneficial effects.

8. Further studies of the effects of orthotic intervention are urgently required. Although it would be highly desirable to propose Sackett Level I and Sackett Level II studies, it is recognized that the multifactorial nature of cerebral palsy would make this very difficult. Realistically, Sackett Level III studies (probably multiple single-case studies) appear to be indicated, possibly in multicenter collaborations.

9. The conduct of a Sackett Level III type of study requires an adequate experimental design. Unfortunately, many clinical practitioners lack knowledge of research methods and must therefore either obtain training in this subject or seek assistance from qualified colleagues.

10. The data to be collected in such studies must include adequate information regarding the patient's medical history, the type of intervention, and an appropriate measure of the individual's functional status pre- and postintervention, both in the short and the long term.

11. Assessment of the child with cerebral palsy with a view to providing treatment must commence immediately when it is apparent that the child is not able to meet appropriate development milestones.

12. Assessment is a team activity and requires the participation of qualified individuals from the following professions in collaboration with the child's parents or other caregivers:
    - Pediatric medicine
    - Pediatric orthopedics
    - Pediatric neurology
    - Physical therapy
    - Occupational therapy
    - Orthotics
    - Psychiatry

13. The assessment process should be structured in order to obtain objective data regarding the status of the child's neuromuscular skeletal systems, abilities (gait, if appropriate), and quality of life.

14. Following initial assessment, realistic intervention goals need to be established and the appropriate intervention specified (i.e., surgery, therapy, orthotics, or other). Once again, the involvement of the child's parents or caregivers is vital in this process.

15. Regular review/reassessment must take place to evaluate the effect of previous interventions; to establish if the treatment goals have been achieved; and to specify, if appropriate, revised goals and associated further intervention.

16. It is essential that detailed records of the findings of all assessments and/or reviews are maintained with the associated intervention record. Videotape recordings are recognized as having particular value to record gait.

17. It is important to ensure that therapy and orthotic intervention are fully coordinated.

18. Scientific research on biomechanical aspects of lower limb function, the effects of soft tissue adaptation, and motor learning have challenged previous ideas on therapeutic practice. They have also opened up new avenues for the use of orthoses in conjunction with therapy to achieve the various aims.

19. Orthotic designs are probably adequate for the envisaged roles; however, more sophisticated measurement techniques may be required to assess the outcome and to permit fine tuning in a clinical situation.

20. In general, surgical intervention should be considered when there is either a specific pathological indication (e.g., a dislocating joint) or, alternatively, when functional improvement has ceased and therapeutic/orthotic intervention has proved ineffective.

21. Orthotic intervention for children with cerebral palsy may be considered in relation to three levels of function:
    - Pre-standing (For some individuals, this will be the highest level they will ever attain.)
    - Standing
    - Walking

22. The goals of orthotic intervention for the *pre-standing* child include the following:
    - Minimizing or preventing deformity and, hence, maintaining joint ranges of motion
    - Achieving trunk control and, thereby, achieving sitting balance, which will, in turn, promote upper limb and oromuscular function and allow the child to interact with the environment

    The goals of orthotic intervention for the *standing* child include all the objectives defined for the pre-standing child as well as facilitating efficient balanced standing by providing the minimum appropriate support. This will create an environment within which it will be possible to develop optimum control strategies.

    The goals of orthotic intervention for the *walking* child include all the objectives defined for the pre-standing and standing child as well as attaining efficient purposeful gait by facilitating desirable patterns of motion and resisting undesirable joint patterns of motion. This will enable the child to participate in activities of daily living.

23. The following information is required to determine the specific type of orthotic intervention and the most appropriate orthotic design for the *pre-standing* child:
    - The child's medical and social history
    - The child's diagnosis
    - The child's functional gross motor status and any specific motor or sensory impairments
    - The child's skeletal abnormalities
    - The child's home, school, and other relevant environments
    - Behavioral features (e.g., compliance and tolerance to proposed form of intervention)
    - Associated relevant conditions (e.g., gastroesophageal reflux, epilepsy)

    In terms of the *standing* child, all of the information already specified for the pre-standing child is required. In addition, the child's standing posture and a balance assessment are required to determine the specific type of orthotic intervention that is appropriate.

    In terms of the *walking* child, all of the information already specified for the pre-standing and standing child is required. In addition, a gait assessment (the Gage criteria for efficient gait was recognized as an appropriate tool for this purpose.) is required to determine the specific type of orthotic intervention that is appropriate (Gage, 1991).

24. The specification of the orthotic intervention that is most appropriate to achieve the defined goals requires the following information:
    - The joints and segments to be encompassed by the orthosis
    - The intersegmental orientation of the segments

- The type of control to be applied to the joints encompassed by the orthoses
- The form of any sensory input
- The type of control that is intended to be exerted on any joints not encompassed by the orthoses (e.g., the effect of a floor reaction orthosis on knee joint motion)

25. A range of orthotic designs is available that, when appropriately prescribed and correctly fabricated and fitted, will satisfy the range of clinical and functional objectives considered as being necessary.

26. The evidence for any specific tone reducing or tone inhibiting effect of an orthosis is inconclusive; however, it is clear that a close fit with accurate anatomical contouring will optimize the function that is attainable.

27. The care provided for people with cerebral palsy needs to be multidisciplinary. Ideally, it should be community based, goal oriented, and agreed on by all interested parties. Orthotic care cannot effectively be provided in isolation.

28. ISPO should act to obtain improved evidence of the effect of orthotic intervention by any of the following methods:
    - Coordinating the development of a standardized protocol to record the requisite information regarding patient status, type of orthotic intervention, and outcome of intervention
    - Establishing a multicenter orthotic treatment evaluation project based on the above mentioned protocol

29. ISPO should examine the feasibility of conducting multidisciplinary instructional courses designed to disseminate the principles of treatment agreed by the conference allied to practical instruction on all forms of intervention by recognized experts from all the concerned disciplines.

Creating Opportunities for the Child with Cerebral Palsy: Preventing Handicap

CHAPTER 17

The Family

Symme W. Trachtenberg and Christine F. Rouse

As of 1998, the term *family* is more broadly defined in the United States than it has ever been in years past. Family members can be related by blood or by nature of their intimate relationships. They may be supportive, unavailable, or confrontational. People tend to be very clear about who are the members of their family, especially in times of crisis and celebration. For the purposes of this chapter, the term *family* refers to the biological or the adoptive parent(s) and the family members who provide daily care to children with disabilities. Families are structured in many different ways: the traditional two-parent family, the single-parent family (Boyce, Miller, White, & Godfrey, 1995), the biological parent and partner family, the adoptive family, the gay and/or lesbian family, and the intergenerational family. The family unit, regardless of its composition, serves as the focal point for transmitting familial traditions and for keeping ethnic and cultural heritage alive. These traditions provide family members with stability, support, comfort, strength, guidance, and culturally specific strategies for coping with the demands of daily life (McCubbin, Thompson, Thompson, McCubbin, & Kaston, 1993).

INITIAL FAMILY REACTIONS AND
ADAPTATIONS TO HAVING A CHILD WITH A DISABILITY

Regardless of their structure, most families experience a progression of typical stages within the development of the family unit (Carter & McGoldrick, 1980); these stages may be thought of as analogous to the typical stages of the life cycle of an individual. The adjustments made during various stages of the child's development may be stressful for any family. In terms of the family that has a child with a disability, this stress may be amplified, especially if the child's life cycle remains incomplete or if developmental milestones are not achieved when typically expected (e.g., communion, bar or bat mitzvah, leaving for college). The child with a disability may remain dependent throughout his or her life. When expected life-cycle changes do not occur, family members may experience the reemergence of the sadness they experienced when their child's disability was first diagnosed, which is known as *chronic sorrow* (Tunali & Power, 1992; Wikler, Wasow, & Hatfield, 1983).

Christine's Story

"I was born with cerebral palsy because during the birth I was in a breech position, and the cord was wrapped around my neck, and I experienced a lack of oxygen. I was diagnosed when I was a year old. My family had different reactions to my diagnosis. My grandfather is a doctor and was there when I was born. Because of his medical background, he suspected there would be problems, and he was not surprised by the diagnosis. My grandmother was annoyed that the doctors had not delivered me by C-section but realized that even doctors are only human and can make mistakes. My dad was in shock because his father had multiple sclerosis and he could not believe that he had another family member with a disability to care for. My dad is very religious, though, and that helped him to deal with my cerebral palsy. My mom was very upset and was in shock. She was upset with the doctors who delivered me because they did not do enough to prevent it from happening. She wanted to believe it was just a delay and I would catch up, but her gut feeling was to start therapy because she was concerned with how my development compared to my brothers'.

"My brother Bill was 4 years old when he found out. He was my best support. He played with me in ways that helped me to sit straighter and that helped my hand muscles. He encouraged me to try everything.

(continued)

Christine's Story–continued

He treated me like anyone else and never pitied me. My other brother, Mike, was 8 years old when he found out, and he was very worried and concerned. He asked my parents a lot of questions, such as 'Will she die? Will she be in a wheelchair? and Will she be smart?' All of my family have found ways to encourage me. My aunt Carol says that my whole family has a level of respect and compassion for life. She has seen an inner strength in me that helps me to persist despite adversity and to see a purpose from God in my life.

"I am so grateful to my parents because they provided me with excellent therapies and have always given me support throughout my life. They got me involved in therapeutic horseback riding, swimming, gymnastics, and tennis. I loved riding because it gave me a lot of self-confidence and responsibility. It also helped my balance and posture. I felt close to many of my therapists; they were like my friends. My therapists and I did more than just therapy; we talked about issues that concerned me. They were really supportive and cared about me."

When parents first learn that their child has cerebral palsy, their lives undergo immediate change. Suddenly, they must readjust their expectations of their child, a host of professionals and services enter the family setting, unexpected financial burdens emerge, and isolation may occur. As a result of these stresses, there may be significant changes in family roles, relationships, and organization.

Christine's story emphasizes that every individual and family differs in its initial response and its ability to cope with the diagnosis of cerebral palsy. The reaction may depend on the parents' previous experiences; the family's religious and cultural backgrounds; or whether the disability was identified prenatally, shortly after birth, or later in the child's life (Davis, 1987; Leyser, 1994). Other factors that may influence familial reactions to the diagnosis of cerebral palsy include perceptions and attitudes regarding disabilities, health and healing techniques, motivation, and the tolerance to allow others to assist with care (Hanline & Daley, 1992; Lynch & Hanson, 1998; McCubbin et al., 1993). For example, some parents with strong religious beliefs may feel that God chose them to care for a child with a disability, whereas other parents may feel that they are being punished for things they did earlier in their lives. By the time the child receives a diagnosis, some parents may feel relieved to finally get answers and help for their child, whereas other parents may feel anger toward the professionals who did not provide interventions as early in the child's life as they could have or reassured them that their child would "grow out of it."

The most common response of parents being told that their child has a disability such as cerebral palsy is a combination of shock, disbelief, guilt, and an overwhelming feeling of loss (Singer & Irvin, 1989; Trachtenberg, 1997). Families must have time to grieve for the loss of their "typical" child. Kübler-Ross (1969) described the stages of grieving that are experienced by many families as they learn to cope with the impact of a disability. These stages include denial, depression, anger and guilt, bargaining, and acceptance. These stages are not bound by time nor are they orderly in their progression; some elements may be combined or omitted (Schleifer & Klein, 1985). There is controversy as to whether this model is generally applicable: Although research does not fully support the model, anecdotal experience suggests that parents often do cope with their child's diagnosis in these stages. Table 17.1 presents typical ways in which families may demonstrate their reactions to grief.

With the passage of time and the support of family, friends, parents of other children with disabilities, and community resources, most parents learn to cope with their child's challenges. Many parents find that confiding in a friend or contacting a professional who has been helpful in the past provides a release for voicing their feelings about a current dilemma, examining their feelings, or getting another viewpoint to help them move on. There is an active "network" among family members of children with disabilities; this "networking" can be very empowering and can help parents to educate one another, often becoming

Table 17.1. Typical responses of parents to stages of grieving

Stage of grieving	Common parent reactions
Denial	Disbelief in the diagnosis; multiple consultations in an effort to find a more optimistic diagnosis or prognosis
Depression	Symptoms of depression, including fatigue, insomnia, over- or undereating, irritability, and problems with sexuality; episodic feelings of sadness or despair, often triggered by life-cycle events
Anger	Blaming self or others for the child's disability; attributing disability to an avoidable act on the part of the parent
Guilt	Expressing anger toward someone "safe" rather than toward the person to whom anger is felt; using anger as an expression of frustration when advocating for the child; upset with the professional who gives the diagnosis or who is unable to cure the child
Bargaining	Turning to nonconventional forms of intervention in an effort to find a cure; making a deal with God to do good deeds in exchange for the child improving in function

more effective than professional support in making recommendations for intervention for the child. For many parents, speaking to a fellow parent or receiving supportive counseling is all that is needed. However, psychotherapy may be beneficial if feelings of depression or anger interfere with the parents' ability to work or to care for their child or if a cognitive approach to problem solving will improve family functioning.

After a period of time, most parents can effectively cope with their child's disability. In fact, family experts have found evidence of improved family cohesion and hardiness; increased understanding and compassion among family members; and, in some families, a more enriched and meaningful life (Cadman, Rosenbaum, Boyle, & Offord, 1991; Featherstone, 1980; Leyser, 1994; Turnbull & Turnbull, 1986; Wikler et al., 1983). It is impossible to predict how a particular family will deal with the child who has severe or mild disabilities. What may be considered a minor stressor for one family may be considered a major stressor for another.

EFFECTS OF A DISABILITY ON THE CHILD'S DEVELOPMENT

For the purposes of this section, it is important to keep in mind that every child is unique and is different in his or her own way; it also is important to remember that the child with cerebral palsy may feel particularly "different" from other children because of his or her disability. Christine describes some of her feelings about being "different" in these terms:

"I went to regular school all my life. In elementary school, my classmates saw me for who I was and not just my cerebral palsy. My friends from elementary school have always looked beyond my body and got to know me for who I am on the inside. These are still my best friends today. The real shock came when I had to change schools for high school. For the first time in my life I experienced how ignorant people can be to someone who is "different." I felt rejected and ignored and finally left the school because I couldn't stand being treated like a nobody. That experience nearly destroyed my life. I started to hate cerebral palsy and hate myself. Fortunately, my friends and family were very supportive. I also started counseling, which was very helpful. Gradually, I learned to accept my cerebral palsy. I came to realize that what happened at that school was not my problem, but the school's problem. I came to my own conclusion that the reason my classmates did not accept me was because they were never educated about my disability."

Preschool (1 1/2–6 years of age)

Prior to school age, the child with a disability may not realize that he or she is "different" from other children. This is particularly true if the child has been in an early intervention program with other children with disabilities (Harvey & Greenway, 1982) rather than an inclusive program.

School Age (6–11 years of age)

By school age, most children with disabilities are aware of their disability and may need help dealing with feelings of being "different" (Kaufman, 1988). Providing the child with knowledge about his or her disability and allowing him or her to examine and express his or her feelings in regard to having a disability is critical. The understanding gained from this process enables the child to take "ownership" of the disability and to develop the motivation and investment needed to cope with his or her personal issues.

The first step toward self-acceptance is acceptance in the home. Children such as Christine, whose parents and siblings view them as worthwhile, generally have a good self-image. It is important for the child with a disability to be included in family activities (e.g., religious activities, recreational activities, vacations), to participate as much as possible in developmentally appropriate responsibilities, and to be able to discuss his or her disability openly. Discussing and practicing how to handle difficult situations in the home also improves the child's potential for social success.

Acceptance outside of the home can be difficult for the child with a disability to attain (e.g., Christine's experience when she entered high school). Classmates may tease the child who has a disability and schoolwork may be difficult for the child, especially if teachers and other school personnel are not knowledgeable about and sensitive to the specific needs of children with disabilities. In addition, children with limited communication and social skills may have difficulty with interpersonal interactions. The child who is not accepted by others may have doubts about his or her self-worth and may exhibit depression or other behavioral problems.

Whenever the child with a disability enters a school that has no previous experience with children with disabilities, it is important for personnel to plan and prepare the class and the school. This can be accomplished with the child's parents explaining the disorder and collaborating with the school's personnel to make the necessary adaptations for the teacher and the students. When the child has been newly diagnosed, however, parents may be less able to take such an active role. Programs that offer disability awareness workshops for children with developmental disabilities in hospitals and in communities may be able to help.

The key to developing self-confidence in any child is to encourage a range of experiences with activities in which he or she can succeed. Children with disabilities may be more accepted by their peers when they are provided with special assistance that enables them to participate in the same typical group activities (e.g., playground, camps) as their peers. This practice is known as *inclusion* and helps children without disabilities to appreciate people with differences and prepares them for a future of living, working, and having friendships with people with disabilities (Davern & Schnorr, 1991). Another approach to improving self-esteem in children with disabilities is to facilitate involvement in activities for people with disabilities, such as Special Olympics or other sports for children with physical impairments.

Adolescence (12–18 years of age)

Adolescence can be difficult for all children; for children with disabilities, adolescent difficulties often can be magnified (Hill, 1993). Children with cerebral palsy, like other adolescents, may become preoccupied with how they compare with their peers. However, sameness and peer approval in areas of physical development and self-image may be unattainable for children with cerebral palsy because of a physical or an intellectual disability (Dossetor & Nicol, 1989). Adolescents with disabilities who have strong peer groups or who have come to terms with being "different" may have less difficulty.

The issue of sexuality is usually confronted during adolescence. Adolescents with disabilities should be recognized as sexual human beings and encouraged to talk about their sexuality (Rousso, 1985). Adolescents should be provided with opportunities to be exposed to appropriate materials regarding intimate relationships and safe sex. They also should be given the chance to discuss these issues with peers and adults in a way and at a level that they can understand.

Although dating and sexual liaisons are sometimes an issue during adolescence, a more common problem is social isolation. Because of the limitations imposed by their disabilities, lack of self-esteem, and the attitudes and reactions of those around them, adolescents with disabilities may feel socially isolated (Hill, 1993). Adolescents with communication difficulties may have social skills that are not well developed and, as a result, may feel awkward in social interactions. They may appear to be uncomfortable around other people who, in turn, may feel equally uncomfortable around them. Adolescents with disabilities may benefit from continued professional support to find areas and activities in which they can be successful (e.g., listening to music, horseback riding, watching movies); this may help to maximize their ability to socialize. The normalization of social experiences reduces social isolation and increases feelings of self-worth and productivity (Blum, Resnick, Nelson, & St. Germaine, 1991).

Adolescence is a critical time for predicting a teenager's ability to function as an adult; those who are dependent throughout adolescence tend to remain dependent as adults (Ludlow, Turnbull, & Luckasson, 1988). Adolescents with disabilities who have difficulty with issues of independence, separation, and individuation need assistance during these developmental stages. Parents should be encouraged to give their children the necessary freedom to become independent. This includes taking reasonable risks at times. When parents persist in managing their child's life or the way their child deals with his or her disability (e.g., speaking for the child at the doctor's office, taking over responsibilities that the child is capable of handling alone), they give the adolescent the message that he or she is incompetent.

Young Adulthood (18–25 years of age)

The transition to young adulthood is rarely easy. Christine describes some of the plans she has for her future in these terms:

"My dating experience has been challenging in my life. I dated one boy during college, and this was a wonderful experience, but now we are just good friends. My future plan is that I would like to have a boyfriend and someday get married, but I am not in any hurry because I want to meet the right person at the right time. I feel this is possible because many people with disabilities are married."

Making the transition from adolescence to young adulthood is particularly difficult for individuals with disabilities as well as for their parents. When the young adult moves from the family home to an independent living arrangement, an appropriate level of supervision or assistance is required. In Christine's case, she hopes someday to live in her own apartment with minimal assistance from a friend who would help with making meals, with cleaning, and with other daily activities. Moving out of a parentally protected environment provides the young adult with important socialization opportunities within the community that contribute to his or her personal development, competence, maturity, and adaptive functioning (Whitman, 1995). This important developmental milestone is dependent on either the family's personal resources (i.e., parent-supported living arrangements with paid caregivers) or on publicly funded programs providing the necessary support.

The young adult's ability to cope and become independent depends on the degree of disability and how effective the family is in emotionally, financially, and concretely managing their child's health care needs (Howe, Feinstein, Reiss, Molock, & Berger, 1993; Turnbull, Turnbull, Bronicki, Summers, & Roeder-Gordon, 1989). The current focus on person-centered planning provides a model for assisting the child with disabilities to maximize his or her potential by having a circle of supportive family members, friends, and community agencies that can help him or her plan for the future. This process allows for combining resources and creatively developing an individualized functional plan that requires the supporters to commit to providing concrete and emotional assistance.

THE EFFECT OF THE CHILD'S DISABILITY ON FAMILY MEMBERS AND FRIENDS

When a child is diagnosed with cerebral palsy, it can be extremely stressful on his or her entire family. Reactions can vary from anger or denial to guilt or grief. However, with strong familial cohesion and communication, families can become closer rather than more distant as a result of the diagnosis.

Effects on Parents

Parents of children with disabilities encounter a wide array of problems that may produce stress. The most common problems include the following:

- The physical effects and the time-consuming demands of in-home care
- Medical, educational, and therapy appointments, which require coordination of family members' time as well as service coordination
- Financial concerns
- An inability to change jobs as a result of the need for uninterrupted medical insurance or service provision
- An inability or a need to change residences as a result of accessibility of housing or the location of medical or educational services
- A lack of information and resources, including respite care, recreational programs, legal services, and transportation (Herman & Thompson, 1995; Leyser, 1994; Marcenko & Smith, 1992; Trachtenberg & Lewis, 1996)

The ability to cope with a child's disability is dependent on many factors, including marital status, support systems, and related life experiences (Leyser, 1994). In general, couples with strong marital relationships, harmony in parenting, well-developed problem-solving skills, financial security, and supportive social networks usually cope well, especially if both parents have similar views of their child's disability and abilities (Leyser, 1994; Tunali & Power, 1992). Coping mechanisms that produce the highest degree of family functioning are mastery of the child's health care and developmental needs, emphasis on promoting self-esteem and positive communication styles, and overall family hardiness (Failla & Jones, 1991; Snowdon, Cameron, & Dunham, 1994). Strong religious affiliation as well as structure and effective behavior interventions in the home also are associated with effective coping (Leyser, 1994; Leyser & Dekel, 1991). It is interesting to note that related life experiences may have different effects on the family's ability to cope. Research shows that, although experience with a chronic illness or a disability in another family member may increase competence for handling the child who has recently been diagnosed with a disability, it also may result in *burnout*. Burnout is a state of distress that can be caused by the daily pressures of parenting the child who has physical and other associated limitations (e.g., feeding, movement). Parents who experience burnout often show signs of fatigue, emotional exhaustion, frustration, and generalized dissatisfaction with their lives. Support groups, clinical intervention, or respite care, all of which provide opportunities for parents to talk or to get help with caring for their child, may help parents feel better as well as improve their energy and ability to care for their child (Trachtenburg & Trachtenburg, 1996).

Parents often react differently to having a child with a disability. For example, a mother caring for the child with multiple disabilities (e.g., mental retardation and vision or hearing loss) who requires total care is at high risk for increased stress caused by feelings of depression and despair; however, she also may experience increased mastery of the child's care and competence, which contributes to positive family functioning (Miller, Gordon, Daniele, & Diller, 1992; Saddler, Hillman, & Benjamins, 1993; Timko, Stovel, & Moos, 1992). Another mother may become so immersed in the care of her child who has a disability that she has nothing left to give to her partner, to her other children, or to herself. A father may focus on financial issues or may avoid the reality of the child's disability by working excessively. Some fathers choose not to participate at all in child care responsibilities, neither for the child with a disability nor for the other children in the family (Cobb & Hancock, 1984; Timko et al., 1992). In some families, illness-related avoidance behaviors or other maladaptive responses by one parent decrease the other parent's ability to adequately adapt to the daily demands of the child with disabilities (Sloper & Turner, 1993; Timko et al., 1992).

Equal participation in child care provides greater parental satisfaction, sharing of problems and joys, and improvement of co-parenting skills. During the 1990s, fathers are assuming greater child care responsibilities and at times reverse roles with the mother (Willoughby & Glidden, 1995). Although some marriages are strengthened by the challenges associated with having a child with a disability, other marriages deteriorate, especially if the relationship was not previously strong (Goldfarb, Brotherson, Summers, & Turnbull, 1986). Support networks of family, friends, and community services can be helpful if marital or co-parental support is emotionally or physically absent, but they cannot replace the need for an active co-parent (Simons, Lorenz, Wu, & Conger, 1993). Every individual, couple, or family must find the option that works best for them. With the support of family and professionals, parents can become empowered to gather the services that their child needs, creating a true parent–professional partnership that ensures high-quality, family-centered care.

Some families experience so much stress as a result of the demands of caring for the child with a disability and the demands of their social or economic situation that they show signs of either being unable to care for the child, thus neglecting the child's medical and therapeutic needs, or, in the most extreme situations, abusing the child. Any child who appears to be neglected or abused must be referred to the local child welfare agency for protection, intervention, and support.

Effects on Siblings

The siblings of the child with a disability have special needs and concerns that vary according to age, birth order, and temperament (Breslau & Prabueki, 1987; Simeonsson & McHale, 1981). Their concerns also are affected by situational variables such as whether their own needs are being met, how their parents are emotionally handling the diagnosis, what they are told, and how much they understand.

Having a child with a disability in a family does not necessarily adversely affect the development of the siblings. In fact, there is some evidence that siblings in these families may have increased maturity, a sense of responsibility, a tolerance for "being different," a sense of closeness in the family, and enhanced feeling of self-confidence and independence. Many siblings of individuals with disabilities ultimately enter helping professions (Lobato, 1990).

In working to achieve healthy development in homes that have children with disabilities, the first point to remember is that children follow their parents' lead. If parents are upset, then children will be upset as well, even if they don't understand why. Parents who, in addition to being proud of the accomplishments of their child with disabilities and accepting him or her as a part of the family, acknowledge their own pain, set the tone for the siblings. Care must be given to "balance" the parenting efforts, support, and concern so that a sibling who does not have a disability is not forced into second place.

In a study of young children (ranging in age from 3 to 6 years, 9 months) who have a sibling with a disability compared with those who do not, researchers found that the children with a sibling with special needs were more involved in parallel play and social play and were more nurturing. (These children did demonstrate just as much aggressive, commanding, and directive behavior as the comparison group.) The study also found that mothers of children with disabilities were more likely to put demands on the siblings who were unaffected and were more likely to reprimand them as well (Lobato, Miller, Barbour, & Hall, 1991).

It is important to acknowledge that children may have mixed feelings toward their sibling with a disability (Ellifritt, 1984). Although these children may be glad that they are not affected, they may feel guilty at the same time because they do not have a disability. These children may worry that they will "catch" the disability or that they actually caused it by having bad thoughts about their sibling. Adolescents may question whether they will pass a similar disability on to their own children. Because of the extra care and the time required by the child with a disability, children who do not have disabilities may think that their parents love their brother or sister more than they love them. In order to get attention, some children may act out or get in trouble, whereas other children may withdraw, not wanting to ask for attention from their overly stressed parents (Powell & Gallagher, 1993). Parents must recognize and accept that their children who do not have disabilities often feel torn between protecting their brother or sister, whom they love, and being accepted by children outside the family, who may tease them and their sibling.

At some time, all children who have siblings with disabilities must be able to ask questions, sort out their feelings, and spend time alone with their parents. Siblings do best psychologically when their parents' marriage is stable and supportive, when feelings are discussed openly, when the disability is explained honestly, and when they are not expected to perform excessive child care responsibilities (Lobato, 1990; Schleifer, 1987).

Some parents do not discuss the issues related to the child's disability until the sibling and the child with a disability reach adulthood and the parents approach old age. It is then that the designated sibling(s), self- or parent-appointed, is informed of his or her possible responsibilities for caring for his or her sibling. It is important for parents to inform either one of the siblings of his or her responsibilities or have an estate plan, guardianship arrangement, or a written will outlining their preferences for their child with developmental disabilities. These preferences should be written early in the child's life, and adjustments to the plan should be incorporated every few years as life circumstances change.

Effects on Grandparents, Extended Family, and Friends

Grandparents also are affected by the presence of the child with disabilities in the family. For grandparents, grandchildren are a source of joy, comfort, and satisfaction (Schleifer, 1988). When the child is born with a disability, grandparents grieve for their own loss and for the pain that their child is experiencing (George, 1988). However, grandparents also can be a strong source of emotional and financial support, or they can provide respite care in the home that may be crucial for maintaining the child who has a severe disability. Although some grandparents need help in understanding how they can be helpful, denial may cause others to interfere with the parents' adaptation to the disability. Counseling, support groups for grandparents, and information given directly to them or via the parents can often help them deal with the reality of the child's disability and assist them to become more involved in supporting the family.

Extended family members and friends also can help or hinder the parents' ability to cope. Some family members may have their own issues that interfere with their ability to be supportive (e.g., parents' siblings having concerns regarding genetically based conditions and their own risks, family and friends' sadness or discomfort with the diagnosis). Professionals can suggest ways to discuss these issues with family and friends and should encourage parents to fill gaps in support systems with support groups, other parents, and available community service agencies.

THE ROLE OF SOCIETY AND COMMUNITY

The focus of this chapter is the internal dynamics of the family. However, the family's social context also plays an important role in determining the outcome of its members. In the United States, there is greater appreciation than in many other parts of the world for people who are "different." There are more educational, vocational, transportation, and housing services. Federally mandated entitlements ensure educational and societal compliance with standards set to provide equal services for people with disabilities (see Chapters 18 and 19). The effects of these mandated programs are visible: Many sidewalks have direct curb access so that wheelchairs can be used, some buses are equipped with wheelchair lifts, buildings must have wheelchair access, and theater and sporting events must be able to accommodate individuals with disabilities.

Although laws are important, they must be combined with a change in the public's perception of individuals with disabilities, which also seems to be occurring in the United States, perhaps as a result of "inclusion" that began in the mid-1970s (see Chapter 18). Young adults who have attended schools with children with disabilities are more sensitive to the needs of individuals with disabilities and are more cognizant of these individuals' abilities (Fortini, 1987). Individuals with disabilities are seen in movies, on television, and in magazine advertisements. Finally, there has been an increase in "volunteerism," with religious organizations, civic groups, and social-recreational groups championing the cause of individuals with disabilities (Schalock & Kiernan, 1990).

Christine had always been in inclusive school and recreational settings. Many times this went well, but at other times she experienced the pain of being "different." As a result, she developed a program that promotes social inclusion by underscoring how people with disabilities are just like everyone else (perhaps with a few more challenges). As she explains, "My desire to help others understand what it means to have a disability inspired me to create 'Kids are Kids,' which is a disability awareness educational program that I present to children of all ages in schools, camps, and colleges. 'Kids are Kids' helps me to know that I have a purpose in life and that I am making a difference with my cerebral palsy."

Parents, family members, friends, and professionals need to be alert to governmental shifts in the planning for allocation of funds and services for people with disabilities. Educating lawmakers and speaking out against changes that could negatively affect people with disabilities is essential. Parent–professional partnerships that effectively advocate for the rights of people with disabilities can help keep society focused on doing the right thing for these individuals.

Children, adolescents, and adults with disabilities are in contact with many individuals in their lives. Therefore, knowing who not to trust may be difficult. Individuals with disabilities may be vulnerable to exploitation and at risk for being influenced by people who offer alcohol, drugs, and sex. Therefore, training in prevention of substance, child, and sexual abuse is necessary. Understanding safe sex, both for prevention of acquired immunodeficiency syndrome (and other sexually transmitted diseases) and unwanted pregnancy, is essential for everyone. People with disabilities may need training tailored to their ability to learn and must be included in the outreach efforts to educate the world's youth.

Transition services have been mandated in the United States but still are limited in number and in quality (see Chapter 20). These services involve teaching skills necessary for competitive or supported employment as well as skills for leisure and living independently in the community. The goal of these services is a quality life that provides the opportunity to live, to work, and to play in the community and to have meaningful personal relationships (Hayes, 1991). Building an inclusive community in which children with developmental disabilities interact with children without disabilities throughout their lives will lead to individual success and benefit society as a whole.

Although U.S. society has made itself more accessible to individuals with disabilities, much more needs to be done. Supplemental Security Income provided by the Social Security Administration, medical assistance, and food stamps help parents and eventually help the child with a disability when he or she turns 18 years of age. However, many of these entitlement programs are being challenged and, as a result, are being changed. Insurance, and especially managed care, have uncovered costs (e.g., medications, house alterations, wheelchair-accessible van) that families cannot afford. In addition, the costs for medical care and education per child are high (Waitzman, Romano, & Scheffler, 1994). Additional educational programs and skills training are needed. Cost-effective care models must be developed that promote high-quality, outcome-oriented services that build on the strengths of the children, the children's families, and the professionals who know the children best. (See Chapter 3 for more detailed discussion of specific recommendations for the role of professionals.)

SUMMARY

As a family progresses through life, its members face various changes and adjustments; these are magnified for the family that has a child with a disability. The child and his or her parents, siblings, extended family members, and friends are all affected by the diagnosis of cerebral palsy. Over an extended period of time, a child and his or her parents' coping strategies and resources improve. Parents gradually learn to master their child's care and learn to effectively advocate in the medical, educational, and social systems in which they participate. Many families develop the increased strengths needed to cope effectively in order to manage the stresses associated with having a child with a disability (Hanline & Daley, 1992; Miller et al., 1992; Snowdon et al., 1994; Tunali & Power, 1992). Professionals who participate in the interdisciplinary team process and work closely with the child with a disability and his or her parents can play a critical role in helping these families and may be instrumental in determining the prognosis for the child as well as the outcome for the entire family.

REFERENCES

Blum, R.W., Resnick, M.D., Nelson, R., & St. Germaine, A. (1991). Family and peer issues among adolescents with spina bifida and cerebral palsy. *Pediatrics, 88*(2), 280–285.

Boyce, G.C., Miller, B.C., White, K.R., & Godfrey, M.K. (1995). Single parenting in families of children with disabilities. *Marriage and Family Review, 20*(3–4), 389–409.

Breslau, N., & Prabueki, K. (1987). Siblings of disabled children: Effects of chronic stress in the family. *Archives of General Psychiatry, 44,* 1040–1047.

Cadman, D., Rosenbaum, P., Boyle, M., & Offord, D.R. (1991). Children with chronic illness: Family and parent demographic characteristics and psychological adjustment. *Pediatrics, 87*(6), 884–889.

Carter, E.A., & McGoldrick, M. (Eds.). (1980). *The family life cycle: A framework for family therapy.* New York: Gardner Press.

Cobb, L.S., & Hancock, K.A. (1984). Development of the child with a physical disability. *Advances in Developmental and Behavioral Pediatrics, 5,* 75–107.

Davern, L., & Schnorr, R. (1991). Public schools welcome students with disabilities as full members. *Children Today, 20*(2), 21–25.

Davis, B.D. (1987). Disability and grief. *Social Casework, 6,* 352–357.

Dossetor, D.R., & Nicol, A.R. (1989). Dilemmas of adolescents with developmental retardation: A review. *Journal of Adolescence, 12,* 167–185.

Ellifritt, J. (1984). Life with my sister—Guilty no more. *Exceptional Parent, 14,* 16–21.

Failla, S., & Jones, L.C. (1991). Families of children with developmental disabilities: An examination of family hardiness. *Research in Nursing and Health, 14*(1), 41–50.

Featherstone, H. (1980). *A difference in the family: Life with a disabled child.* New York: Basic Books.

Fortini, M.E. (1987). Attitudes and behavior toward students with handicaps by their non-handicapped peers. *American Journal of Mental Deficiency, 92,* 78–84.

George, J.D. (1988). Therapeutic intervention for grandparents and extended family of children with developmental delays. *Mental Retardation, 26,* 369–375.

Goldfarb, L.A., Brotherson, M.J., Summers, J.A., & Turnbull, A.P. (1986). *Meeting the challenge of disability or chronic illness: A family guide.* Baltimore: Paul H. Brookes Publishing Co.

Hanline, M.F., & Daley, S.E. (1992). Family coping strategies and strengths in Hispanic, African-American, and Caucasian families of young children. *Topics in Early Childhood Special Education, 12*(3), 351–366.

Harvey, D., & Greenway, P. (1982). How parent attitudes and emotional reactions affect their handicapped child's self-concept. *Psychological Medicine, 12,* 357–370.

Hayes, A. (1991). What the future holds. In M.L. Batshaw (Ed.), *Your child has a disability* (pp. 308–321). Boston: Little, Brown.

Herman, S.E., & Thompson, L. (1995). Families' perceptions of their resources for caring for children with developmental disabilities. *Mental Retardation, 33*(2), 73–83.

Hill, A.E. (1993). Problems in relation to independent living—A retrospective study of physically disabled school leavers. *Developmental Medicine and Child Neurology, 35*(12), 1111–1115.

Howe, G.W., Feinstein, C., Reiss, D., Molock, S., & Berger, K. (1993). Adolescent adjustment to chronic physical disorders: I. Comparing neurological and non-neurological conditions. *Journal of Child Psychology and Psychiatry and Allied Disciplines, 34*(7), 1153–1171.

Kaufman, S.Z. (1988). *Retarded isn't stupid, Mom!* Baltimore: Paul H. Brookes Publishing Co.

Kübler-Ross, E. (1969). *On death and dying.* New York: Macmillan.

Leyser, Y. (1994). Stress and adaptation in orthodox Jewish families with a disabled child. *American Journal of Orthopsychiatry, 64*(3), 376–386.

Leyser, Y., & Dekel, G. (1991). Perceived stress and adjustment in religious Jewish families with a child who is disabled. *Journal of Psychology, 125,* 427–438.

Lobato, D.J. (1990). *Brothers, sisters, and special needs: Information and activities for helping young siblings of children with chronic illnesses and developmental disabilities.* Baltimore: Paul H. Brookes Publishing Co.

Lobato, D.J., Miller, C.T., Barbour, L., & Hall, L.J. (1991). Preschool siblings of handicapped children: Interactions with mothers, brothers and sisters. *Research in Developmental Disabilities, 12*(4), 387–399.

Ludlow, B.L., Turnbull, A.P., & Luckasson, R. (Eds.). (1988). *Transitions to adult life for people with mental retardation—Principles and practices.* Baltimore: Paul H. Brookes Publishing Co.

Lynch, E.W., & Hanson, M.J. (Eds.). (1998). *Developing cross-cultural competence: A guide for working with children and their families.* Baltimore: Paul H. Brookes Publishing Co.

Marcenko, M.O., & Smith, L.K. (1992). The impact of a family-centered case management approach. *Social Work in Health Care, 7*(1), 87–100.

McCubbin, H.I., Thompson, E.A., Thompson, M.S., McCubbin, M.A., & Kaston, A.J. (1993). Culture, ethnicity and the family: Critical factors in childhood chronic illnesses and disabilities. *Pediatrics, 91*(5), 1063–1070.

Miller, A.C., Gordon, R.M., Daniele, R.J., & Diller, L. (1992). Stress, appraisal, and coping in mothers of disabled and non-disabled children. *Journal of Pediatric Psychology, 17*(5), 587–605.

Powell, T.H., & Gallagher, P.A. (1993). *Brothers & sisters: A special part of exceptional families* (2nd ed.). Baltimore: Paul H. Brookes Publishing Co.

Rousso, H. (1985). Fostering self-esteem: Part two. What parents and professionals can do. *The Exceptional Parent, 15,* 9–12.

Saddler, A.L., Hillman, S.B., & Benjamins, D. (1993). The influence of disabling condition visibility on family functioning. *Journal of Pediatric Psychology, 18*(4), 425–439.

Schalock, R., & Kiernan, W. (1990). *Habilitation planning for adults with disabilities.* New York: Springer-Verlag.

Schleifer, M.J. (1987). I'm not going to be John's baby sitter forever: Siblings, planning and the disabled child. *Exceptional Parent, 17,* 60–64.

Schleifer, M.J. (1988). I wish our parents would help us more. Understanding grandparents of children with disabilities. *Exceptional Parent, 18,* 62–68.

Schleifer, M.J., & Klein, S.D. (Eds.). (1985). *The disabled child and the family: Understanding and treatment.* Boston: The Exceptional Parent Press.

Simeonsson, R.J., & McHale, S.M. (1981). Review: Research on handicapped children: Sibling relationships. *Child: Care, Health and Development, 7,* 153–171.

Simons, R.L., Lorenz, F.O., Wu, C.I., & Conger, R.D. (1993). Social network and marital support as mediators and moderators of the impact of stress and depression on parental behavior. *Developmental Psychology, 29*(2), 368–381.

Singer, G.H.S., & Irvin, L.K. (Eds.). (1989). *Support for caregiving families: Enabling positive adaptation to disability.* Baltimore: Paul H. Brookes Publishing Co.

Sloper, P., & Turner, S. (1993). Risk and resistance factors in the adaptation of parents of children with severe physical disability. *Journal of Child Psychiatry and Allied Disciplines, 34*(2), 167–188.

Snowdon, A.E., Cameron, S., & Dunham, K. (1994). Relationships between stress, coping resources, and satisfaction with family functioning in families of children with disabilities. *Canadian Journal of Nursing Research, 26*(3), 63–76.

Timko, C., Stovel, K.W., & Moos, R.H. (1992). Functioning among mothers and fathers of children with juvenile rheumatic disease: A longitudinal study. *Journal of Pediatric Psychology, 17*(6),705–724.

Trachtenberg, S.W. (1997). Coping and caring: The family of a child with developmental disabilities. In M.L. Batshaw (Ed.), *Children with disabilities* (4th ed., pp. 743–756). Baltimore: Paul H. Brookes Publishing Co.

Trachtenberg, S.W., & Lewis, D.F. (1996). Case management. In L. Kurtz, P.W. Dowrick, S.E. Levy, & M.L. Batshaw (Eds.), *Children's Seashore House handbook of developmental disabilities: Resources for interdisciplinary care* (pp. 203–208). Rockville, MD: Aspen Publishers, Inc.

Trachtenberg, S.W., & Trachtenberg, J.I. (1996). Prevention of burnout for parents and professionals. In L. Kurtz, P.W. Dowrick, S.E. Levy, & M.L. Batshaw (Eds.), *Children's Seashore House handbook of developmental disabilities: Resources for interdisciplinary care* (pp. 593–597). Rockville, MD: Aspen Publishers, Inc.

Tunali, B., & Power, T.G. (1992). Creating satisfaction: A psychological perspective on stress and coping in families of handicapped children. *Journal of Child Psychology and Psychiatry, 34*(6), 945–957.

Turnbull, A.P., & Turnbull, H.R. (1986). *Families, professionals, and exceptionality: A special partnership* (2nd ed.). Columbus, OH: Charles E. Merrill.

Turnbull, H.R., Turnbull, A.P., Bronicki, G.J., Summers, J.A., & Roeder-Gordon, C. (1989). *Disability and the family: A guide to decisions for adulthood.* Baltimore: Paul H. Brookes Publishing Co.

Waitzman, N.J., Romano, P.S., & Scheffler, R.M. (1994). Estimates of the economic costs of birth defects. *Inquiry, 31,* 188–204.

Whitman, C. (1995). Heading toward normal: Deinstitutionalization for the mentally retarded client. *Marriage and Family Review, 21*(1–2), 51–64.

Wikler, L., Wasow, M., & Hatfield, E. (1983). Measuring strengths in families of developmentally disabled children. *Social Work, 28,* 313–315.

Willoughby, J.C., & Glidden, L.M. (1995). Father's helping out: Shared child care and marital satisfaction of parents of children with disabilities. *American Journal on Mental Retardation, 99*(4), 399–406.

CHAPTER 18

The School

Susan K. Effgen

During the 18th century, educators in the United States began to recognize the need to provide education and training for children with disabilities; as a result, many large cities established special schools to meet the unique needs of these children. The children who attended these special schools usually had a variety of disabilities, including polio and cerebral palsy (Cable, Fowler, & Foss, 1936), and the services provided varied based on the individual school's resources. Some schools were fortunate and, as a result of the charitable donations of a few leading families in the community, could provide a wide range of services in addition to education (e.g., medical care, nursing care, nutritional counseling, psychological counseling, physical therapy [PT], occupational therapy [OT]). Cities such as Philadelphia and Atlanta were fortunate to have wealthy families that were able to establish schools and foundations for children with physical disabilities.

The number of services for children with disabilities began to increase during the 1960s. President John F. Kennedy's personal interest in individuals with disabilities helped encourage some state and local education agencies to provide support for the education of children with cerebral palsy. In the late 1960s and early 1970s, a number of landmark court cases established the right of individuals with disabilities to receive a free, appropriate public education (FAPE). As a result of these court cases, in 1975, the federal government finally intervened on behalf of the needs of all children with disabilities across the nation. In October of that year, the U.S. Congress passed the Education for All Handicapped Children Act of 1975 (PL 94-142), which mandated a FAPE for all children with disabilities. This meant that all children, no matter where they lived or how severe their disability, would receive special education and related services (e.g., physical therapy, occupational therapy, speech-language therapy) as part of their individualized education program (IEP). Prior to the passage of PL 94-142, children with disabilities frequently did not receive any education, and large numbers of children with cerebral palsy were systematically excluded from the educational system if they could not walk or use the bathroom independently.

Since the enactment of PL 94-142, enormous strides have been made in the United States in the education of children with cerebral palsy. Children with cerebral palsy are being educated in their local schools with age-appropriate peers and are receiving the related services and adaptive equipment they need to fully benefit from their special education. Infants, toddlers, and preschoolers with disabilities also are receiving a variety of services to enhance their development. In many local educational systems, parents also are welcomed partners in the educational process.

These great strides must continue. Assisting individuals with cerebral palsy to become productive members of society benefits not only the individual but also society as a whole. Services provided early to individuals with disabilities save society money and hardship later. Continued reauthorization of these important laws and the services they guarantee is essential to ensure that children with cerebral palsy achieve their potential.

ROLE OF THE FEDERAL GOVERNMENT IN THE EDUCATION OF CHILDREN WITH CEREBRAL PALSY

PL 94-142 and its later reauthorizations, the Education of the Handicapped Act Amendments of 1986 (PL 99-457), the Education of the Handicapped Act Amendments of 1990 (PL 101-476; which in its first sentence is retitled the Individuals with Disabilities Education Act [IDEA] of 1990), the Individuals with Disabilities Education Act Amendments of 1991 (PL 102-119), and the Individuals with Disabilities Education Act Amendments of 1997 (PL 105-17), have a number of important key elements (see the Appendix at the end of this chapter).

School-Age Children

According to the federal laws previously mentioned, every child receiving special education must have an IEP that guides his or her program of special education and related services. The IEP is developed after the child has had a comprehensive evaluation using more than one measurement device. Within

30 days after the determination that the child might need special education and related services, an IEP meeting is held. The meeting is attended by the child's parents, a representative of the local education agency, a special education teacher, a general education teacher, and an individual who can interpret the child's evaluation. Related-services personnel are not required to attend this meeting, but good practice dictates that they should attend all meetings regarding the children whom they assist. Parents also can request the attendance of any additional individuals. Figure 18.1 presents the definition and guidelines for all IEPs (as mandated by PL 105-17).

In terms of teachers or school personnel being held responsible for the success of students with disabilities,

> The IEP sets forth in writing a commitment of resources necessary to enable a child with a disability to receive needed special education and related services.... IDEA does not require that teachers or other school personnel be held accountable if a child with a disability does not achieve the goals and objectives. (*Federal Register,* 1992, p. 44833)

Good faith in attempting to achieve these objectives is expected.

In order to be eligible for special education and related services, a child must fit into one of the federal categories of definitions for children with disabilities. Children with cerebral palsy are usually included in the category of orthopedic impairments. If these children have additional impairments, they also may be included in the categories of autism, deaf-blindness, deafness, hearing impairment, mental retardation, multiple disabilities, other health impairment, serious emotional disturbance, specific learning disabilities, speech or language impairments, traumatic brain injury, or visual impairments (*Federal Register,* 1992). Occasionally, the child with cerebral palsy is listed in one of these separate categories—other than orthopedic impairment—in order to qualify for more services or for the state in which he or she lives to qualify for additional funding.

Infants, Toddlers, and Preschoolers

PL 99-457, enacted in October 1986, was an extension of PL 94-142 to include infants, toddlers, and preschoolers with disabilities and their families. Part H (now referred to as Part C in PL 105-17) outlined the provision of services to infants and toddlers (from birth to 36 months of age) with disabilities. According to this legislation, early intervention services

> are designed to meet the developmental needs of an infant or toddler with a disability in any one or more of the following areas:
> (i)   physical development,
> (ii) cognitive development,
> (iii) communication development,

(A) INDIVIDUALIZED EDUCATION PROGRAM — The term 'individualized education program' or 'IEP' means a written statement for each child with a disability that is developed, reviewed, and revised in accordance with this section and that includes—

(i) a statement of the child's present levels of educational performance, including—

(I) how the child's disability affects the child's involvement and progress in the general curriculum; or

(II) for preschool children, as appropriate, how the disability affects the child's participation in appropriate activities;

(ii) a statement of measurable annual goals, including benchmarks or short-term objectives, related to—

(I) meeting the child's needs that result from the child's disability to enable the child to be involved in and progress in the general curriculum; and

(II) meeting each of the child's other educational needs that result from the child's disability;

(iii) a statement of the special education and related services and supplementary aids and services to be provided to the child, or on behalf of the child, and a statement of the program modifications or supports for school personnel that will be provided for the child—

(I) to advance appropriately toward attaining the annual goals;

(II) to be involved and progress in the general curriculum in accordance with clause (i) and to participate in extracurricular and other nonacademic activities; and

(III) to be educated and participate with other children with disabilities and nondisabled children in the activities described in this paragraph;

(iv) an explanation of the extent, if any, to which the child will not participate with nondisabled children in the regular class and in the activities described in clause (iii);

(v)(I) a statement of any individual modifications in the administration of State or districtwide assessments of student achievement that are needed in order for the child to participate in such assessment; and

(II) if the IEP Team determines that the child will not participate in a particular State or districtwide assessment of student achievement (or part of such an assessment), a statement of—

(aa) why that assessment is not appropriate for the child; and

(bb) how the child will be assessed;

(vi) the projected date for the beginning of the services and modifications described in clause (iii), and the anticipated frequency, location, and duration of those services and modifications;

(vii)(I) beginning at age 14, and updated annually, a statement of the transition service needs of the child under the applicable components of the child's IEP that focuses on the child's courses of study (such as participation in advanced-placement courses or a vocational education program);

(continued)

Figure 18.1. The guidelines set forth by the Individuals with Disabilities Education Act (IDEA) Amendments of 1997 (PL 105-17) for the development of all individualized education programs (IEPs) (PL 105-17, Section 614).

Figure 18.1. *(continued)*

> (II) beginning at age 16 (or younger, if determined appropriate by the IEP Team), a statement of needed transition services for the child, including, when appropriate, a statement of interagency responsibilities or any needed linkages; and
>
> (III) beginning at least one year before the child reaches the age of majority under State law, a statement that the child has been informed of his or her rights under this title, if any, that will transfer to the child on reaching the age of majority under section 615(m); and
>
> (viii) a statement of—
>
> (I) how the child's progress toward the annual goals described in clause (ii) will be measured; and
>
> (II) how the child's parents will be regularly informed (by such means as periodic report cards), at least as often as parents are informed of their nondisabled children's progress, of—
>
> (aa) their child's progress toward the annual goals described in clause (ii); and
>
> (bb) the extent to which that progress is sufficient to enable the child to achieve the goals by the end of the year.

(iv) social or emotional development or

(v) adaptive development (PL 105-17, Section 631)

A multidisciplinary team, which includes the parent or the guardian of the infant with a disability, evaluates the infant across all five domains. Because eligibility requirements for services in the United States are determined by individual states, there is variability in qualifications for services from state to state and sometimes variability even within an individual state. In order to be eligible for services, infants and toddlers with cerebral palsy commonly must score 1.5 standard deviations below the mean on a standardized test or have a 25% or a 6-month delay in one or more of the developmental domains. The early intervention services that are provided to infants and toddlers can be extensive (see Figure 18.2).

The plan for services is developed in a meeting with the multidisciplinary team. The team develops an individualized family service plan (IFSP) according to the requirements stipulated in PL 102-119 (see Figure 18.3). Based on the needs of the infant or the toddler, the IFSP must be evaluated once a year and reviewed either at 6-month intervals or more often. Children with complex needs (e.g., those associated with cerebral palsy) may need more frequent evaluations. The degree of services provided to infants or to toddlers varies with location; some locations provide as many comprehensive services as are necessary to meet the individual needs of the infant or the toddler and his or her family, whereas other locations might limit services to a maximum of 2 hours

---

   (i)   family training, counseling, and home visits;
   (ii)   special instruction;
  (iii)   speech-language pathology and audiology services;
  (iv)   occupational therapy;
   (v)   physical therapy;
  (vi)   psychological services;
 (vii) service coordination services;
(viii) medical services only for diagnostic or evaluative purposes;
  (ix)   early identification, screening, and assessment services;
   (x)   health services necessary to enable the infant or toddler to benefit from the other early intervention services;
  (xi)   social work services;
 (xii) vision services;
(xiii) assistive technology devices and assistive technology services; and
(xiv) transportation and related costs that are necessary to enable an infant or toddler and the infant's or toddler's family to receive another service.

Figure 18.2. The early intervention services that may be provided to all infants and toddlers (as mandated by the Individuals with Disabilities Education Act [IDEA] Amendments of 1997, PL 105-17, Section 631).

per week or set a cost limit. Some states, such as Pennsylvania, have even considered returning Part H (PL 99-457) funds to the federal government, thereby freeing themselves of the responsibility to follow the federal guidelines in serving infants and toddlers (Brian, 1996).

Services must be provided by "qualified personnel." During early intervention, any one of the professionals involved with an infant or a toddler may assume the primary responsibility for providing the most direct services. This individual may be the service coordinator; for infants and toddlers with cerebral palsy, the service coordinator or the primary service provider also may be the therapist.

Under IDEA and its amendments, children 3–5 years of age are eligible for preschool services. Every child receiving special services must have an IEP; however, the state also has the option of allowing the more comprehensive IFSP. Every child must require educational services in order to receive related services, unless the education agency has chosen to allow the IFSP. In this situation, therapy may not have to be provided solely to meet the educational needs of the child. If the preschool child with cerebral palsy does not need educational services but does need related services, then these frequently can be obtained if there is a developmental delay in any domain of the child's development (generally in physical development). Under PL 105-17, developmental delay is one of the diagnostic categories that preschoolers can use to qualify for preschool and related services and is an accepted category of eligibility for school-age children up to 9 years of age.

The IFSP must be in writing and contain
(1) a statement of the infant's or toddler's present levels of physical development, cognitive development, communication development, social or emotional development, and adaptive development based on acceptable objective criteria;
(2) a statement of the family's resources, priorities, and concerns relating to enhancing the development of the family's infant or toddler with a disability;
(3) a statement of the major outcomes expected to be achieved for the infant or toddler and the family, and the criteria, procedures, and timeliness used to determine the degree to which progress toward achieving the outcomes is being made and whether modifications or revisions of the outcomes or services are necessary;
(4) a statement of specific early intervention services necessary to meet the unique needs of the infant or toddler and the family, including the frequency, intensity, and the method of delivering services;
(5) a statement of the natural environments in which early intervention services shall appropriately be provided, including a justification of the extent, if any, to which the services will not be provided in a natural environment;
(6) the projected dates for initiation of services and the anticipated duration of the services;
(7) the identification of the service coordinator from the profession most immediately relevant to the infant's or toddler's or family's needs (or who is otherwise qualified to carry out all applicable responsibilities under this part) who is responsible for the implementation of the plan and coordination with other agencies and persons; and
(8) the steps to be taken supporting the transition of the toddler with a disability to preschool or other appropriate services.

Figure 18.3. The requirements set forth by the Individuals with Disabilities Education Act (IDEA) Amendments of 1997 (PL 105-17) for the development of all individualized family service plans (IFSPs) (PL 105-17, Part C, Section 636).

As with school-age children, services to infants, toddlers, and preschoolers must be provided in the least restrictive environment (LRE). This means that not only is the home one of the major locations of service delivery but the local child care center also is a main locale. Court cases in the 1990s have mandated that private, for-profit child care providers must include children with disabilities. In order to comply with the LRE mandate, related services should always come to the child (i.e., be provided in the general classroom) rather than the child going to the related services (i.e., in a resource room or a separate school).

IDEA emphasizes that at each stage of the child's education, plans must be made for successful transition to the next level of educational or vocational services. This must be started long before the actual transition is to occur to allow for a smooth, seamless transition.

Section 504 of the Rehabilitation Act of 1973 (PL 93-112)

Preschool and school-age children with cerebral palsy whose disabilities do not adversely affect their educational performance and, as a result, who are not eligible for special education and related services under IDEA may still qualify for related services and other supports under Section 504 of the Rehabilitation Act of 1973 (PL 93-112). The definition of "qualified handicapped person" in Section 504 is broader than it is in IDEA. According to Section 504, the child with a disability must have the following characteristics:

- A physical or a mental impairment that substantially limits one or more major life activities
- A record of having a physical or a mental impairment that substantially limits one or more major life activities
- Regarded as having such an impairment

Thus, a child who does not require special education but who is a "qualified handicapped person" may be able to receive all the aids and the accommodations necessary to receive a FAPE under Section 504 (National Information Center for Children and Youth with Disabilities, 1991).

RECOMMENDED PRACTICES FOR CHILDREN WITH DISABILITIES IN SCHOOLS

A review of the literature on the delivery of services to children with disabilities reveals a number of characteristics that describe the "recommended practices" that help students with disabilities (including those with cerebral palsy) to benefit from their early intervention and educational programs (Campbell, 1987; Dunn, 1991; Effgen & Klepper, 1994; Giangreco, 1995; Hanft & Place, 1996; McEwen & Sheldon, 1995; Orelove & Sobsey, 1996; Rainforth & York-Barr, 1997). Although the hope was that these characteristics would precede the formulation of enlightened federal laws, IDEA has actually taught many people how to create recommended practice and state-of-the-art services. Advocates for individuals with disabilities have done an outstanding job in guiding practice, and one hopes that their vision will continue to be acted on at the state level as states gain more control of the practices that meet the educational and the health care needs of children with disabilities.

The major elements of IDEA are the keystones of what is considered recommended practice in the educational environment. Not every school system is doing its most to use recommended practice; however, many states and local education agencies provide excellent educational opportunities for children with cerebral palsy. The key elements that must be met in order to provide recommended practices are inclusive education, educational and early intervention teams, early intervention, assistive technology, and transition planning.

Inclusive Education

A very important key element in PL 94-142 and later amendments of IDEA is that a child's education is to be provided in the LRE (e.g., in a general classroom with age-appropriate peers in his or her local school). Public agencies are to ensure "that to the maximum extent, appropriate children with disabilities, including children in public or private institutions or other care facilities, are educated with children who are not disabled" (PL 105-17, Section 612). In 1975, this was considered a rather radical concept, and, in 1997, it is still considered radical by some individuals. No other element of IDEA has caused as much discussion and litigation.

Following the passage of PL 94-142, many areas in the United States that did not have special schools found it relatively easy and inexpensive to comply with the law and to include children with disabilities in their local schools. States would either enroll children in their age-appropriate classroom or develop special classes within the local school. School systems that had already established segregated programs and schools for children with disabilities found it especially difficult to place children in local schools; they did not believe these children would be able to obtain the same services in local schools as they were able to obtain in the segregated settings. This was particularly true for children with cerebral palsy because therapies were provided at the specialized schools, whereas many local schools could not or would not provide therapy to the children with disabilities. Since 1980, many children with disabilities have been moved out of institutions and segregated special schools. The move toward inclusive educational environments has been slowest in the northeast region of the United States, where special schools were more common than in other parts of the country (U.S. Department of Education, 1995).

Children in special segregated classes are slowly being included in general classes; however, it is important to remember that these students also go to resource classes where they receive one-to-one or group instruction in specific areas of need. Children with cerebral palsy who have no cognitive difficulties may spend all of their time in the general class and may receive resource assistance in the general classroom. Providing the amount of resource assistance needed is an evolving process. Frequently, by middle school, a child either no longer needs as many resource or special services, or he or she requires a significant increase in his or her resource services. As the pace of the educational process quickens in the general classroom, it frequently becomes more difficult for the child with a disability to maintain the same learning pace as his or her classmates; this is especially true for the child with both cerebral palsy and mental retardation. The transition to more or less resource assistance or, if necessary, a change in the location of services in middle school must be properly planned well before the actual transition in order for the change to be successful.

Educational and Early Intervention Teams

A team of professionals is required by law to perform an initial assessment of the child using multiple assessment tools. The IEP or IFSP then is developed based on this evaluation. An IEP or IFSP generally is not implemented by a single individual; rather, a team of professionals and members of the child's family typically implement them. This is usually the situation with a child who has cerebral palsy and who requires not only educational services but also the support of related-services personnel (e.g., a speech-language pathologist, an occupational therapist, a physical therapist, a psychologist, a nutritionist, a nurse). The team must work together to maximize the services and to obtain the best possible outcomes for the child while being careful not to "overdo" related services. Giangreco (1995) suggested that the "more-is-better" approach to service provision is misguided and confuses quantity of care with quality of care; instead, he recommended that the "only-as-special-as-necessary" approach be followed in order "to avoid the inherent drawbacks of well-intended over service" (p. 58). There must be a balance in the amount of services provided and a recognition that school is not a medical setting but is a place where the child is to receive an education and learn the social skills necessary for life.

Although IDEA uses the terminology "multidisciplinary teams," there are many other names given to these groups of professionals who work together in an integrated, coordinated manner (e.g., interdisciplinary, transdisciplinary, integrated, collaborative). The broad concept is that no single individual or professional is able to provide comprehensive evaluations and services to the child with a disability, especially the child with cerebral palsy; rather, an interdisciplinary team made up of professionals from several fields can best promote the well-being of the child (see Chapter 3). Developing an effective team can be a difficult process. The major elements of collaborative teamwork are outlined in Table 18.1. Equal participation, respect, and consensus decision making result in more successful service delivery.

Early Intervention

In 1975, the U.S. Congress discussed the importance of addressing the needs of all children during the earliest ages of life. The data from Head Start, the U.S. Bureau of Education of the Handicapped, and other projects supported various benefits of early intervention for children from families of low socioeconomic status and children with disabilities (Guralnick, 1991; Hunt, 1975; Martin, Ramey, & Ramey, 1990). Even in 1975, many members of Congress wanted the range of coverage in PL 94-142 to begin at birth. This, however, was too great a change for some members of Congress and perhaps for the nation. Therefore, Congress compromised and started with school-age children. It was not until 1986 when the Education of the Handicapped Act Amendments was passed that infants, toddlers, and preschoolers (i.e., birth to 5 years of age) were included in the provisions. The lessons learned from PL 94-142 helped in the

Table 18.1. Defining the characteristics of collaborative teamwork

1. Equal participation in the collaborative teamwork process by family members and the educational service providers on the educational team

2. Equal participation by all disciplines determined to be necessary for students to achieve their individualized educational goals

3. Consensus decision making about the type and the amount of support required from related services personnel

4. Consensus decision making about priority educational goals and objectives related to all student functioning at school, at home, and in the community.

5. Attention to motor, communication, and other embedded skills and needs throughout the educational program and in direct relevance to accomplishing priority educational goals

6. Infusion of knowledge and skills from different disciplines into the design of educational methods and interventions

7. Role release to enable team members who are involved most directly and frequently with students to develop the confidence and competence necessary to facilitate active learning and effective participation in the educational program

8. Collaborative problem solving and shared responsibility for student learning across all aspects for the educational program

From Rainforth, B., & York-Barr, J. (1997). *Collaborative teams for students with severe disabilities: Integrating therapy and educational services* (2nd ed., p. 23). Baltimore: Paul H. Brookes Publishing Co.; reprinted by permission.

development of PL 99-457 (Martin, 1989), and, as a result, states were given more freedom in choosing how to serve young children with disabilities. However, PL 99-457 also led to a great variability in eligibility for services and availability of services in different states.

The benefits of early intervention for children with disabilities and their families are numerous (Connolly, Morgan, Russell, & Richardson, 1980; Connolly & Russell, 1976; Guralnick, 1991; Palisano, 1991; Warren & Kaiser, 1988). Early intervention not only helps children to achieve optimal development in all domains but also is believed to help prevent deformity, abnormal movement patterns, abnormal behavior patterns, aberrant adaptive behavior, and other secondary problems. In addition, early intervention services help parents learn how best to meet their child's and their own needs (Dunst, Trivette, & Deal, 1993; Sparling, Kolobe, & Ezzelle, 1994). By assisting children and their families at an early age, special services might not be necessary later in the child's life (Bowe, 1995).

Assistive Technology

The Technology-Related Assistance for Individuals with Disabilities Act of 1988 (PL 100-407) was reauthorized in 1994 (as PL 103-218) and provided the terminology and concepts for assistive technology provisions. In 1991, as part of PL 102-119, assistive technology devices and assistive technology services were outlined as services provided under IDEA. Children with cerebral palsy became eligible for extensive technology-based assistance to help them benefit from their education. A technology-based assistive device was broadly defined as

> any item, piece of equipment, or project system whether acquired commercially off the shelf, modified, or customized, that is used to increase, maintain, or improve the functional capabilities of children with disabilities.... Assistive technology services means any service that directly assists a child with a disability in the selection, acquisition, or use of assistive technology device. (*Federal Register,* 1992, p. 44801)

Assistive technology services incorporate the processes of evaluating a child, selecting and purchasing the device, and coordinating team members who are participating in the development of the child's IEP or IFSP. Communication devices and computer systems make up a major area of assistive technology (see Chapter 15). These devices directly affect the ability to educate many children with cerebral palsy. It is not unreasonable to assume that every child with cerebral palsy who needs a computerized communication device should be provided with one at school. In addition to communication devices, all devices that may help a child meet his or her educational needs should be considered. Adaptive seating may help the child function more efficiently and safely at school (see Chapter 12). Ambulation devices may allow the child to explore his or her environment, get to class, or go to the bathroom; or they may expand his or her options for educational and vocational training. Power mobility devices may allow the child with severe functional limitations to gain access to the school building and grounds independently and, thus, minimize his or her disability while broadening his or her opportunities.

There must be consistency in the use of assistive technology across settings. The child should not be expected to use different types of computers or seating devices in different classrooms and during different activities. The child also needs access to similar technology at home in order to do homework. In addition, assistive technology devices should travel with the child to new settings. When the child moves to a new school, it is very common for the school to have to order new equipment for the child's use. This can be costly, and critical learning time will be lost if the equipment is not there at the beginning of the new school year. Moreover, if different types of devices arrive, time will be lost while the child and related-services personnel learn to use the new system. Most individuals—with or without a disability—find it difficult to continually learn new computer programs or systems.

The extent of services and the purchasing of assistive technology devices vary among school systems. The law, however, is quite generous in its provisions, and, when tested through due process, the child usually receives the needed device. For example, in 1995, the U.S. Office of Special Education Programs (OSEP) informed a special education director that if a student with a visual impairment required eyeglasses to receive a FAPE and the student's IEP indicated the need for the eyeglasses, then the school had to provide the glasses at no cost to the student's parents (*OSEP explains,* 1996). When there is both an educational and a medical need for the assistive technology, the issue of provisions is not as clear because the school system is not obligated to provide medical services beyond those required for evaluative purposes (Golden, 1996).

Transition Planning

In order for the child to have the most successful and appropriate transition to a new setting, there must be ongoing transition planning. In early intervention, there must be planning for preschool. Parents should be prepared for changes in the service delivery system that might occur in the preschool setting. Therapies may or may not be provided, and the preschool service delivery system is likely to be quite different from early intervention. The child must be prepared to spend the entire day or part of the day away from home (and may need to be prepared to travel on a school bus), and the parent will not have as much contact as before with related-services personnel. The earlier preparations can be made, the more likely it is that the transition will go smoothly and successfully.

The move from preschool to school is a major transition. In an ideal situation, the child with cerebral palsy will attend the local school where siblings and neighbors are enrolled. A sense of familiarity and community often helps to ease the transition process for both the child and his or her family. Arrangements should be made for children and their families to visit the school before the school year begins. The IEP meeting held before the transition should include not only the preschool teachers and appropriate related-services personnel but also the teachers and staff from the new school. If only the federally mandated minimum attendees plan to attend the IEP meeting, then the child's parents have the right to request the presence of additional personnel.

If the child is going to attend school in a new building, then the new building must be accessible according to the letter of the law and it should be made "user friendly." The child should be able to enter the front door, use all or at least most of the bathrooms, and gain access to the auditorium and cafeteria. Arrangements must be made so that the adaptive equipment and assistive technology devices the child uses will be available when the child starts attending the new school. It is frustrating for all involved when a child has to wait for a communication device to arrive at the new school before his or her educational program can begin. It is equally frustrating when the child has to wait for the appropriate wheelchair before being able to go with his or her classmates to the cafeteria. These frustrating and demoralizing delays can easily be prevented with advance planning.

There will be additional transitions throughout the child's educational program depending on his or her needs as well as the structure of the school system he or she attends. All transitions, if possible, should be planned years in advance. For example, physical therapists need to know while the child is attending middle school how far and how fast the child will have to walk to get to class on time in high school. Knowing this information in advance helps not only to determine appropriate objectives for the child but also to motivate the child to achieve new, meaningful goals. School nurses need to be aware of the child's medical problems and needs before the child arrives at school, especially now that children with cerebral palsy and serious health care needs are attending general classrooms (Rapport, 1996). Transition planning for leaving school should begin by 14 years of age, or earlier if necessary (see Chapter 20).

SERVICE DELIVERY MODELS

There is an array of service delivery models that have a wide range of confusing and sometimes conflicting terminology. When selecting a model of service delivery, the objective is to assist the child to achieve educational and developmental objectives in preparation for independent life; however, there is not one service delivery model that will meet all the needs of every child or every system.

The provision of services to infants, toddlers, and most preschoolers who have disabilities has historically been based on a team approach. The leader of the team varies depending on the setting and the needs of the child. If a classroom model is used, the teacher is frequently the team leader; if a home-based model is used, the professional with the most frequent contact with the child and family may be the team leader. As mandated by PL 102-119, the service coordinator must come from the discipline most relevant to the needs of the child and his or her family. Unfortunately, in many parts of the United States, service coordinators are not from the disciplines most relevant to the individual children's needs; rather, the service coordinator is often the member of the child's team whose time is least costly.

For the school-age child, the teacher is clearly the team leader and all other personnel are there to provide related services, which are given solely to meet the educational needs of the child. The teacher who assumes the role of team leader varies. This role may be taken by the general educator or by a consulting special education teacher with a background in meeting the needs of children with disabilities. Other professionals on the team work with the teachers and the child's parents to assist in promoting the child's development.

Therapists can provide direct (i.e., hands-on treatment) and indirect (i.e., consultation or supervision) services to the child in numerous environments. For many children, especially younger children and those with severe impairments, services should ideally be provided in the classroom or another natural environment where the therapist can encourage activities indigenous to the setting; this is in keeping with the legal requirement outlined in IDEA that education must be provided in the LRE. For example, a physical therapist provides gait training while the child is walking around class or to the cafeteria, the occupational therapist works on the child's writing skills during class sessions, and the speech-language therapist addresses the child's language skills during classroom learning activities. When children are fully included in the LRE for all of their education, there may be times, especially for older children or highly distractible children, when specialized equipment is necessary and direct service must be provided in a separate setting. Direct service in an isolated area should be reserved for the most extreme situations when a separate setting is the best environment in which a child can learn a specific task. Frequent practice in multiple settings has been shown to be the best way to generalize learning to multiple environments (Brown, 1994; Horner, Dunlap, & Koegel, 1988; McEwen & Sheldon, 1995).

During the 1990s, there has been a trend toward an integrated model of service delivery, which has various forms and names. In general terms, in an integrated model of service delivery, a team coordinates goals and objectives and all individuals serving the child are instructed in how to achieve the objectives. For example, if the objective is for the child to feed him- or herself independently in the cafeteria, the physical therapist may determine the appropriate seating system and position, the occupational therapist may provide the best eating utensils and suggest the most appropriate perceptual-motor strategies for getting the food from the table to the child's mouth, and the speech-language therapist may assist in food selection and instructing other team members in the correct oral-motor activities for the child to chew and swallow the food. The parent may play a part in service delivery as well by indicating the foods that the child has the most and least success in eating. The child indicates what he or she wants to eat. The teacher and paraeducator would be instructed by the physical therapist, the occupational therapist, and the speech-language therapist because these individuals are involved in every step of the eating process. Therapists may not need to provide direct, one-to-one therapy to the child if they are comfortable with the teacher's ability to safely follow their instructions. However, if therapists decide that they want to try a different eating utensil or an oral desensitization technique, then they may try the new utensil or new technique directly with the child in an isolated setting. There should be no rigid boundaries in an integrated approach; if the child needs direct service or service in a special setting, then this should be an option. The essence of an integrated model is that the goals and objectives for the child are functional and directed toward helping him or her function optimally in his or her real-life, natural environment.

A variant of the integrated model is the collaborative model or the collaborative teaming design (Rainforth & York-Barr, 1997) (see Table 18.1). Many professionals believe that elements of the collaborative process should be found in every service delivery system. "Collaboration is the sine qua non of successful integration efforts" (Hanson & Widerstrom, 1993, p. 149).

In the consultative model, service is usually provided in the learning environment, and the implementor of the activities is the teacher, the parent, the paraeducator, or another team member. The consultant is asked to address specific issues and generally is not involved in the overall programming for the child. The amount of service is intermittent and based on the needs of the team (Effgen, 1994). "Inclusion of children with disabilities in regular classrooms has highlighted the need for collaborative consultation between special educators, regular educators and therapists" (Hanft & Place, 1996, p. 1).

Therapists assume the responsibility for overseeing the child in the monitoring model. Within this model, the therapist and the team have decided that direct or indirect service is no longer required; rather, the therapists believe that it is best to check on the child periodically. Maintaining this contact, though infrequent, is especially important during periods of rapid growth, puberty, school transitions, and following hospitalizations or surgery. Ideally, monitoring would be listed in the child's IEP with a frequency of perhaps once a month or twice a year. Having a monitoring schedule in the child's IEP not only provides accountability but also reduces the paperwork that is necessary in order to get permission to reevaluate or treat a child if changes are observed mid-year (Effgen, 1994).

Educators and related-services personnel must collaborate to provide the best possible education for children with cerebral palsy. Parents also must remember that the primary function of an educational environment is education, not therapy. Therapy is designed to assist with the child's education; if it is not serving this purpose—regardless of whether the child needs it for noneducational reasons— it must be obtained outside of the educational setting. In addition, as opposed to a lifetime of structured therapy sessions, parents and children also should consider the therapeutic benefits of such physical activities as swimming, horseback riding, martial arts, arts and crafts, and other recreation activities.

SUMMARY

All children spend a significant amount of their childhood in school. Professionals working with children in schools have an obligation to make the experience as successful and as meaningful as possible. If the child does not learn to be independent and self-functioning during school, he or she will not learn these traits after leaving. Insightful federal laws in the United States have guaranteed the right to a FAPE for all children with cerebral palsy. It is the joint responsibility of families and professionals to ensure that this education is appropriate and effective.

REFERENCES

Assistance to States for the Education of Children with Disabilities Program and Preschool Grants for Children with Disabilities. (1992). 34 CFR, Parts 300, 301.

Bowe, F.G. (1995). *Birth to five: Early childhood special education.* New York: Delmar.

Brian, X. (1996, February 20). Pa. governor proposes quitting IDEA's. *Education Daily,* pp. H1, H3.

Brown, D.A. (1994). *Acquisition and generalization ability following physical therapy in persons with significant physical and mental disabilities.* Unpublished doctoral dissertation, Hahnemann University, Philadelphia.

Cable, O.E., Fowler, A.F., & Foss, H.S. (1936). The crippled children's guide of Buffalo, New York. *Physical Therapy Review, 16,* 85–88.

Campbell, P.H. (1987). The integrated programming team: An approach for coordinating professionals of various disciplines in programs for students with severe and multiple handicaps. *Journal of The Association for Persons with Severe Handicaps, 12,* 107–116.

Connolly, B., Morgan, S., Russell, F.F., & Richardson, B. (1980). Early intervention with Down syndrome children: Follow-up report. *Physical Therapy, 60,* 1405–1408.

Connolly, B., & Russell, F. (1976). Interdisciplinary early intervention program. *Physical Therapy, 56,* 155–158.

Dunn, W. (1991). Integrated related services. In L.H. Meyer, C.A. Peck, & L. Brown (Eds.), *Critical issues in the lives of persons with severe disabilities* (pp. 353–377). Baltimore: Paul H. Brookes Publishing Co.

Dunst, C., Trivette, C.M., & Deal, A. (1993). *Supporting and strengthening families: Methods, strategies, and outcome.* Cambridge, MA: Brookline Books Inc.

Education for All Handicapped Children Act of 1975, PL 94-142, 20 U.S.C. §§ 1400 *et seq.*

Education of the Handicapped Act Amendments of 1986, PL 99-457, 20 U.S.C. §§ 1400 *et seq.*

Effgen, S.K. (1994). The educational environment. In S.K. Campbell (Ed.), *Physical therapy for children* (pp. 847–872). Philadelphia: W.B. Saunders.

Effgen, S.K., & Klepper, S. (1994). Survey of physical therapy practice in educational settings. *Pediatric Physical Therapy, 6,* 15–21.

Giangreco, M.F. (1995). Related services decision-making: A foundational component of effective education for students with disabilities. *Physical & Occupational Therapy in Pediatrics, 15,* 47–67.

Golden, D.C. (1996). Assistive technology: It's the law, but how do you do it? *The Special Educator, 11*(14), 6–7.

Guralnick, M.J. (1991). The next decade of research on the effectiveness of early intervention. *Early Education and Development, 58*(2), 174–183.

Handicapped Children's Protection Act of 1986, PL 99-372, 20 U.S.C. §§ 1415 *et seq.*

Hanft, B., & Place, P. (1996). *Consultation in schools.* Tucson, AZ: Therapy Skill Builders.

Hanson, M.J., & Widerstrom, A.H. (1993). Consultation and collaboration: Essentials of integration efforts for young children. In C.A. Peck, S.L. Odom, & D.D. Bricker (Eds.), *Integrating young children with disabilities into community programs: Ecological perspectives on research and implementation* (pp. 149–168). Baltimore: Paul H. Brookes Publishing Co.

Horner, R.H., Dunlap, G., & Koegel, R. (1988). *Generalization and maintenance: Lifestyle changes in applied settings.* Baltimore: Paul H. Brookes Publishing Co.

Hunt, J.M. (1975). Reflections on a decade of early education. *Journal of Abnormal Psychology, 3*(4), 275–330.

Individuals with Disabilities Education Act (IDEA) of 1990, PL 101-476, 20 U.S.C. §§ 1400 *et seq.*

Individuals with Disabilities Education Act Amendments of 1991, PL 102-119, 20 U.S.C. §§ 1400 *et seq.*

Individuals with Disabilities Education Act Amendments of 1997, PL 105-17, 20 U.S.C. §§ 1400 *et seq.*

Martin, E.W. (1989). Lessons from implementing PL 94-142. In J.J. Gallagher, P.L. Trohanis, & R.M. Clifford (Eds.), *Policy implementation and PL 99-457: Planning for young children with special needs* (pp. 19–32). Baltimore: Paul H. Brookes Publishing Co.

Martin, S.L., Ramey, C.T., & Ramey, S. (1990). The prevention of intellectual impairment in children of impoverished families: Findings of a randomized trial of educational day care. *American Journal of Public Health, 80*(7), 844–847.

McEwen, I.R., & Sheldon, M.L. (1995). Pediatric therapy in the 1990s: The demise of the educational versus medical dichotomy. *Physical & Occupational Therapy in Pediatrics, 15,* 33–45.

National Information Center for Children and Youth with Disabilities. (1991). Related services for school-aged children with disabilities. *News Digest, National Information Center for Children and Youth with Disabilities, 1*(2), 8.

Orelove, F., & Sobsey, D. (1996). *Educating children with multiple disabilities: A transdisciplinary approach* (3rd ed.). Baltimore: Paul H. Brookes Publishing Co.

OSEP explains duty to provide eyeglasses for certain students. (1996). *The Special Educator, 11*(1), 17.

Palisano, R. (1991). Research on the effectiveness of neurodevelopmental treatment. *Pediatric Physical Therapy, 3*(3), 143–148.

Rainforth, B., & York-Barr, J. (1997). *Collaborative teams for students with severe disabilities: Integrating therapy and educational services* (2nd ed.). Baltimore: Paul H. Brookes Publishing Co.

Rapport, M.J. (1996). Legal guidelines for the delivery of special health care services in schools. *Exceptional Children, 62,* 537–549.

Rehabilitation Act of 1973, PL 93-112, 29 U.S.C. §§ 701 *et seq.*

Sparling, J.W., Kolobe, T.H.A., & Ezzelle, L. (1994). Family-centered intervention. In S.K. Campbell (Ed.), *Physical therapy for children* (pp. 824–846). Philadelphia: W.B. Saunders.

Technology-Related Assistance for Individuals with Disabilities Act of 1988, PL 100-407, 29 U.S.C. §§ 2201 *et seq.*

Technology-Related Assistance for Individuals with Disabilities Act Amendments of 1994, PL 103-218, 29 U.S.C. §§ 35 *et seq.*

U.S. Department of Education. (1995). To assure the free appropriate public education (FAPE) of all children with disabilities. *Seventeenth Annual Report to Congress on the Implementation of The Individuals with Disabilities Education Act.* Washington, DC: Author.

Warren S.F., & Kaiser, A.P. (1988). Research in early language intervention. In S.L. Odom & M.B. Karnes (Eds.), *Early intervention for infants and children with handicaps: An empirical base* (pp. 89–108). Baltimore: Paul H. Brookes Publishing Co.

Key Elements of the Individuals with Disabilities Education Act

The Individuals with Disabilities Education Act (IDEA), PL 94-142, was passed in 1990 and amended in 1992 and 1997. Entries in this appendix are from the original law (PL 94-142) as well as its amendments.

Assistive technology An assistive technology device is "any item, piece of equipment, or product system whether acquired commercially off the shelf, modified, or customized, that is used to increase, maintain, or improve the functional capabilities of children with disabilities." Assistive technology services are "any service[s] that directly assist a child with a disability in the selection, acquisition, or use of assistive technology device." (*Federal Register,* 1992, p. 44801)

Individualized education program (IEP) Every school-age child receiving special education must have an IEP, which is a comprehensive program outlining the specific special educational and related services the child is to receive, including the child's annual goals and objectives. The IEP is developed annually at an IEP meeting attended by the child's parents, a representative of the local education agency, the child's teacher, and an individual involved in the child's evaluation.

Individualized family service plan (IFSP) The IFSP is developed for infants and toddlers and their families, and in some states for preschool-age children and their families. The IFSP is developed and reviewed every 6 months by an interdisciplinary team, which must include the child's parent(s) or guardian(s). The family is central to the development and objectives of the IFSP.

Least restrictive environment (LRE)   Public agencies are to ensure "that to the maximum extent appropriate children with disabilities, including children in public or private institutions or other care facilities, are educated with children who are nondisabled." (PL 105-17, 1997, Section 612)

Nondiscriminatory evaluation   Nondiscriminatory tests are to be used to evaluate children; however, no one test can be the sole criterion used for placement.

Parent participation   The active participation of parents is encouraged. Parents are the individuals responsible for the continuity of services for their child and should be the child's biggest advocates. Parents are major decision makers in the development of their child's IEP and IFSP. They must give permission for an evaluation, they can restrict the release of information, they have access to their child's records, and they can request due process hearings.

Related services   Related services, such as transportation, speech-language pathology, audiology, psychological services, PT, OT, recreation, and medical and counseling services, must be provided "as may be required to assist a child with a disability to benefit from special education." (PL 105-17, 19, Section 602)

Right to due process   Parents have the right to an impartial hearing, the right to be represented by counsel, and the right to a verbatim transcript of a hearing and written findings. They can appeal the evaluation findings and educational recommendations for their child and get an independent evaluation. Under the Handicapped Children's Protection Act of 1986 (PL 99-372), parents may be reimbursed for legal fees if they prevail in court.

Transition   Early intervention and school personnel are to plan for the successful transition of a child to the next level of service. Transition plans must be included in the IEP and IFSP. "The coordinated set of activities shall be based upon the individual student's needs taking into account the student's preferences and interests and shall include instruction, community experiences, development employment, and other postschool adult living objectives, and when appropriate acquisition of daily living skills and functional vocabulary evaluation." (PL 101-476, 20 U.S.C. §§ 1400 *et seq.*)

Zero reject   All children are to receive an education regardless of how severe or profound the disability.

CHAPTER 19

Public Policy

Disability-Related Legislation

Linda Hock-Long

Societal obstacles can unfairly limit the range of opportunities available to individuals with cerebral palsy and other developmental disabilities. In fact, the term *handicap* is included in the *International Classification of Impairments, Disabilities, and Handicaps* to characterize the inequities associated with architectural barriers, inadequate educational services, discriminatory hiring practices, and other environmental and attitudinal forces (World Health Organization, 1980; see Chapter 3). Although the National Center for Medical Rehabilitation Research replaced "handicap" with "societal limitation" in its model of the disabling process, both frameworks underscore the negative consequences of societal obstacles.

Social welfare legislation plays an important role in counteracting the effects of societal limitations. Consequently, this chapter presents an overview of federal disability-related social welfare legislation in the United States. Information is provided regarding traditional approaches to social welfare in the United States; the incremental expansion of the federal government's social welfare role; and the processes surrounding the development, implementation, and evaluation of public policy. The final section contains an overview

467

of current statutes in the areas of civil rights, income maintenance, health care, technology-related assistance, and vocational rehabilitation. (see Chapter 18 for a detailed discussion of educational regulations.)

THE UNITED STATES AND SOCIAL WELFARE

When broadly defined, *social welfare* refers to "all social interventions intended to enhance or maintain the social functioning of human beings" (Dolgoff, Feldstein, & Skolnik, 1993, p. 4). Because disability-related legislation can enhance the functioning of individuals with disabilities, it represents a critical social welfare function.

Social welfare is generally considered to be the joint responsibility of a nation's government as well as its market economy, its voluntary organizations, and its families. The level of responsibility each sector assumes is determined by a number of dynamic philosophical, political, cultural, social, environmental, and temporal factors. A common model frequently used to characterize governmental social welfare interest breaks involvement into two categories: residual approaches and institutional approaches. Adherents of the residual approach believe that the government should provide a temporary safety net when an individual's needs are not met by the market economy, by his or her family, or by voluntary organizations. In contrast, proponents of the institutional approach believe that government should offer broad-based, ongoing protections. The U.S. response to social welfare is rooted in the residual perspective, a perspective that supports principles such as individual freedom and decentralization of sovereign powers that are basic to the country.

The Elizabethan Poor Law, enacted in England in 1601, provided the framework for the residual social welfare policies and practices in the British colonies. The significance of these nearly 400-year-old laws cannot be overestimated; they continue to shape U.S. social welfare responses. For instance, debate regarding whether an individual or a group is "deserving" of services and whether these services should be offered in homes and communities or in institutional settings has continued since Colonial times. Other elements of the Elizabethan Poor Laws that influence social welfare practices in the United States are the expectation that the family is responsible for the well-being of its members and the belief that, whenever possible, assistance should be provided at the local level (Katz, 1995).

THE U.S. PUBLIC POLICY PROCESS

A multiplicity of complex issues fostered the gradual expansion of U.S. federal social welfare legislation. As a result, many policies now reflect an institutional orientation. The process for developing, enacting, and implementing incremental legislative changes has typically included five phases: problem identification, policy development, legislative action, implementation, and evaluation (see Figure 19.1) (DiNitto, 1991).

Problem Identification

The legislative process is initiated when a problem or a need that has widespread implications is identified. For instance, inadequate educational services for students with learning differences and employment practices discriminating against individuals with disabilities provided the impetus for important disability-related statutes in U.S. legislative history, such as the Individuals with Disabilities Education Act (IDEA) of 1990 (PL 101-476) and the Americans with Disabilities Act (ADA) of 1990 (PL 101-336).

Policy Development

Congress is responsible for making laws. For instance, in order to improve home- and community-based services, a bill may be proposed in either the House of Representatives or the Senate. The congressional committee responsible for health-related legislation then fosters the development of the bill through activities such as public hearings and committee reviews. Although lobbyists and other stockholder groups play pivotal roles in recommending legislative solutions, the committee is ultimately responsible for the bill's destiny. Consequently, because of unresolved internal conflicts, some bills may never leave committees, whereas other bills may fail at the level of their original supporters.

Legislative Action

When a bill receives a majority of votes in Congress, presidential action is required within 10 days. The bill becomes a law if the president approves it or takes no action during this 10-day period. In the case of a presidential veto, the

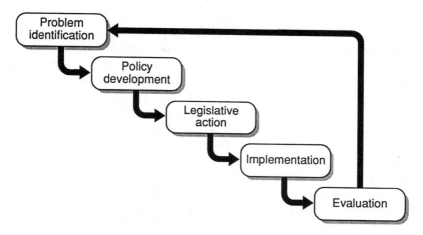

Figure 19.1.   Typical phases of the public policy process.

bill is sent back to the house where it originated. Options available to Congress at this juncture include referring the bill back to the congressional committee for further consideration, postponing action, or taking steps to overturn the veto. In order to overturn a presidential veto, the bill must be passed by a two-thirds majority vote in both houses of Congress.

Implementation

During the implementation phase, resources are appropriated by Congress, and programs, policies, and regulatory mechanisms are developed by executive agencies such as the Department of Education and the Department of Health and Human Services.

Evaluation

The evaluation phase consists of assessing the effectiveness of policies and practices with methods such as public hearings, projects, site visits, quasi-experimental research, and judicial review. When gaps or problems are identified, previous steps in the policy process may be repeated in order to revise existing statutes. For instance, the Supreme Court's ruling in *Sullivan v. Zebley* (1990), which found that adult-oriented disability criteria discriminated against children, provided the impetus for amendments to Supplemental Security Income (SSI) legislation.

HISTORICAL OVERVIEW OF U.S. SOCIAL WELFARE LEGISLATION: 1776–1935

The U.S. government had limited administrative and financial resources prior to the 20th century. Consequently, the family, local community, and charitable organizations assumed primary responsibility for social welfare throughout the 18th and 19th centuries. Because community-based services predominated until the 1820s, institutional care then became the preferred venue for many individuals who were poor or had disabilities because of the belief that institutions offered curative approaches that could not be replicated in the community. However, by the turn of the 20th century, the efficacy of institutional care came under dispute. Social and economic factors were in part responsible for this reversal. For instance, instead of offering therapeutic services that cured people, many facilities provided custodial care that often was of dubious quality. In addition, the cost-effectiveness of institutional care was questioned during the periods of economic distress that followed the Civil War. Thus, steps were taken to provide more humane, less costly alternatives (e.g., community-based services).

By the latter part of the 19th century, the U.S. economy was shifting from an agricultural to an industrial base. The social changes accompanying industrialization resulted in a heightened demand for social welfare services. As a result of the limited resources of the family, the local community, and private charities, increased state and federal support was required. Several noteworthy child welfare, health, and vocational policies enacted between 1900 and 1935 illustrate the evolving role of the federal sector.

A major development in the area of child health and welfare was the first White House Conference on Children in 1909. This conference emphasized the superiority of family care over institutional care and resulted in the creation of the Children's Bureau in 1912. Despite resistance to governmental involvement in family rights, the mission of the Children's Bureau was to ensure that children received humane treatment and adequate care. Data gathered by the Children's Bureau supported later federal initiatives on behalf of children and families, such as the 1921 Sheppard Towner Act for the Promotion of the Welfare and Hygiene of Maternity and Infancy (PL 67-97) and Title V of the Social Security Act of 1935 (PL 74-271).

The Sheppard Towner Act authorized the first national health care program for civilians in the United States. Under this law, states received federal grants-in-aid to support maternal and child health initiatives; a limited portion of the appropriated funds was earmarked for services for children with disabilities. Despite the Sheppard Towner Act's narrow scope and limited resources, it had a number of powerful opponents who viewed government-sponsored health care as a threat to their self-interests. As a result of the lobbying efforts of the American Medical Association, health insurance organizations, and other stakeholders, the Sheppard Towner Act's funding was repealed in 1929.

Two significant vocational laws, Smith-Sears and Smith-Fess, also were enacted during the period between 1900 and 1935. Smith-Sears, the Soldiers Rehabilitation Act of 1918 (PL 65-178), mandated the creation of vocational training programs for veterans injured during World War I. Then, Smith-Fess, the National Rehabilitation Act of 1920 (PL 66-236), expanded benefits to include individuals in the general public with physical disabilities. With its increased scope of coverage, Smith-Fess represented a major accomplishment in the evolution of vocational rehabilitation policy.

The federal government's residual approach to social welfare continued until the 1930s. However, as a result of an economic downturn extending from 1929 to the early 1940s (i.e., the Great Depression), the resources of many families, voluntary organizations, and states were depleted. U.S. President Franklin D. Roosevelt appointed the Committee on Economic Security to design a comprehensive national response to the Great Depression and the resulting unparalleled level of need. One of the major assumptions influencing the committee's work was the belief that the federal government should offer limited, ongoing social welfare protections when individuals encounter problems beyond their control. The culmination of its efforts was the Social Security Act of 1935.

The Social Security Act of 1935 firmly established the federal government's involvement in social welfare and reflected a shift toward an institutional social welfare approach with provisions such as Title V—Maternal and Child Welfare (see Table 19.1). In addition, the exclusion of healthcare protections from the Social Security Act of 1935 underscored the incremental course of U.S. social welfare legislation. For instance, a national health care plan was excluded from the final version of the bill presented to Congress because of opposition from the lobbyists responsible for the downfall of the Sheppard Towner Act.

U.S. SOCIAL WELFARE LEGISLATION SINCE 1970

The United States has no specific disability policy. Instead, disability-related policies are contained in multiple legislative categories, including civil rights, income maintenance, health, technology-related assistance, and vocational rehabilitation. Although numerous federal statutes have been enacted since the Social Security Act of 1935, information in this section is limited to an overview of federal statutes enacted since the early 1970s.

Civil Rights

The civil rights of individuals with disabilities have received incremental legislative protections. Key developments include the Rehabilitation Act of 1973 (PL 93-112), the Developmental Disabilities Assistance and Bill of Rights Act of 1975 (PL 94-103), the ADA of 1990, and the Civil Rights Act of 1991 (PL 102-166). See Table 19.2 for an outline of these statutes.

Section 504 of the Rehabilitation Act of 1973   Section 504 of the Rehabilitation Act of 1973 represents landmark legislation because it provided the first civil rights safeguards for individuals with disabilities.

Table 19.1.   Title V of the Social Security Act of 1935

Part	Objective
Part 1—Maternal and Child Health Services	Promote health of mothers and children, especially in rural areas and areas suffering from economic distress
Part 2—Services for Crippled Children	Extend and improve services for locating "crippled" children and providing medical, surgical, corrective, and other services and facilities
Part 3—Child Welfare Services	Establish, extend, and strengthen services for the protection and care of homeless, dependent, and neglected children
Part 4—Vocational Rehabilitation Services	Extend and strengthen state vocational rehabilitation programs for individuals with physical disabilities

No otherwise qualified handicapped individual in the United States shall, solely by reason of his handicap, be excluded from the participation in, be denied the benefits of, or be subjected to discrimination under any program or activity receiving federal financial assistance. (PL 93-112, 1974, §§ 87, p. 394).

Section 504 closely resembles Title VI of the Civil Rights Act of 1964 (PL 88-352) in that both prohibit recipients of federal funds from discriminating on the basis of race, color, or national origin. In addition, Section 504 underscores the critical role of the implementation phase of the public policy process. Although the addition of Section 504 was not questioned when Congress passed the Rehabilitation Act of 1973 nor when President Richard Nixon signed it into law, political debates on issues such as the definition of "disability" delayed regulatory approval for 4 years (Scotch, 1982).

The Developmental Disabilities Assistance and Bill of Rights Act of 1975 Precedents for the Developmental Disabilities Assistance and Bill of Rights Act of 1975 include the Mental Retardation Facilities and Community Mental Health Centers Construction Act of 1963 (PL 88-164) and the Developmental Disabilities Services and Facilities Construction Act of 1970 (PL 91-517). These laws provided federal support for construction of residential centers, community service facilities serving people with mental retardation, and University Affiliated Facilities. Subsequent expansions occurred with the Developmental Disabilities Assistance and Bill of Rights Act of 1975, which stipulated that in order to receive federal funds states must develop protection and advocacy systems for individuals with developmental disabilities.

The Mental Retardation Facilities and Community Mental Health Centers Construction Act of 1963 was amended by The Developmental Disabilities

Table 19.2. Disability-related civil rights legislation

Statute	Provision
Rehabilitation Act of 1973 (PL 93-112)	Authorized the first civil rights for individuals with disabilities
Developmental Disabilities Assistance and Bill of Rights Act of 1975 (PL 94-103)	Mandated states to develop protection and advocacy systems for individuals with developmental disabilities
Americans with Disabilities Act (ADA) of 1990 (PL 101-136)	Provided civil rights protection in four primary areas: employment, public accommodations, public transport services, and telecommunications
Civil Rights Act of 1991 (PL 102-166)	Authorized payment of compensatory and punitive damages for intentional discrimination under the ADA and the Rehabilitation Act of 1973

Assistance and Bill of Rights Act of 1994 (PL 103-230). The primary mission of this legislation is 1) to promote the development of comprehensive, culturally competent, and consumer- and family-centered service systems that facilitate independence, productivity, integration, and inclusion and 2) to provide civil rights protections, especially for individuals residing in residential facilities. The following is an excerpt from the 1994 law that describes the federal government's position regarding the rights of individuals with developmental disabilities:

1) Individuals with developmental disabilities have the right to appropriate treatment, services, and habilitation.
2) Treatment, services, and habilitation should be designed to maximize an individual's potential and be provided in the least restrictive setting.
3) The Federal government and States have an obligation to ensure that public funds are not provided to any institution or other residential program that does not provide services appropriate to the needs of individuals with developmental disabilities and does not meet the following standards: provision of a nourishing, well-balanced diet; provision of sufficient medical and dental services; prohibition of the use of physical restraints; prohibition of the excessive use of chemical restraints; and permission of close relatives to visit at reasonable hours without prior notice. (PL 103-230, 1994, 42 U.S.C. §§ 6009).

The Developmental Disabilities Assistance and Bill of Rights Act of 1994 defines *developmental disability* as a severe, chronic disability of an individual (5 years of age or older) that is

- Attributable to a mental and/or a physical impairment
- Manifested before 22 years of age
- Likely to continue indefinitely
- Manifested in substantial functional limitations in three or more areas of daily living
- Resultant in an extended or a lifelong need for special services

Federal funds are used to support efforts such as state-level Developmental Disabilities Planning Councils and protection and advocacy systems as well as university affiliated programs (UAPs). In order to receive Developmental Disability Act funds, states are required to have a Developmental Disability Planning Council. Federal priorities guide council activities, which include identifying areas of need, engaging in outreach and advocacy efforts, assisting communities to develop informal and formal supports and networks, and providing community education programs. State protection and advocacy systems have the authority to take legal and administrative action to protect the rights of individuals with developmental disabilities. These systems must be separate from any agency providing services to individuals with developmental disabilities, including Developmental

Disability Planning Councils. The mandate for UAPs includes providing interdisciplinary preservice training programs for students and advanced trainees and conducting state-of-the-art community service activities.

The Americans with Disabilities Act of 1990   The legislative significance of the ADA is comparable to that of the Rehabilitation Act of 1973, the Social Security Act of 1935, and the Smith-Fess Act of 1920 (i.e., the National Rehabilitation Act of 1920). Issues identified in the ADA's problem identification phase included

- The persistence of discrimination against individuals with disabilities in critical areas such as employment, housing, public accommodations, transportation, communication, recreation, health services, voting, and accessibility to public services
- The lack of sufficient protections to redress discrimination
- The continuing existence of unfair and unnecessary discrimination and prejudice denies people with disabilities the opportunity to compete on an equal basis (PL 101-336, 1990, 42 U.S.C. §§ 12101)

Individuals with a wide range of conditions receive protection under the ADA as a result of its broad definition of the term *disability:*

The term *disability* refers to individuals who
A)   have a physical or mental impairment that substantially limits one or more major life activities of such individual;
B)   have a record of such an impairment;
C)   are being regarded as having such an impairment. (PL 101-336, 1990, 42 U.S.C. §§ 12102)

In summary, the ADA prohibits discrimination in the areas of employment, public transportation, public accommodations and services, and telecommunications.

Title I—Employment   Employers with 15 or more employees cannot discriminate against an individual with disabilities in terms of application procedures; hiring, advancement, and termination practices; employee compensation; job training; or other terms, conditions, and privileges of employment. Employers are to provide reasonable accommodations for employees with disabilities; such accommodations include making workplace facilities readily accessible and usable, job restructuring, and the acquisition and modification of equipment.

Title II—Public Services   Individuals with disabilities must be able to obtain access to and use newly purchased fixed route buses, rail, and other vehicles; communities with fixed route transportation systems also must provide a paratransit system for individuals who are unable to use the fixed route services. In addition, newly constructed public transportation facilities (e.g., rail stations) must be accessible; major structural modifications to existing structures must ensure accessibility; and commuter rail systems must have a minimum of one accessible car per train.

Title III—Public Accommodations and Services Operated by Private Entities Public and private entities may not discriminate against individuals with disabilities through activities such as failure to provide goods, services, or accommodations. Services must be provided in the most integrated setting possible to meet the needs of the individual with a disability. In addition, the following are prohibited: failure to make reasonable accommodations in policies, practices, or procedures and failure to remove architectural, communication, and transportation barriers in which removal is readily achievable. The term *accommodation* refers to structures such as hotels or motels, restaurants, entertainment and sports facilities, convention centers, grocery stores and shopping centers, laundry facilities, banks, pharmacies, hospitals, and other service establishments. Also included under the accommodation mandate are public transportation terminals and stations, museums and libraries, zoos and amusement parks, schools, child care centers, senior citizen centers, homeless shelters, other social services establishments, and exercise and recreation establishments (e.g., bowling alleys).

Title IV—Telecommunications Telecommunication companies offering services to the general public must provide intrastate and interstate services for people with hearing and speech impairments (unless the services are offered via a statewide relay program). In addition, televised public service announcements that are produced or funded by a federal government agency must be closed captioned.

Title V—Miscellaneous Provisions Miscellaneous provisions specify that the ADA cannot reduce the scope of coverage or the standards applicable to federal agencies and recipients of federal assistance under the Rehabilitation Act of 1973; the provisions of the ADA are fully applicable to state governments; acts of retaliation or coercion against people with disabilities who are exercising their rights under the ADA are prohibited. The prevailing party in litigation under the ADA may recover reasonable legal fees and the Architectural and Transportation Barriers Compliance Board must issue minimum accessibility guidelines.

The Civil Rights Act of 1991 The history of the civil rights legislation dates back to the Civil Rights Act of 1866. Despite the progress made through the Rehabilitation Act of 1973 and the ADA, additional protections against unlawful employment discrimination were needed as of 1990. Therefore, the Civil Rights Act of 1991 authorized payment of compensatory and punitive damages for intentional discrimination under the ADA and Section 504 of the Rehabilitation Act of 1973. As a result, individuals with disabilities found to be the victims of unlawful discrimination can now receive limited monetary awards.

Social Security Act Amendments: Health Legislation   Important health-related services for individuals with cerebral palsy and other developmental disabilities have emerged through incremental expansions to the Social Security Act of 1935. Social Security amendments have authorized the establishment of Title V–Maternal and Child Health Block Grant of 1989 (in the Omnibus Budget Reconciliation Act [OBRA] of 1981, PL 97-35), Title XVIII–Medicare (in the Social Security Act Amendments of 1965, PL 89-97), and Title XIX–Medicaid (also in PL 89-97), which offers the widest range of services to individuals with cerebral palsy and other disabilities. The U.S. Department of Health and Human Services is the executive agency responsible for all three programs: The Maternal and Child Health Bureau administers the Maternal and Child Health Services Block Grant and the Health Care Financing Administration (HCFA) administers Medicare and Medicaid (see Table 19.3).

Title V–Maternal and Child Health Block Grant   Title V is now referred to as the Maternal and Child Health Services Block Grant and includes the following: Services for Children with Special Health Care Needs; Maternal, Infant, Child, and Adolescent Health Services; Healthy Start; and Systems, Education, and Science services. Title V grant funds support state Maternal and Child Health (MCH) programs. State-level MCH responsibilities include activities such as needs assessment, program planning, and development; service delivery, coordination, and financing; standard setting and monitoring; and technical assistance.

The original Crippled Children's Services (CCS), renamed the Children with Special Health Care Needs (CSHCN) program in 1985, was the first federal health care program specifically designed for children with disabilities and chronic health conditions. The Committee on Economic Security sought the assistance of the Children's Bureau in shaping CCS because of the Bureau's commitment to maternal and child health. In the 1930s, the polio epidemic was a major public health concern. One of the serious consequences of this epidemic was a growing number of children with physical disabilities, many of

Table 19.3.   Provisions of Social Security amendments

Title	Statute	Executive administrative agency
V	Maternal and Child Health Services Block Grant	Department of Health and Human Services Maternal and Child Health Bureau (MCHB)
XVIII	Medicare	Department of Health and Human Services, Health Care Financing Administration (HCFA)
XIX	Medicaid	Department of Health and Human Services, Health Care Financing Administration (HCFA)

whom had difficulty obtaining specialty care because of a paucity of services in rural areas or because of inadequate financial resources. As a result, the needs of this group influenced the direction of the original CCS programs.

Although Social Security legislation stipulated that state health departments must administer MCH programs, no clear guidelines regarding CCS oversight were established. In addition, states had a great deal of latitude in choosing the groups they served and the services offered through CCS. As a result of these administrative and programmatic differences, the structure and the scope of state CCS programs have varied (Hutchins & McPherson, 1989; Ireys & Nelson, 1992).

Until 1981, Title V services were organized through separate federal grants-in-aid programs like CCS. However, a major structural change occurred with the authorization of the MCH Block Grant Program contained in the OBRA of 1981. This law reflected the Reagan administration's desire to reduce the level of federal government involvement in social welfare by merging separate services into single programs and shifting greater administrative authority to the states. Through OBRA of 1981, the following Title V services were centralized:

- CCS
- MCH Services
- SSI Disabled Children's Services
- Hemophilia
- Sudden infant death syndrome
- Lead-based paint poisoning prevention
- Genetic diseases
- Adolescent pregnancy programs

As a result of OBRA legislation, Title V funding was decreased and states gained greater programmatic control in terms of priority setting, resource allocation, and service structures.

The Omnibus Budget Reconciliation Act of 1989 (PL 101-239) reauthorized the MCH Block Grant Program. This statute had special significance for children with disabilities and their families because it contained stricter administrative requirements and mandated the inclusion of family-centered care principles and practices in state plans. The stricter administrative requirements specified that states must

- Spend at least 30% of their Title V funds on CSHCN services
- Develop generic systems that serve children who have a broad range of conditions
- Collect demographic and socioeconomic information routinely regarding children with special health needs

- Conduct needs assessment surveys in order to prioritize areas of need
- Develop service systems based on findings from needs assessment surveys

A major impetus for passage of the Omnibus Budget Reconciliation Act of 1989 was the fact that multiple delivery systems for children with disabilities existed as a result of Medicaid and education legislative developments (Ireys & Nelson, 1992). Recognizing that separate administrative structures can result in duplicative or fragmented service systems, the MCH Bureau encourages states to

- Provide rehabilitation services that are not provided through Medicaid to children under 16 years of age who are blind or have a disability
- Provide family-centered, community-based, coordinated care for children with special health care needs
- Facilitate the development of community-based systems of services

State CSHCN programs provide specialty clinic services; diagnostic treatment and follow-up services; and service coordination, care coordination, and family support services.

Medicare   Medicare was instituted through the Social Security Act Amendments of 1965. It is federally funded and administered and provides health insurance for 1) people 65 years of age or older, 2) workers who become disabled and meet Federal Insurance Contributions Act (FICA) requirements that are determined by the individual's history of work and wage tax payment, 3) children 18 years of age or older who are dependent and have parents who meet FICA requirements by having a disability or being deceased, and 4) widows and widowers 50 years of age or older with disabilities. The two primary Medicare benefits—Hospital Insurance (HI) and Supplementary Medical Insurance (SMI)—are available to dependent children with disabilities 24 months after they first become eligible for Social Security Disability Insurance (SSDI). Part A of Medicare (i.e., HI) covers costs associated with inpatient hospital care; Part B (i.e., SMI) provides supplemental benefits for physician and other ambulatory services. Recipients must pay a small monthly premium in order to receive SMI coverage. Medicare offers limited long-term care benefits, such as part-time or intermittent home health services and hospice care.

Medicaid   Medicaid also was established through the 1965 Social Security Act Amendments. It is a jointly funded federal–state program administered at the state level. Although Medicaid programs vary from state to state, each state must provide "mandated" services for individuals under 21 years of age, including physician services; laboratory and X ray services; inpatient hospital care; skilled nursing facility care; family planning services; and early and periodic screening, diagnosis, and treatment (EPSDT) services. In addition, with federal approval, states can include optional services in their Medicaid plan. For instance, for individuals who have qualifying diagnoses, some states subsidize physical, occupational, and speech-language therapy as well as "targeted" service coordination services.

The model for Medicaid was the Social Security Act Amendments of 1950 (PL 81-734), which authorized federal assistance to help states underwrite medical care for recipients of Old Age Assistance. In 1962, eligibility requirements expanded to include individuals who were blind or who were permanently and totally disabled. The 1965 Medicaid legislation further increased the scope of the 1950 Social Security Act Amendments by providing grant support to establish state medical assistance programs for individuals receiving public assistance and individuals who were "medically needy" and who had income levels above the eligibility limits for public assistance. Although no special provisions for individuals with disabilities were included in the 1965 Medicaid legislation, the Social Security Act Amendments of 1971 (PL 92-223) authorized Medicaid reimbursement for interim care facilities (ICFs). The amendments permitted public institutions serving individuals with mental retardation to receive ICF certification if their primary purpose was to provide active medical and rehabilitation services and if the states in which they were located maintained their previous level of funding support.

The Early and Periodic Screening, Diagnosis, and Treatment Program The EPSDT Program became a mandatory Medicaid service through the Social Security Act Amendments of 1967 (PL 90-248). As a result, children and youth who are eligible for Medicaid can receive EPSDT benefits, which include comprehensive health and developmental screening services, vision services, dental care, hearing services, and other services to "correct or ameliorate" illnesses and conditions identified through screening services.

As a result of the perceived gap in medical services, the original objective of the EPSDT Program was to provide preventive treatment and outreach services. Unfortunately, the EPSDT Program is an example of a program that experienced problems during its implementation phase due to ambiguous guidelines, uncoordinated services, unwieldy eligibility requirements, and a perceived lack of public commitment. Some of these problems were rectified with the Omnibus Budget Reconciliation Act of 1989, which mandated that any "medically necessary" service identified through EPSDT screening must be available to children covered by Medicaid, regardless of whether the state's Medicaid plan includes that service. In order to receive EPSDT coverage, children must be examined by a medical provider enrolled in the EPSDT Program.

Home- and Community-Based Services Medicaid provided limited home care benefits prior to 1981. However, as a result of factors such as spiraling health care costs, the range of reimbursable services increased with the authorization of the Home- and Community-Based Care Waiver Program, a component of OBRA of 1981. Waivers allow states to provide services that are exceptions to typical Medicaid practices and rules as long as they do not exceed institutional care costs. In order to initiate a waiver program, state plans must be approved by HCFA.

The range of reimbursable home care services was expanded with subsequent legislation such as the Tax Equity and Fiscal Responsibility Act (TEFRA) of 1982 (PL 97-248) and the Consolidated Omnibus Budget Reconciliation Act (COBRA) of 1985 (PL 99-272). As a result of these laws, states can provide some or all of the following home and community services: service coordination, homemaker assistance, home health aides, adult day care, and respite care. In addition, individuals with developmental disabilities may be eligible to receive Community Support Living Arrangement Services, such as personal assistance, training and habilitation, assistive technology, or adaptive equipment.

Managed Care Medicaid was originally based on a fee-for-service delivery model; in other words, beneficiaries could obtain services from Medicaid-approved providers of their choice. However, in response to steadily rising health care costs, a number of states have introduced managed care programs for some or all of their Medicaid beneficiaries. In order to implement managed care systems, states must first obtain Social Security Act Section 1915(b) waivers or Section 1115 waivers from HCFA.

As of 1997, the majority of states have implemented managed care programs with Section 1915(b) waivers. Mandatory Medicaid services must be included in 1915(b) waiver programs. States have generally offered three alternatives to beneficiaries under 1915(b) waivers:

1. Voluntary enrollment in a health maintenance organization (HMO) or utilization of services on a fee-for-service basis
2. Mandatory enrollment in an HMO with the provision that beneficiaries have the ability to choose among competing organizations
3. Voluntary or mandatory enrollment in a preferred provider organization or physician gatekeeper system

In many cases, beneficiaries can choose to disenroll from Section 1915(b) HMO programs after a period of 1 month. However, if the HMO meets certain federal requirements, beneficiaries may be "locked" in a managed care organization for 6 months.

During the period from 1993 to 1995, 12 states obtained Section 1115, or "demonstration and research" waivers. In order to qualify for this waiver program, states must show that proposed services will 1) be cost neutral (i.e., not result in increased Medicaid costs), 2) expand Medicaid eligibility criteria to include individuals without health care coverage, and 3) provide services not previously covered by Medicaid. In addition, states are required to develop ongoing quality assurance programs for evaluating activities related to Section 1115.

States have greater flexibility under Section 1115 waivers. For example, HMOs do not need to offer all of the mandatory Medicaid services, beneficiaries can be required to stay in an HMO for up to 12 months, and managed care systems can be developed to serve targeted populations such as individuals with disabilities. Although incremental social welfare change is the standard in the United States, it has been suggested that vehicles such as Section 1115 are more likely to "reform" health care than are broad-based initiatives such as national health care legislation.

Income Maintenance: Social Security Act Amendments

The two primary federal income maintenance programs for individuals with disabilities (i.e., SSDI and SSI) have been authorized through Social Security Act amendments. SSDI is a social insurance program; SSI is a means-tested program. Thus, eligibility for SSDI is based on disability and work history requirements. Because SSI eligibility is determined through means-testing, individuals must meet disability and financial criteria (see Figure 19.2).

Social Security Disability Income   SSDI was established through the Social Security Act Amendments of 1956 (PL 84-880). It is an income maintenance program available to unmarried, dependent children who have disabilities that were acquired before 22 years of age and whose parents are retired, have disabilities, or are deceased. Similar to Medicare, eligibility for SSDI depends on parental work history and the level of contributions paid to the Social Security Trust Fund through wage tax deductions. The SSDI and SSI programs use the same disability criteria for determining the individual's entitlement to benefits.

Supplemental Security Income   SSI was established through the Social Security Act Amendments of 1972 (PL 92-603). It is an income maintenance program for individuals with disabilities whose financial resources do not exceed the federal benefit rate (FBR). Monthly payments are based on factors such as income level, resources, and place of residence. For example, if the

Eligibility criteria	SSDI	SSI
Disability	X	X
Parental disability	X	
Parental work history	X	
Income		X

Figure 19.2.   Eligibility requirements for Social Security Disability Insurance (SSDI) and Supplemental Security Income (SSI) for individuals with developmental disabilities.

individual receiving SSI lives in someone else's household in which food and shelter are provided, his or her FBR is reduced by one third. As of 1996, maximum monthly federal SSI benefits were $470 per individual and $705 per married couple (if both people met eligibility criteria).

SSI legislation consolidated the Old Age Assistance, Aid for the Blind, and Aid for the Disabled programs. The former categorical programs received federal support but were administered by the states; thus, benefits varied a great deal. One objective of SSI was to standardize eligibility requirements and income guidelines by shifting administrative responsibilities to the federal government. Although minimum income benefits are established at the federal level, states can offer supplemental support. Because the states formulate eligibility requirements and payment levels for supplemental programs, monthly SSI benefits continue to vary.

Many states offer Medicaid and food stamps to individuals receiving SSI. In terms of Medicaid, states can choose to base Medicaid eligibility on either SSI or Medicaid criteria. The majority of states provide Medicaid to all SSI participants. In approximately 12 states, stricter state Medicaid standards are used. However, SSI recipients in these states must be allowed to *spend down* to become eligible for Medicaid, regardless of whether the state has a "medically needy" program. (The term *spend down* refers to the process used to determine Medicaid eligibility when SSI participants do not automatically receive medical benefits. The state is responsible for devising its spend-down formula, which is based on a comparison of out-of-pocket medical expenditures with allowable income. When expenditures exceed allowable income levels, the individual becomes eligible for Medicaid.)

The following disability and income criteria are used in determining SSI eligibility:

> Individuals over 18 years of age are considered to be disabled if a medically determinable physical or mental impairment, or combination of impairments, prevents them from working and is expected to last for a continuous period of at least 12 months or to result in death. Children under the age of 18 are generally considered to be disabled if they have a medically determinable physical or mental impairment that results in marked and severe functional limitations and that can be expected to result in death or to last for a continuous period of 12 months or more. (PL 104-193, 42 USC §§ 1382)

Prior to the enactment of the Personal Responsibility and Work Opportunity Reconciliation Act of 1996 (PL 104-193), an individualized functional assessment (IFA) could be used to determine SSI eligibility for children younger than 18 years of age. IFAs were instituted as a response to the Supreme Court's ruling in *Sullivan v. Zebley* (1990), which found that the SSI evaluation and the determination process discriminated against children because it was based solely on adult disability criteria. Because the number of children entering the SSI system dramatically increased as a result of the *Sullivan v. Zebley* verdict, concerns arose regarding the associated costs. As a result, the Personal Responsibility and Work Opportunity Reconciliation Act of 1996 included a narrower definition of "disability" and eliminated the IFA. The actual impact of these changes for children is yet to be determined.

Financial Requirements For children and youth younger than 18 years of age, SSI financial eligibility and payment amounts are generally based on parental income and assets through a process known as *deeming*. With deeming, deductions for parents and siblings living in the household are subtracted from total parental income and assets; the child's eligibility for SSI then is based on remaining resources. Deeming is not applicable if the child meets disability criteria and is hospitalized for 30 days or more. In such instances, the child may receive a monthly SSI payment of $30 after being discharged from the hospital if he or she continues to meet disability eligibility requirements. In addition, the child's own assets may be excluded from the determination process if the assets are held in a discretionary trust administered by a guardian who is legally appointed.

For individuals 18 years of age or older, earned and unearned income and other assets are used to determine financial eligibility for SSI and monthly payment amounts. Earned income may include wages, net income from self-employment earnings, and sheltered workshop earnings. Examples of unearned income are interest from savings accounts or money market funds; some child support and alimony payments; and Social Security, veteran's, or unemployment benefits. As of 1994, assets valued at more than $2,000 for an individual or $3,000 for a couple are considered in the SSI application process. These resources include cash, bank accounts, stocks, personal property, and other possessions that could be exchanged for cash and used to pay for food, clothing, and shelter.

Some of the items excluded from SSI financial eligibility determinations are applicants' homes, food stamp benefits, Agent Orange settlements, and applicants' resources held in trust funds administered by a legally appointed guardian. The value of one household car also may be excluded if it is 1) used for transportation to a job or to obtain regular medical treatments, 2) modified for use by an individual with disabilities, or 3) necessary to perform essential activities.

In general, individuals residing in institutional settings are not eligible for SSI. However, possible exceptions to this rule include

- Recipients living in publicly operated community residences, which are alternatives to institutional settings and serve no more than 16 people
- Recipients residing in public institutions for the purpose of attending an approved educational or vocational training programs
- Recipients living in public emergency homeless shelters for no more than 6 months during any 9-month period

- Physician certification that a recipient's stay in a medical facility is unlikely to exceed 3 months and SSI benefits are needed to cover expenses at home

Federal monthly benefits may be reduced to $30 following the first full month of the individual's stay in a hospital or in another medical institution when Medicaid pays for half or more of the charges related to the stay. This reduced benefit is known as the personal needs allowance.

The SSI program offers several work-related incentives. Some individuals who work can continue to receive Medicaid benefits—even though a portion of their earnings exceeds SSI income limits—if their ability to work is dependent on these benefits. In addition, expenses for necessary work-related supports (e.g., attendant care) may be deducted from earnings. SSI was intended to be a program that ensured a minimal level of income as a last resort, and, as a result, the original legislation included a work incentive program: the Plan to Achieve Self Sufficiency (PASS). With PASS, an individual receiving SSI or SSDI submits a written plan outlining job training or employment goals to the local Social Security office. If the plan is approved, the recipient will receive higher monthly benefits by excluding non-SSI income and resources that are used to pursue work goals from eligibility and benefit calculations. For example, the individual may use his or her earnings to purchase adaptive equipment, pay tuition for school or job-training programs, or cover transportation costs. Unfortunately, PASS is another example of a program that has been hindered by nebulous standards and goals, lack of training and guidance for staff in local Social Security offices, and inadequate dissemination efforts (Ross, 1996).

Technology-Related Assistance

The recognition that technological advances had come to play a critical role in the United States was a major impetus for passage of the Technology-Related Assistance for Individuals with Disabilities Act of 1988 (PL 100-407). The primary mission of this law was to provide financial assistance to states in order to develop and implement statewide technology-related assistance programs and to identify federal policies that facilitate and impede payment for technology-related assistive devices and services. This statute defines the term *assistive technology device* as any item, piece of equipment, or product used to increase, maintain, or improve functional capabilities of individuals with disabilities.

The planning process for the Technology-Related Assistance for Individuals with Disabilities Act of 1994 (PL 103-218) uncovered a number of continuing obstacles, including

- Difficulty gaining access to existing telecommunication and information technologies
- Lack of financial resources to cover the cost of assistive devices and services

- Inadequate technology training resources
- Lack of coordination among federal agencies

As a result, the Technology-Related Assistance Act of 1994 authorized funding for the development and the evaluation of model delivery systems, such as income-contingent loan programs and lending programs that provide technological devices to individuals, employers, public agencies, or private organizations that attempt to meet ADA and Rehabilitation Act requirements.

Vocational Rehabilitation

Early vocational rehabilitation legislation was enacted to support veterans with war-related disabilities. Services next became available to civilians with physical disabilities under the Smith-Fess Act of 1920. As a result of later incremental expansions, individuals with a broad range of disabilities became eligible for vocational rehabilitation.

Each state is responsible for administering its vocational rehabilitation system. Unlike the health and income maintenance programs described previously, vocational rehabilitation services are not entitlements; the term *entitlement* refers to services that must be provided to any individual who requests them and who is eligible to receive them. Because vocational rehabilitation is not an entitlement, the level of demand may exceed the level of available services as a result of inadequate program funds or other factors. When faced with this dilemma, individuals with the most severe disabilities must be given priority. Individuals with severe disabilities are defined as

> a) having a physical or mental impairment which seriously limits one or more functional capacities—mobility, communication, self-care, self-direction, work tolerance, or work skills—in terms of employment outcome; b) needing multiple vocational rehabilitation services over an extended period; and c) having one or more disabilities associated with conditions such as arthritis, autism, cerebral palsy, muscular dystrophy, or spinal cord injuries. (PL 93-112, 1973, 29 U.S.C. §§ 706)

The Rehabilitation Act of 1973 continues to inform vocational rehabilitation programs and practices. In addition to the civil rights protections contained in Section 504, this law included

- An expanded definition of the term "handicapped individual" to include people with a wider range of disabilities
- An emphasis on the need to develop independent living supports for individuals who might not be able to fully participate in the competitive marketplace
- The creation of the Rehabilitation Services Administration

The law also required states to develop individualized written rehabilitation programs for people participating in rehabilitation services.

The civil rights movement during the 1960s influenced the development of the independent living movement for individuals with disabilities, as reflected in the Rehabilitation Act of 1973. The Rehabilitation, Comprehensive Services, and Developmental Disabilities Amendments of 1978 (PL 95-602) authorized the establishment of more definitive comprehensive services for independent living. Consequently, employment-related training funds could be used to promote independent living through wheelchair repair and ramp construction, personal attendant training, accessible housing and employment information and referral, and other similar services (Scotch, 1989).

Although the Rehabilitation Act of 1973 has been amended on multiple occasions, its scope and content have not changed significantly. The Rehabilitation Act Amendments of 1992 (PL 102-569) contains the most extensive changes to the 1973 mandate. One of the primary purposes of the 1992 legislation (see Table 19.4 for summary of the eight titles found within the Rehabilitation Act Amendments of 1992) is to empower individuals with disabilities to maximize employment opportunities, economic self-sufficiency, independence, and integration into society. These goals can be achieved through comprehensive vocational rehabilitation programs, independent living centers and services, research and demonstration projects, and the guarantee of equal opportunity.

SUMMARY

Social welfare legislation offers a powerful mechanism for modifying or eliminating societal handicaps that unfairly restrict the range of opportunities available to individuals with disabilities. Although the United States has no comprehensive "disability policy," disability-related social welfare legislation is contained in a number of areas, including civil rights, income maintenance, health, technology-related assistance, and vocational rehabilitation. Disability-related legislation holds the promise that individuals with cerebral palsy and other developmental disabilities may enjoy richer lives. However, in terms of eligibility criteria, type and range of available services, funding levels, and accessibility, one must carefully investigate the programs and the services that are developed and implemented as a result of legislative actions.

The approach to social welfare in the United States has been influenced by the Elizabethan Poor Law enacted in England in 1601 and Constitutional principles such as decentralization of sovereign powers. Although the Elizabethan Poor Laws are nearly 400 years old, Poor Law assumptions continue to affect social welfare practices and policies: Individuals must be "deserving" in order to receive assistance, families are primarily responsible for the well-being of

Table 19.4.   Overview of Rehabilitation Act Amendments of 1992

Title	Summary
I–Administration and Vocational Rehabilitation Services	Details federal standards for state Vocational Rehabilitation programs, such as the need to include transition, personal assistance, and supported employment services
II–Research and Training	Authorizes the National Institute on Disability and Rehabilitation Research (NIDRR). NIDRR's primary purpose is to support rehabilitation research
III–Training and Demonstration Projects	Provides funds to support training activities for vocational rehabilitation personnel, individuals with disabilities, family members, and other individuals involved in caring for the child
IV–National Council on Disability	Supports the activities of the National Council on Disability, the federal agency responsible for assessing disability-related statutes and developing policy recommendations
V–Rights and Advocacy	Promotes civil rights supports with programs such as the Architectural and Transportation Barriers Compliance Board and the Protection and Advocacy of Individuals' Rights
VI–Employment Opportunities for Individuals with Disabilities	Provides three employment-related services: Community Service Employment Pilot Program for Individuals with Disabilities, Projects with Industry, and Supported Employment Services for Individuals with Severe Disabilities
VII–Independent Living Services and Centers for Independent Living	Supports independent living for individuals with disabilities through services such as information and referral, life skills approaches, mobility training, recreation, and transportation
VIII–Special Demonstration and Training Projects	Fosters development of innovative direct service and training projects

their members, and services should be provided at the local level whenever possible.

There has been ongoing debate regarding the level of social welfare responsibility that federal, state, and local authorities should assume. The federal government's social welfare role started to expand in the late 19th century, with the most rapid period of growth occurring between the passage of the Social Security Act in 1935 and the early 1970s. Since the 1980s, however, the trend has reversed, with greater responsibility shifting back to state and local governments. A prime example of this reversal is the expansion of Medicaid managed care programs that offer states greater autonomy in terms of determining the nature and the scope of available services. In addition, because it contains a narrower definition of "disability" and eliminates the individualized functional assessment, the Personal Responsibility and Work Opportunity Reconciliation Act of 1996 has critical implications for determining a child's eligibility for SSI. Although it is too early to assess the effect of these changes, they do reflect the Elizabethan Poor Law perspective that assistance should be restricted to those who are "deserving."

The dilemma of meeting an infinite level of need with finite resources is a major social welfare challenge. Given the fact that the legislative process is influenced by a number of contingencies (e.g., politics, special interest groups, economic trends), it is essential that individuals with cerebral palsy, their families, and professionals have the information necessary to identify gaps in programs and services and to assist in shaping future policies.

REFERENCES

Americans with Disabilities Act (ADA) of 1990, PL 101-336, 42 U.S.C. §§ 12101 et seq.

Civil Rights Act of 1964, PL 88-352, 42 U.S.C. §§ 1981 et seq.

Civil Rights Act of 1991, PL 102-166, 42 U.S.C. §§ 1981 et seq.

Consolidated Omnibus Budget Reconciliation Act (COBRA) of 1985, PL 99-272, 42 U.S.C. §§ 1396 et seq.

Developmental Disabilities Assistance and Bill of Rights Act of 1975, PL 94-103, 42 U.S.C. §§ 6101 et seq.

Developmental Disabilities Assistance and Bill of Rights Act of 1994, PL 103-230, 42 U.S.C. §§ 6000 et seq.

Developmental Disabilities Services and Facilities Construction Act of 1970, PL 91-517, 42 U.S.C. §§ 6000 et seq.

DiNitto, D.M. (1991). Social welfare: Politics and public policy (3rd ed.). Upper Saddle River, NJ: Prentice-Hall.

Dolgoff, R., Feldstein, D., & Skolnik, L. (1993). Understanding social welfare (3rd ed.). New York: Longman.

Hutchins, V.L., & McPherson, M. (1989). Roots of current perspectives. In R.E.K. Satin (Ed.), Caring for children with chronic illness: Issues and strategies (pp. 3–15). New York: Springer-Verlag.

Individuals with Disabilities Education Act (IDEA) of 1990, PL 101-476, 20 U.S.C. §§ 1400 et seq.

Ireys, H.T., & Nelson, R.P. (1992). New federal policy for children with special health care needs: Implications for pediatricians. Pediatrics, 90, 321–327.

Katz, M.B. (1995). Improving poor people: The welfare state, the "underclass," and urban schools as history. Princeton, NJ: Princeton University Press.

Mental Retardation Facilities and Community Mental Health Centers Construction Act of 1963, PL 88-164, 42 U.S.C. §§ 2670 et seq.

National Rehabilitation Act of 1920, PL 66-236.

Omnibus Budget Reconciliation Act (OBRA) of 1981, PL 97-35, 42 U.S.C. §§ 701 et seq.

Omnibus Budget Reconciliation Act (OBRA) of 1989, PL 101-239, 42 U.S.C. §§ 701 *et seq.*

Personal Responsibility and Work Opportunity Reconciliation Act of 1996, PL 104-193, 42 U.S.C. §§ 1382 *et seq.*

Rehabilitation Act Amendments of 1992, PL 102-569, 29 U.S.C. §§ 701 *et seq.*

Rehabilitation Act of 1973, PL 93-112, 29 U.S.C. §§ 701 *et seq.*

Rehabilitation, Comprehensive Services, and Developmental Disabilities Amendments of 1978, PL 95-602, 29 U.S.C. §§ 701 *et seq.*

Ross, J.L. (1996). *SSA disability: Program redesign necessary to encourage return to work.* (GAO/HEHS Report No. 96-62). Gaithersburg, MD: General Accounting Office.

Scotch, R.K. (1982). *From good will to civil rights: Transforming federal disability policy.* Philadelphia: Temple University Press.

Sheppard Towner Act for the Promotion of the Welfare and Hygiene of Maternity and Infancy (1921), PL 67-97, Chapter 135.

Social Security Act Amendments of 1950, Chapter 809.

Social Security Act Amendments of 1956, PL 84-880, 42 U.S.C. §§ 401 *et seq.*

Social Security Act Amendments of 1965, PL 89-97, 42 U.S.C. §§ 1396 *et seq.*

Social Security Act Amendments of 1967, PL 90-248, 42 U.S.C. §§ 1396 *et seq.*

Social Security Act Amendments of 1971, PL 92-223, 42 U.S.C. §§ 1396 *et seq.*

Social Security Act Amendments of 1972, PL 92-603, 42 U.S.C. §§ 1381 *et seq.*

Social Security Act of 1935, PL 74-271, 42 U.S.C. §§ 301 *et seq.*

Soldiers Rehabilitation Act of 1918, PL 65-178, 29 U.S.C. §§ 31 *et seq.*

Sullivan v. Zebley, 110 S.C.T. 885, February 20, 1990.

Tax Equity and Fiscal Responsibility Act (TEFRA) of 1982, PL 97-248, 42 U.S.C. §§ 1396 *et seq.*

Technology-Related Assistance for Individuals with Disabilities Act of 1988, PL 100-407, 29 U.S.C. §§ 2201 *et seq.*

Technology-Related Assistance for Individuals with Disabilities Act of 1994, PL 103-218, 29 U.S.C. §§ 2201 *et seq.*

World Health Organization. (1980). *International classification of impairments, disabilities and handicaps.* Geneva, Switzerland: Author.

CHAPTER 20

Transitions to Adulthood

The Adult with Cerebral Palsy

Adadot Hayes

Similar to many pediatricians, Dr. Adadot Hayes was drawn to issues related to child development during her residency in pediatrics and, as a result, decided to pursue specialty training in child development and child developmental disabilities. After completing her training in California, Dr. Hayes practiced as a neurodevelopmental pediatrician for 12 years in private practice in Scranton, Pennsylvania. It was during this time that she met Robert Walsh.

Robert was a teenager at the time and, as described in this chapter, had encountered many physicians under a variety of circumstances, both before and after meeting Dr. Hayes. Dr. Hayes was among the first professionals to recognize Robert's true potential behind the "screen" of his physical disability. Dr. Hayes's initial foresight and Robert's trust in her as a friend have fostered a relationship that extends more than 10 years and continues to influence both parties.

As a young adult, Robert has strong opinions about professionals and their interactions with people with disabilities. In Robert's opinion, Dr. Hayes represents an exception to the typical distance he feels with most professionals with which he has come into contact with over the years. For Dr. Hayes, the friendship with Robert has significantly influenced her perceptions of developmental disabilities as they are experienced by adults. Similar to many neurodevelopmental pediatricians (and similar to many other professionals who work with children with developmental disabilities), Dr. Hayes has needed to expand her interests and activities beyond the usual scope of the pediatrician. Although most professionals tend to specialize in working with either adults or with children, professionals working in the field of developmental disabilities are called on to take a life-span perspective.

Dr. Hayes continues to work in the field of developmental disabilities and has taken a special interest in the way that public policy issues affect the lives of children and adults who have developmental disabilities. This chapter represents a collaborative effort between Robert and Dr. Hayes; it is an attempt to provide contrasting viewpoints on the subject of developmental disabilities in adulthood. In the following sections, Dr. Hayes takes the narrative position and uses Robert's comments as a springboard for reflections on the state of affairs for adults with developmental disabilities. Robert's views are presented as extracts.

BACKGROUND

Robert "Bob" Walsh was born to a 16-year-old mother in 1971. Difficulties at birth left him with cerebral palsy, and he was placed in a small institution. It was not until one of the staff members at the center recognized Bob's potential and later adopted him that he found a home. I met Bob when he was entering adolescence and fighting to get into an inclusive class in middle school. During the past 10 years, I have watched him graduate with honors from both middle school and high school, and he graduated from Marywood College (Scranton, Pennsylvania) with a Bachelor of Science in Computer Science in May of 1997.

> I was born in 1971 with cerebral palsy, not being able to talk, walk, or use my hands. From the time that I was born, I was considered a disaster. I didn't breathe right away, which was the cause to set my path for the future. I was doomed. " Just keep him comfortable and try to make life as easy as possible for him," was the general advice given by most. At first, I felt that I was a prisoner in my own body. I tried very hard to communicate verbally, which was very frustrating for me. At the age of 10, I received a word board. At last, I could ask for a drink or tell how I was feeling. It was not until I finally met Dr. Hayes, who was trained to take care of people like me and who had experience in this type of care, that the wealth of opportunities, both medical and nonmedical, opened up to me. This made my mother feel more comfortable.

Bob, as he will tell you, has not received proper medical care during most of his life. On many occasions, professionals have felt that he was not "worth it."

One day an orthopedic doctor came to my school to evaluate all the students. My mother wanted to see if my legs could be straightened out so that I could at least sit correctly in my wheelchair. I was placed on the floor where this doctor proceeded to look me over. He didn't touch my body and remarked to my mother that "nothing could be accomplished with this kid." He even made statements such as "He will never go any place, just let him go." However, his attitude did not stop my mother, who proceeded to take me to several other orthopedists and finally found one who would treat me. After I had my surgery, I was back in school and walking with a walker when I ran into the former physician who just laughed. The joke was on him. Maybe his attitude might have changed about helping guys like me after that, but he sure didn't make my day brighter.

In other situations, professionals did not understand Bob's medical problems.

One day I took too big a bite of hamburger, and it got stuck in my throat. I could not breathe and my mother rushed me to the hospital. They decided that I had aspirated. Three days later, I really felt like I was dying. I knew the piece of hamburger was still in my throat, but no one would listen to me. I was getting sicker and the surgeon was afraid to operate on me, but he had no choice and a big piece of hamburger was found at the opening of my stomach blocking everything. The amazing thing was that my first meal that was sent to me after surgery was a hamburger.

In many situations, professionals did not examine Bob or did not even know how to examine him.

When I was 9 years old, I developed a 103-degree fever. My mother called our doctor, but because he was off for the weekend, I saw another one. On arriving, the doctor asked what was the problem, and I could tell right away that he was very uneasy with my presence. The doctor handed my mother a thermometer and told her to take my temperature. He did not touch me, look at my throat, or check my heart; he finally asked my mother what he should do. She proceeded to tell him to give me an antibiotic along with Tylenol. "Okay, good," he acknowledged; then he said, "That will be $20.00." I felt like my mother should have been the doctor. I did get better but not because of that doctor.

Another time, I needed glasses because I worked with computers a great deal. I arrived for my appointment, and they had everybody in the building looking at me as if I was from Mars. As usual, my mother had to tell them that I could answer with my communication device, but they didn't listen. They were upset and couldn't do an examination, and with all of the confusion, I lost memory in my computer that I would usually use to communicate.

Because of these experiences, both Bob and his family have lost respect for professionals who should be able to help them. Although knowledge and experience are changing (as demonstrated by the information within this book), the changes have occurred mostly in relation to developmental disabilities in childhood. The issues related to adults have not been adequately addressed, and people like Bob Walsh have developed aversions to medical care that may not be overcome easily.

Individuals rarely die of cerebral palsy, but they have an increased risk of ongoing health concerns leading to discomfort and interference with a typical lifestyle. Many of these problems are treatable, sometimes quite early; some, if not treated, can lead to premature death. Most of these problems are complications of cerebral palsy, many of which can be avoided if children receive care described in the prior chapters of this book. Research has clearly shown that individuals with cerebral palsy have decreased access to preventive care and care for minor problems, which often is related to lack of knowledgeable and lack of adequate care and may even contribute to increased mortality (Strauss, Eyman, & Grossman, 1996; Strauss & Kastner, 1996). Some of the difficulties experienced by individuals who are quite severely affected and institutionalized have led to the involvement of the Department of Justice in state developmental centers. This involvement has revealed a high number of serious unrecognized problems such as severe gastroesophageal reflux (GER) and osteoporosis. GER often is found with signs of significant complications such as pulmonary problems secondary to significant aspiration and pneumonia, bleeding and anemia, and secondary intestinal problems (e.g., severe constipation, obstruction), all of which have the potential for death. Osteoporosis is caused by a combination of long-term nonweight bearing; nutritional compromise; and administration of antiepileptic medications, which may lead to secondary pathological fractures and pain or loss of skills. Problems with seizure control also have been recognized, but they are the most likely to be addressed with treatment.

In a study of individuals who were not institutionalized, Bax, Smyth, and Thomas (1988) found that young adults with physical disabilities living in England in the early 1980s were in a poor state of health. Fifty-nine percent of the individuals with problems severe enough to warrant attention but remained unaddressed even under the free medical system. These problems included emaciation (60%), bowel and bladder problems (53%), kyphoscoliosis (26%), lower extremity contractures (71%), skin care problems (31%), and communication problems (60%).

In a more recent study, Murphy, Molnar, and Lankaskey (1995) demonstrated significant unmet health needs in Oakland, California, although most of these were a less serious nature than the disabilities found in England. In addition to the range of general health problems that were similar to what might be seen in the age range of the group (i.e., 19–74 years, mean of 42 1/2 years), there also were several striking features. For instance, a high percentage of the individuals had problems with urinary tract infections related to poor perineal hygiene or use of an external collecting device, whereas others were affected by overflow incontinence often related to infrequent opportunities for urination and to physical and environmental factors. Incontinence often could be relieved if toileting was regular. The frequent use of fluid restriction (to avoid daytime wetting) often led to constipation and its complications. Twenty-six percent of the adult individuals had lost the ability to ambulate in adulthood. Inadequacy of wheelchair equipment and its association with postural back pain was common (43% had back pain; 50% had cervical pain). Thirty percent of individuals had fractures that were much more common in ambulatory individuals. The lack of preventive care was a major concern. Over 90% of the individuals did not have regular periodic examinations or screening tests (e.g., Pap smears, breasts exams, rectal exams, cardiac evaluations).

Impairments that interfere with daily living also were common. Ninety percent of the individuals had ambulatory equipment (e.g., crutches, wheelchairs) in disrepair; 25% had visual impairments, most of which were uncorrected; and 10% had hearing impairments. Back pain was common in 23%, whereas hand paresthesia, which is similar to carpal tunnel syndrome, was common in 10%. Lower extremity contractures were found in 64% of the individuals. Only 2% had augmentative and alternative communication devices. Disorders thought to be extremely severe in individuals within the institutional setting were not cited as major problems (18% had seizures, zero instances of GER). Whether these issues were unrecognized or the individuals at high risk had died was not addressed. In general, care was suboptimal and fragmented. The authors concluded that medical care for adults with cerebral palsy is at best inconsistent and that awareness of medical problems of cerebral palsy in adults among the medical profession was a factor. They also noted that, with few exceptions, an organized system of care for adults, similar to that for children, with cerebral palsy does not exist.

It has been only since the mid-1970s that the field of medicine has begun to conduct research into the pathophysiology and care of cerebral palsy, and this work has been done primarily with children rather than with adults. However, there still remains less information about the long-term effects of cerebral palsy and the care of individuals in adult life. This is further complicated by financial issues, including both medical care and needed equipment (Ware et al., 1986).

> I hate to go to doctors; I feel that doctors should spend more time in school learning about people with special needs. This could prepare them for guys like me. How many times I was taken to the doctor for treatment and, believe me, I felt like I was some kind of freak. Just because body movements are noticeable doesn't mean that a professional should have a nightmare and run for the hills.

Because there is little information about long-term outcome in cerebral palsy and because parents who are primary caretakers are often not present as their children age, many issues often are not addressed. A question that parents ask early but is rarely addressed by adults with cerebral palsy is that of life expectancy. Although there is little data, most studies show that 90% of individuals diagnosed with cerebral palsy live until 10 years of age, and most deaths are related to reduced mobility and severe mental retardation (Eyman, Grossman, Chaney, & Call 1993). Extensive studies in the 1990s are hard to analyze, particularly when considering an individual, but data show that severe mental retardation, inability to feed oneself, and lack of mobility were the chief factors associated with lower life expectancy (Eyman, Grossman, Chaney, & Call, 1990). Also of significance, Crichton, Mackinnon, and White (1995) showed that the presence of epilepsy in mental retardation contributed to overall mortality, but there were no synergistic effects with other associated problems. In this study, the likelihood of surviving to the end of the fourth decade was 85%. Individuals with mental retardation were at the greatest risk for early death (whether or not they had epilepsy); individuals with epilepsy were the second most at risk; the least at risk were those individuals with only a physical disability. This, however, is crude data because approaches to the management of cerebral palsy have changed considerably, and newer factors related to technical advances (e.g., gastrostomy feeding, management of respiratory infections, surgical procedures) also may influence the length of survival.

The issues of sexuality and, in particular, childbearing also are often overlooked or avoided. Although limitations may exist for participation in sex secondary to physical problems, fertility is not typically reduced as a result of cerebral palsy. Pregnancy outcome is thought to be related to the physical status of the mother, but detailed outcome data are not available.

The musculoskeletal complications of cerebral palsy in adults are prevalent. This includes contractures, scoliosis, hip subluxation or dislocation, pathological fractures, and pain (Thometz & Simon, 1988). There is a high incidence of loss of independent skills in adulthood, which is related either to increased energy requirements, pain, joint limitations or to decreased motivation superimposed on the loss of physical skills with aging. It is not known whether these complications are inevitable or whether they may be alleviated with preventive routines.

Medical services for adults with cerebral palsy are not well defined. There are few cerebral palsy clinics for adults and specialty referrals are decreasing as more people are enrolled in managed care organizations. There are no "school therapists" for adults and many insurance companies will not cover preventive or maintenance care. There are limited numbers of physicians who are trained in developmental disabilities and who care for adults, and there is little supporting research. In addition, there also may be significant problems with medical coverage, although managed care organizations may ameliorate this to some extent. There still remains the problem of coverage for "preexisting" illnesses and decreased funding for durable equipment. Although some adults with disabilities are eligible for Social Security Disability Insurance (SSDI) on the basis of their physical limitations (see Chapter 19), the recent changes in the SSDI program may result in some of these individuals losing services.

Another concern for adults with cerebral palsy is the issue of consent. Individuals with cerebral palsy are likely to be nonverbal but may not be mentally retarded. This often is not recognized well by the professional community. Issues of competency and consideration of a guardian should be entertained when significant medical problems arise.

Care for adults with cerebral palsy is often nonexistent or may exist only for acute illnesses and is often fragmented. Young adults addressing disability related issues frequently stay with their pediatrician, and, although this may seem appropriate at the time, it may be inappropriate for dealing with medical issues specific to adults.

With the exception of physical medicine and rehabilitation, most specialists dealing with adults have little experience with a team approach to managed care. This results in fragmentation of care and often in lack of care that may be readily available in many medical settings, such as social service support.

A major concern for adults with cerebral palsy, particularly those who cannot advocate for themselves, is quality of life. In 1972, Flanagan identified 11 domains that contribute to quality of life:

1. Material well-being and financial security
2. Health and personal safety
3. Relationships with a spouse
4. Raising children
5. Relationships with other relatives
6. Helping others (i.e., citizenship)
7. Intellectual development
8. Self-understanding
9. Job roles
10. Creativity and personal experience
11. Socializing in recreation

Other researchers have defined quality of life as the degree of satisfaction with present life circumstances and that which makes life worth living (Buscaglia, 1988; Ludlow, Turnbull, & Luckasson, 1988). Knoll (1990) described 11 quality of life issues most frequently cited by people with developmental disabilities:

1. Real choices in all aspects of daily life
2. Functional skills
3. Interaction with a variety of people
4. Inclusion in generic services and activities
5. Access to community resources
6. Age-appropriateness
7. Use of a range of communication environments
8. Living in a typical neighborhood
9. Meaningful daily activity
10. Nonadversive interventions
11. Relationships with friends

Access to health care, although not cited as one of the most important issues, was noted to be necessary for the enjoyment and integration of all activities.

Changes within the past 10 years and changes in the attitudes of society (e.g., Americans with Disabilities Act [ADA] of 1990, PL 101-336; American Association on Mental Retardation [AAMR]; managed care; deinstitutionalization) also may have a beneficial impact on the lives of adults with cerebral palsy, including changes in health care systems, the "support" movement for developmental disabilities (endorsed by the AAMR), legislative issues (see Chapter 19), and integration of disabled individuals in society as evidenced by more balanced portrayal of developmental disabilities on television and Department of Justice actions in several states.

Issues of medical care often have been related to both attitude and finances. Changes in managed care have the potential to either advance or impair medical care for adults with cerebral palsy. With managed care, every individual potentially has access to a primary care physician. However, several questions arise: Will competition for "bottom line" issues curtail therapies, adaptive equipment, and new treatments? Will the push to get individuals into generic services bypass specialty care in this often medically complicated, infrequently advocated, and vulnerable group of individuals? The potential for a "medical home" and regular and preventive care should contribute to better health care and improved quality of life. Unfortunately, publications in the 1990s raise the issue of less optimal outcomes when older adults and individuals who are chronically ill were examined (Ware, Bayliss, Rogers, Kosinski, & Tarlon, 1996). In addition, recent reports (U.S. General Accounting Office, 1996) relating to the use of Home and Community Based Waiver and Medicaid Managed Care for the disabled note additional risks unless there is quality oversight and careful program design.

The period of transition from childhood with organized medical services, mandated school services, and parents' insurance coverage to the often bewildering world of adult services can be a time of heightening anxiety for both young adults with cerebral palsy and their parents (Thorin, Yovanoff, & Irvin, 1996). The cultural norm mandates that parental control and involvement should diminish during the transition to adulthood, but this may be unacceptable if greater parental advocacy and oversight is necessary. Conflict may develop over who makes choices and what expectations should be during this period. Insufficient funds and lack of program alternatives can create dilemmas for parents and professionals who work to support these adults. (Issues relating to the family, school, society, and daily living are covered in other chapters in this book.) Families can begin to meet the challenge in the medical area even when their children are young. This would include the following:

1. Collecting of all records (Even if actual copies of records are not available, a diary of each visit could be maintained.)

2. Understanding and participating in all transition plans, which may first start with the transition from early intervention to school
3. Asking trained professionals for explanations about cerebral palsy and its effects (This often is important in the adolescent with cerebral palsy who has established a relationship with a professional who can explain what cerebral palsy is, its complications, and its future outcomes.)
4. Understanding preventive and nonacute care
5. Keeping up with changes in the field, which might be accomplished by joining some national organization or by reading publications (e.g., *The Exceptional Parent*)

Robert Walsh and I think differently in terms of adults with cerebral palsy and, in particular, in terms of his future. As a physician, I worry about Robert's health. Having seen many families struggle, I worry about his independence; his future support, both materially and emotionally; and most of all, his chance to be creative and productive and to achieve the rewards associated with accomplishment.

Robert worries about the typical things that a college graduate worries about—a job, a girlfriend, enough time to surf the Internet. He also worries about support for the adaptations that allow him to maintain his everyday lifestyle (e.g., his electric wheelchair, his communicator) and the supports that help him get through each day (e.g., assistance with feeding, transport, talking about the day).

> People with disabilities have to prove to the world that they are human beings and can be productive people in society. All I would like to ask each and every one of you is to give kids with disabilities a chance. Don't judge a person by the way he or she looks. All individuals with or without disabilities are people before they are any of the traits used to describe them. How many times I was discouraged by professionals because I didn't look or act like your average kid. It was only after my family found Dr. Hayes that we were comfortable relying on any medical advice.
> But this wonderful adventure of life has thrown me a challenge. While many caring people often have difficulty working or socializing with a young man who looks up at them from his wheelchair, my crusade is to help others to cope with disabled persons and to help those others feel they are "worth it."

REFERENCES

Americans with Disabilities Act (ADA) of 1990, PL 101-336, 42 U.S.C. §§ 12101 *et seq.*

Bax, M.C.O., Smyth, D.P.L., & Thomas, A.P. (1988). Health care of physically handicapped young adults. *British Medical Journal, 296,*1153–1155.

Buscaglia, L. (1988). *The disabled and their parents* (Rev. ed.). New York: Henry Holt & Co.

Crichton, J.V., Mackinnon, M., & White, C.P. (1995). The life expectancy of persons with cerebral palsy. *Developmental Medicine and Child Neurology, 37,* 567–576.

Eyman, R.K., Grossman, H.T., Chaney, R.H., & Call, T.L. (1990). The life expectancy of profoundly handicapped people with mental retardation. *New England Journal of Medicine, 323,* 584–589.

Eyman, R.K., Grossman, H.T., Chaney, R.H., & Call, T.L. (1993). Survival of profoundly disabled people with severe mental retardation. *American Journal of Disease of Children, 147,* 329–336.

Flanagan, J.C. (1972). A research approach to improving quality of life. *American Psychologist, 33,* 138–147.

Knoll, J.A. (1990). Defining quality in residential services. In V.J. Bradley & A.H. Bersani (Eds.), *Quality assurance for individuals with developmental disabilities: It's everybody's business* (pp. 235–257). Baltimore: Paul H. Brookes Publishing Co.

Ludlow, B.L., Turnbull, A.P., & Luckasson, T. (1988). *Transitions to adult life for people with mental retardation–Principles and practices.* Baltimore: Paul H. Brookes Publishing Company.

Murphy, K.P., Molnar, E.E., & Lankaskey, K. (1995). Medical and functional status of adults with cerebral palsy. *Developmental Medicine & Child Neurology, 37,* 1075–1084.

Strauss, D., Eyman, R., & Grossman, H. (1996). Predictors of mortality in children with severe mental retardation: The effect of placement. *American Journal of Public Health, 86,* 1422–1429.

Strauss, D., & Kastner, T.A. (1996). Comparative mortality of people with mental retardation in institutions and the community. *American Journal of Mental Retardation, 101,* 26–40.

Thometz, J.E., & Simon, S.R. (1988). Progression of scoliosis after skeletal maturity in institutionalized adults who have cerebral palsy. *Journal of Bone and Joint Surgery, FOA, 70A,* 1290–1296.

Thorin, E., Yovanoff, P., & Irvin, L. (1996). Dilemmas faced by families during their young adults transitions to adulthood. *Mental Retardation, 34,* 117–120.

U.S. General Accounting Office. (1996, July). *Medicaid Waiver Program for Developmentally Disabled is promising, but poses some risks* (GAO/HEHS, 96–120). Washington, DC: Author.

Ware, J., Bayliss, M., Rogers, W., Kosinski, M., & Tarlon, A. (1996). Differences in 4-year health outcomes for elderly and poor, chronically ill patients treated in HMO and fee-for-service systems. *Journal of the American Medical Association, 276,* 1039–1047

Ware, J.E., Brook, R.H., Rogers, W.H., Keeler, E., Pavis, A., Sherbourne, C., Goldberg, G., Carup, P., & Newhouse, J. (1986). Comparisons of health outcomes at a health maintenance organization with those fee-for-service care. *Lancet, 1,* 1017–1022.

———————— CHAPTER 21 ————————

Epilogue

John P. Dormans and Louis Pellegrino

There are many different ways to think about cerebral palsy. From a neurological perspective, cerebral palsy is a disorder caused by brain injury or dysfunction that is unchanging (i.e., a *static encephalopathy*). From a broader medical perspective, cerebral palsy is a heterogeneous collection of disorders with different causes, which are grouped together because of similarities in clinical presentation. Cerebral palsy can also be thought of as a disability, characterized primarily by impairments of motor control and mobility. From a societal perspective, cerebral palsy is a condition that may place a person at some disadvantage relative to other members of society. The many ways of viewing cerebral palsy may engender some confusion and may even bring into question the validity of cerebral palsy as a diagnostic term. However, cerebral palsy is not simply a medical diagnosis. Although it is a term that captures a dynamic clinical entity and defies easy classification, it has a clear and recognizable impact on human lives.

In the 20th century, we have learned a great deal about this dynamic clinical entity. As a society, we have also slowly come to grips with the broader implications of disability and have come to recognize individuals with disabilities as a potentially disadvantaged minority with rights that require protection. As we consider what innovative medical and therapeutic advances may be waiting on the horizon for the prevention and treatment of cerebral palsy, we should remember that equally significant advances ought to be anticipated in the realm of cultural attitudes and public policy. If we are to hope for real improvements in the lives of individuals with cerebral palsy, both scientific and cultural advances are needed.

Index

Page numbers followed by "t" or "f" indicate tables or figures, respectively.

approaches to, 298–301
dynamic systems model of, 300–301
environment of, 301
evaluation form for, 198, 199*f*–202*f*
family involvement in, 303
immediate postoperative care,
198–207, 203*t*–205*t*
musculoskeletal assessment in, 285–298
neurodevelopmental treatment model,
300
neuromotor assessment in, 285–298
neurophysiological approach to,
299–300
preoperative evaluation, 194–198
during preschool years, 303
for school age children, 303–304
techniques for, 301–305
treatment goals, 301–305
treatment principles of, 301
Physical therapy assessment form,
285–298, 287*f*–291*f*
Physiological impairments, 26
associated with cerebral palsy, 53
PIAT-R, *see* Peabody Individual
Achievement Test-Revised
Pincer grasp, development of, 43
Pitch, of voice, 358
PL 65-178, *see* Soldiers Rehabilitation
Act of 1918
PL 66-236, *see* National Rehabilitation
Act of 1920
PL 67-97, *see* Sheppard Towner Act for
the Promotion of the Welfare
and Hygiene of Maternity and
Infancy (1921)
PL 81-734, *see* Social Security Act
Amendments of 1950
PL 88-164, *see* Mental Retardation
Facilities and Community
Mental Health Centers
Construction Act of 1963
PL 88-352, *see* Civil Rights Act of 1964
PL 89-97, *see* Social Security Act
Amendments of 1965
PL 90-248, *see* Social Security Act
Amendments of 1967
PL 91-517, *see* Developmental Disabili-
ties Services and Facilities
Construction Act of 1970
PL 92-223, *see* Social Security Act
Amendments of 1971

PL 93-112, *see* Rehabilitation Act of 1973
PL 94-103, *see* Developmental Disabili-
ties Assistance and Bill of
Rights Act of 1975
PL 94-142, *see* Education for All
Handicapped Children Act of
1975
PL 95-602, *see* Rehabilitation, Compre-
hensive Services, and Develop-
mental Disabilities Amend-
ments of 1978
PL 97-35, *see* Omnibus Reconciliation
Act of 1981
PL 97-248, *see* Tax Equity and Fiscal
Responsibility Act of 1982
PL 99-272, *see* Consolidated Omnibus
Budget Reconciliation Act of
1985
PL 99-457, *see* Education of the
Handicapped Act Amendments
of 1986
PL 100-407, *see* Technology-Related
Assistance for Individuals with
Disabilities Act of 1988
PL 101-136, *see* Americans with
Disabilities Act of 1990
PL 101-239, *see* Omnibus Reconciliation
Act of 1989
PL 101-476, *see* Education of the
Handicapped Act Amendments
of 1990; Individuals with
Disabilities Education Act
PL 102-119, *see* Individuals with
Disabilities Education Act of
1991
PL 102-166, *see* Civil Rights Act of 1991
PL 102-569, *see* Rehabilitation Act
Amendments of 1992
PL 103-218, *see* Technology-Related
Assistance for Individuals with
Disabilities Act Amendments
of 1994
PL 103-230, *see* Developmental
Disabilities Assistance and Bill
of Rights Act of 1994
PL 104-193, *see* Personal Responsibility
and Work Opportunity
Reconciliation Act of 1996
PL 105-17, *see* Individuals with
Disabilities Education Act
Amendments of 1997